LIPEDEMA

Principles and Practice of Diagnosis and Treatment

Dedication

To all individuals living with lipedema, whose perseverance and advocacy have brought this disease from obscurity into recognition.

To the scientists, clinicians, surgeons, and pioneers whose dedication and inquiry have laid the scientific and clinical foundation for understanding, diagnosing, and treating lipedema.

And to the global community of practitioners, scientists, and advocates whose collaboration continues to advance knowledge, compassion, and care for all affected.

Your courage and commitment have made this work possible.

LIPEDEMA

Principles and Practice of Diagnosis and Treatment

EDITORS
Stanley G. Rockson, MD
Leslyn Keith, OTD
Catherine Seo, PhD

BOOKS
Hammersmith Health Books
London, UK

First published in 2026 by Hammersmith Health Books
– an imprint of Hammersmith Books Limited
82 Wandsworth Bridge Road, London SW6 2TF, UK
www.hammersmithbooks.co.uk

Disclaimer: This book is designed to provide helpful information on the subjects discussed. It is not meant to be used, nor should it be used, to diagnose or treat any medical condition. For diagnosis or treatment of any medical problem, consult your own physician or healthcare provider. The publisher, editors and authors are not responsible for any specific health or allergy needs that may require medical supervision and are not liable for any damages or negative consequences from any treatment, action, application or preparation, to any person reading or following the information in this book. References are provided for informational purposes only and do not constitute endorsement of any websites or other sources. Readers should be aware that the websites listed in this book may change. The information and references included are up to date at the time of writing but given that medical evidence progresses, it may not be up to date at the time of reading.

British Library Cataloguing in Publication Data: A CIP record of this book is available from the British Library.

Print ISBN 978-1-78161-264-4
Ebook ISBN 978-1-78161-265-1

Commissioning editor: Georgina Bentliff
Designed and typeset by: Julie Bennett of Bespoke Publishing Ltd, UK
Cover design by: Madeline Meckiffe
Cover image: © 2013 Lipedema Simplified LLC
Index: Jan Ross
Production: Anke Ueberberg
Printed and bound by: Short Run Press, Exeter, UK

Contents

In honor and hope we acknowledge

This book is born of courage – of every person who refused to be unseen, of every clinician who chose curiosity over convention, and of every researcher and scientist who followed the science when few were listening.

To the lipedema community around the world – patients, advocates, and families – your collective voice and unwavering spirit have turned pain into purpose and isolation into understanding. You are the reason this work exists, and the heart that guides its mission.

To the global network of scientists, clinicians, and co-authors who have contributed their knowledge, time, and passion to these pages – your dedication illuminates the way forward, transforming what was once invisible into a field of recognized and compassionate care.

With deepest gratitude to our publishing partners at Hammersmith Health Books – Georgina Bentliff, Carolyn White, and Julie Bennett – for your faith in this project, your editorial excellence, and your steadfast care in bringing this vision to life.

A special acknowledgment to Dr. Raymond Perrin, whose belief in this work and introduction to our publishers helped make this collaboration possible.

Heartfelt thanks to the Lipedema Simplified team – Ayla De Vera, Akanksha Daga, Leah Mae Quilaton, and the rest of the dedicated staff – whose tireless effort, creativity, and commitment have supported this project from concept to completion. Your behind-the-scenes care and coordination have made an enduring difference.

To every contributor – authors, editors, reviewers, healthcare providers, and community members – thank you. Together, you have shaped a resource that will serve clinicians and patients for generations to come.

May these pages serve as both an acknowledgment and a promise – that through knowledge, compassion, and collaboration, the future for those with lipedema will be one of healing, dignity, and hope.

Author biographies

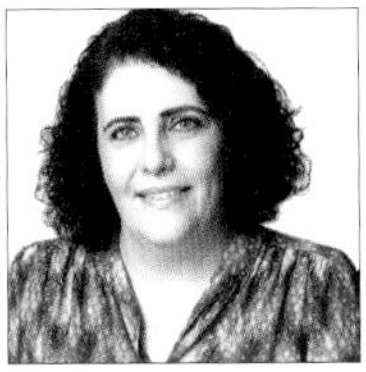

Dr. Sara Al-Ghadban, PhD, is a Senior Research Scientist in the Department of Plastic Surgery at the University of Virginia. She has nine years of expertise in lipedema research, a fat disorder affecting up to 10% of women worldwide. Her work focuses on the complex roles of stem cells, hormones, inflammation, and angiogenesis in the development and progression of lipedema. She is passionate about understanding the lipedema adipose tissue microenvironment and how its alterations drive disease progression. Her work is essential for uncovering the mechanisms of lipedema and guiding the development of targeted therapies.

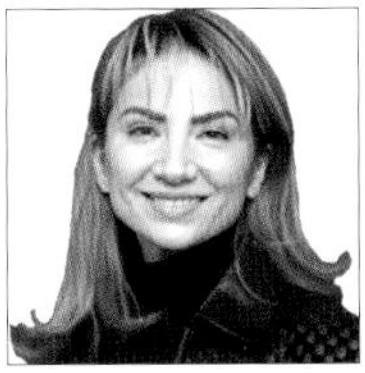

Professor Pınar Borman, MD, PhD, is a leading expert in physical medicine, rehabilitation, and algology, serving at Ankara Medipol University Faculty of Medicine, Dept of PMR Turkey. She is a certified lymphedema specialist and the founder president of the Turkish Lymphedema and Lipedema Association, as well as the Lymphedema Practice and Reserach Center at Hacettepe University. Internationally recognized, she serves on the executive commitee of the International Society of Lymphedema and representative of International Lymphoedema Turkish Framework. Dr Borman is also a founding member of International Lipoedema Association (ILA) and Lipoedema World Alliance (LWA). With over 300 publications and a multidisciplinary approach to pain, rehabilitation and lymphatic care, Professor Borman is a respected clinician, educator, and researcher shaping the future of rehabilitation and lymphatic medicine.

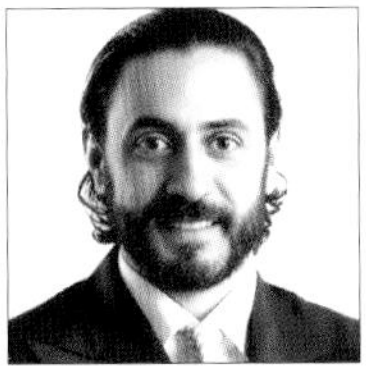

Dr. Corrado Cesare Campisi, MD, PhD, MRM, is a renowned Italian plastic and reconstructive surgeon specializing in lymphatic surgery. He leads the Campisi Clinic in Genoa, a global center for innovative treatments like lymphatic–venous anastomoses and lymphovascular-preserving liposuction. With training from the University of Genoa, the University of Pavia, Columbia University, and the Mayo Clinic, Dr. Campisi blends clinical excellence with surgical innovation. He has authored over 100 publications and currently serves as President of the International Society of Lymphology (2025–2027). His work has reshaped modern approaches to lymphedema and lipedema care worldwide.

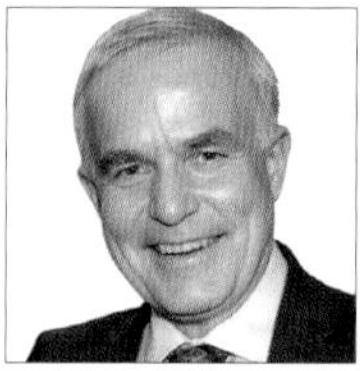

Dr. Matthew Carmody, MD, is a retired board-certified internist and Assistant Professor of Medicine at Harvard Medical School. With over four decades of experience in primary care, he is known for his person-centered approach to chronic and underdiagnosed diseases, particularly lipedema and obesity. He serves as a key medical collaborator with Lipedema Simplified, a global initiative dedicated to advancing education, research, and clinical care for lipedema. A Diplomate of the American Board of Obesity Medicine, Dr. Carmody has contributed to shaping best practices in lipedema diagnosis and treatment through expert panels, academic symposia, and peer-reviewed publications. His work emphasizes the integration of metabolic, inflammatory, and lymphatic health into mainstream clinical practice. Dr. Carmody's contributions reflect a commitment to elevating awareness and improving care for patients living with misunderstood medical conditions.

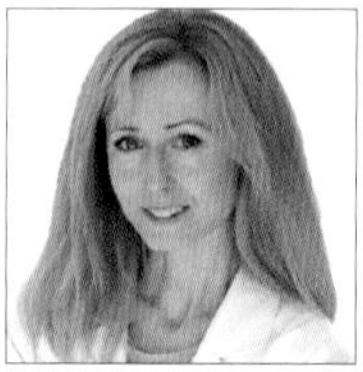

Dr. Angelika Chachaj, MD, PhD, is an Assistant Professor at Wroclaw Medical University in Poland, specializing in internal and vascular medicine. Her research focuses on lymphedema, lipedema, hypertension, and the metabolic and cardiovascular aspects of lymphatic disorders. With over 60 scientific publications, Dr. Chachaj makes significant contributions to lymphatic imaging and disease pathophysiology. She teaches angiology and internal medicine and remains active in clinical care, diagnosing and managing complex vascular conditions. Her work bridges academic research and patient-centered practice, improving both scientific understanding and clinical outcomes in lymphatic medicine.

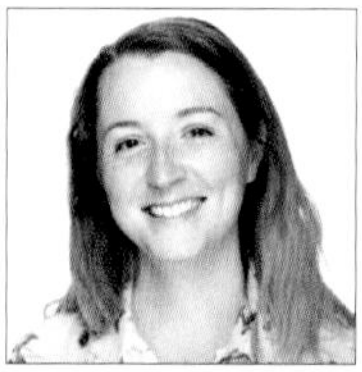

Vanessa Crain, is a Clinical Research Coordinator at the University of Virginia, where she works in Dr. Rachelle Crescenzi's SALT lab. Vanessa supports MRI-based research focused on lymphedema and lipedema, helping develop imaging tools and manage the study's biorepository. She is passionate about creating inclusive spaces in research and advocates for increased LGBTQ+ visibility in science. Vanessa brings a strong clinical foundation and a patient-centered mindset to her work, helping bridge the gap between imaging research and real-world care.

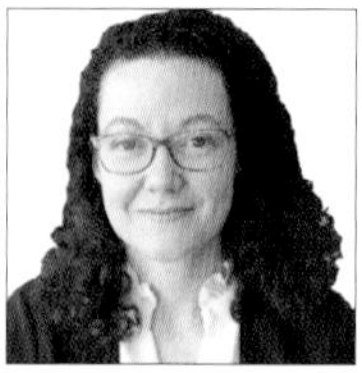

Dr. Rachelle Crescenzi, PhD, is a translational imaging scientist and Associate Professor of Radiology and Medical Imaging at the University of Virginia. Dr. Crescenzi leads the SALT MRI lab, where she develops advanced MRI techniques to study sodium and adipose tissue storage, and lymphatic morphology and function in conditions like lipedema and lymphedema. Her interdisciplinary work bridges radiology, biomedical engineering, and lymphatic research to create non-invasive imaging biomarkers for early diagnosis and treatment monitoring. Dr. Crescenzi's patient-centered approach is advancing the science of lymphatic disorders and paving the way for more targeted and effective therapies.

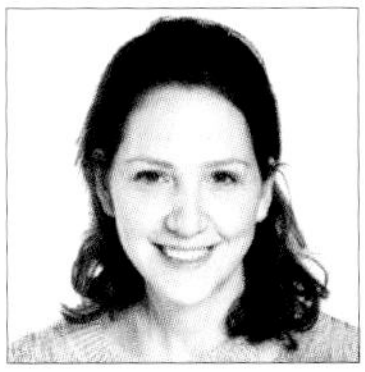

Dr. Sara Dobbins, PhD, is a genetics researcher based in the UK, utilizing large-scale datasets and computational methods to improve our understanding of the genetics of lipedema and lymphedema. As a key member of the Lipoedema Consortium, Dr. Dobbins co-authored the pivotal UK Genome-wide Association Studies (GWAS) on lipedema, exploring the disease's heritability. This work, drawing on innovative genomic methods, highlights her commitment to identifying genetic risk factors that may lead to earlier diagnosis and improved clinical outcomes. Dr. Dobbins employs computational genomics and biostatistical modeling to decode complex datasets, shaping the field's mechanistic insights. Her work relies on clinician-patient partnerships to facilitate the collection of large, high-quality cohorts for analysis, as well as publicly available datasets such as the 100,000 Genomes Project and UK Biobank. Her interdisciplinary work bridges genetic discovery, phenotype association, and population-scale analysis, establishing foundations for targeted screening and precision medicine in lipedema care.

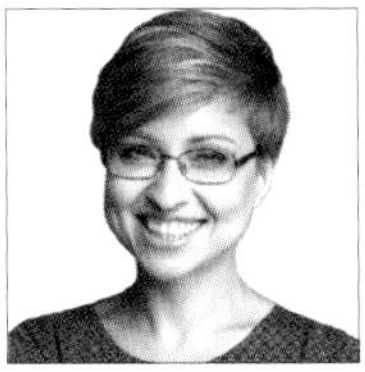

Dr. Joanna Dudek, PhD, is a psychologist, psychotherapist, and Assistant Professor at the SWPS University in Warsaw (Poland). In her clinical practice and research, she focuses on evidence-based treatments, including motivational interviewing, cognitive behavioral therapy, and acceptance and commitment therapy. She has conducted pioneering research on the quality of life and psychosocial functioning of women with lipedema. She co-authored a number of articles about lipedema and delivered numerous conference lectures and workshops on the psychological aspects of functioning with lipedema worldwide. She has been involved in research focused on applying interventions to improve the psychological functioning and well-being of patients. Her goal is to increase awareness and knowledge about lipedema and psychosocial aspects of functioning with this disease, to improve patient care worldwide, and reduce bias and misunderstanding of lipedema.

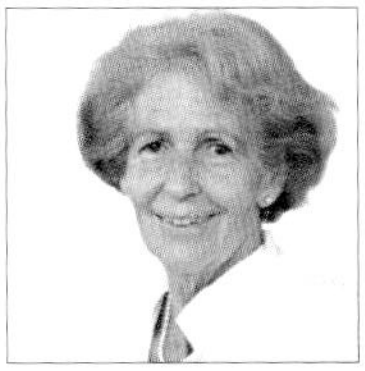

Dr. Gabriele Faerber, MD, PhD, is a German expert in phlebology, lymphology, and nutritional medicine, and has worked at the Vascular Medicine Center in Hamburg-Bahrenfeld since 2001. Her clinical and research work focuses on lipedema, obesity, and metabolic inflammation, with special interest in ketogenic dietary approaches. Dr. Faerber has published widely and lectures internationally. She contributed to the German lipedema guidelines and led their 2020 revision. She has served on the boards of key lymphology and phlebology societies and sits on the editorial board of *Phlebologie*, helping shape standards in vascular and lymphatic care.

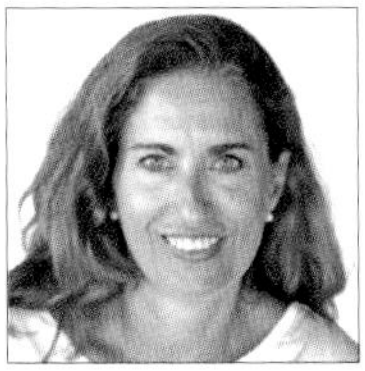

Dr. Isabel Forner Cordero, MD, PhD, is a specialist in Physical Medicine and Rehabilitation and Associate Professor at the University of Valencia. She has worked in the Lymphedema Unit at Hospital La Fe in Valencia, Spain, since 2000. Her clinical and research focus includes lymphology, lipedema, and compression therapy. Dr. Forner Cordero has authored over 50 scientific publications and is active in international lymphology societies. She also teaches at the University of Medicine and mentors medical students and residents. Her work bridges patient care, research, and education, making her a respected leader in the field of lymphatic medicine. She is a founding Member of the Lipedema World Alliance, and the President of the Spanish Group of Lymphology.

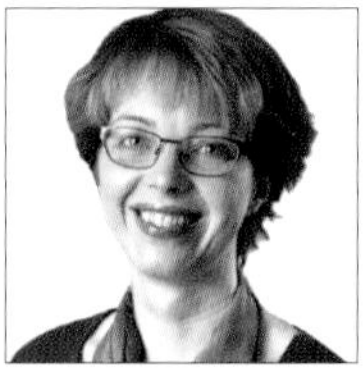

Kate Forster, Chartered FCIPD, is Director of Operations for Europe at BioLegend and a dedicated lipedema advocate. With over 14 years of leadership experience in biotech and medical devices, she combines corporate expertise with grassroots activism. Kate has served on the board of Lipoedema UK since 2016 and helped found the Lipedema World Alliance, where she leads strategic efforts to improve diagnosis, care pathways, and awareness internationally. Known for her powerful storytelling and policy work, she champions the voices of those affected by lipedema and fosters collaboration between patients, clinicians, and healthcare systems.

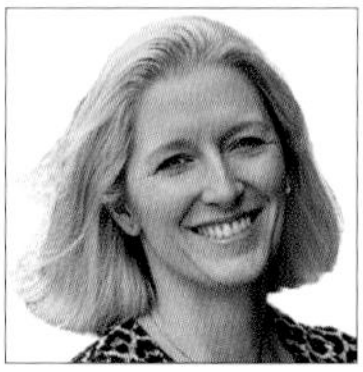

Professor Kristiana Gordon, MBBS, MD(Res), CLT, FRCP, FHEA, is a leading Consultant Dermatologist and Associate Professor in lymphovascular medicine based in London. She serves as Clinical Lead of the National Lymphoedema Service at St George's Hospital, providing specialized care for lymphedema, lipedema, and related diseases. As the UK's first formally qualified physician in lymphovascular medicine, she combines clinical care, genetic research, and advanced imaging. Professor Gordon co-leads major research projects and holds leadership roles in national and international organizations, including Lipoedema UK, the British Lymphology Society, and the International Lipoedema Association.

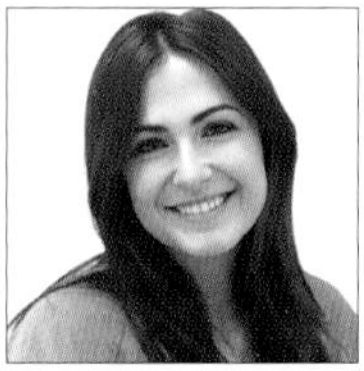

Dr. Luz M. Herrero Manley, MD, PhD, is a Spanish physician and researcher specializing in vascular and lymphatic disorders, with a focus on lymphedema and lipedema. She has contributed to expert guidelines and clinical case studies, including work with the Spanish Group for Lymphology to enhance patient care during complex health challenges, such as the COVID-19 pandemic. Known for her collaborative approach, Dr. Herrero Manley advocates for evidence-based, interdisciplinary strategies that center on patient needs. Her work bridges clinical practice and research to advance awareness, diagnosis, and comprehensive care for lymphatic conditions.

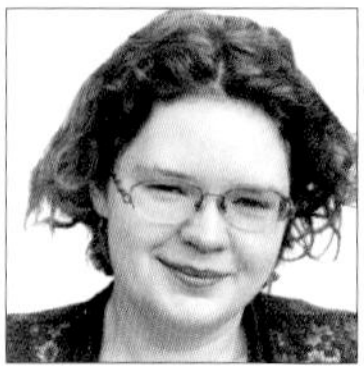

Siobhan Huggins, is an independent researcher focused on therapeutic carbohydrate restriction and metabolic health, as well as the Research Specialist for Lipedema Simplified, a patient advocacy group based out of Boston, MA. Siobhan has dedicated her time to exploring the metabolic underpinnings of lipedema since 2021, resulting in multiple scientific publications focused on both lipedema as well as therapeutic carbohydrate restriction. Her work integrates rigorous science and patient empowerment with the goal of compassionate care.

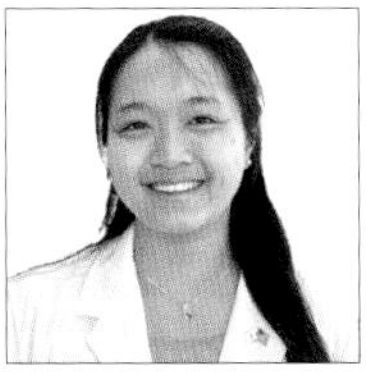

Rachel Huynh, AB, is a medical student at the University of California, San Francisco. She holds a Bachelor of Arts from Brown University, where she completed an independent concentration in 'Food and Health in US American Society'. In medical school, she has contributed to various diabetes- and obesity-related research projects across the fields of endocrinology, vascular surgery, and bariatric surgery. In 2024, she was an NIDDK-funded research student at the McLaughlin Lab at Stanford University, studying tirzepatide's effects on metabolic outcomes and adipocyte health. Having commissioned as an officer through the Patriot Battalion Army ROTC program in Providence, Rhode Island, she will serve as an active-duty US Army physician following medical residency.

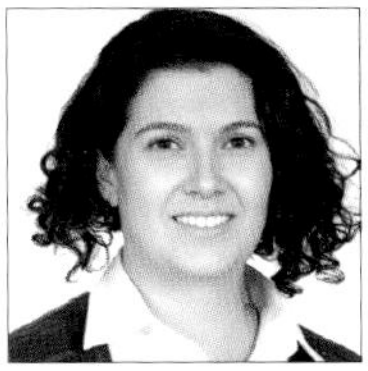

Dr. Ayça Utkan Karasu, MD, serves as an Associate Professor in the Department of Physical Medicine and Rehabilitation at Gazi University in Ankara, Turkey, with a focus on lymphatic diseases, neurological rehabilitation, patient education, and quality of life research. Her work explores the effectiveness of digital resources and compression therapy in the management of lymphedema and lipedema. Dr. Karasu is recognized for her interdisciplinary approach and contributions to advancing patient-centered care in lymphatic medicine.

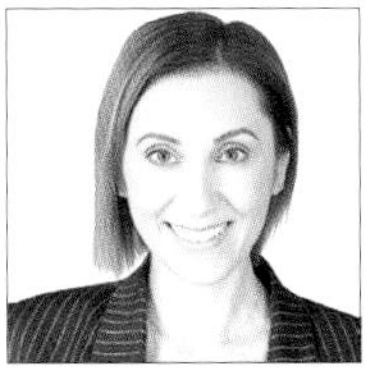

Dr. Tara Karnezis, PhD, is a biomedical scientist and translational researcher based at the O'Brien Institute, St Vincent's Institute of Medical Research in Melbourne, Australia. Her pioneering work spans lymphatic disease, cancer, and lipedema, with over 50 peer-reviewed publications in journals such as *Nature* and *Cancer Cell*. A former postdoctoral fellow at Stanford and co-founder of Gertrude Biomedical, she specializes in the discovery of molecular biomarkers and the development of targeted therapies. Dr. Karnezis collaborates closely with clinicians and advocates to advance understanding of lipedema, blending research innovation with biotech leadership to impact both science and patient care.

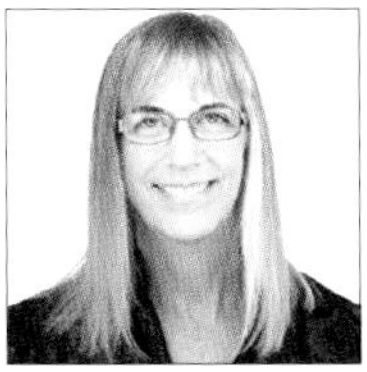

Dr. Leslyn Keith, OTD, CLT, is a leading expert in lymphatic and fat diseases, with over 25 years of clinical experience. She is internationally recognized for her groundbreaking research on ketogenic nutrition for managing lipedema, lymphedema, and obesity. Dr. Keith serves as a consultant for Lipedema Simplified and teaches for Klose Training. An accomplished author, she has written *The Lymphatic Code* and *The Ketogenic Solution for Lymphatic Disorders*, and leads the Lymphatic Lifestyle Solutions program. Her work integrates holistic care with cutting-edge science to empower patients and improve outcomes.

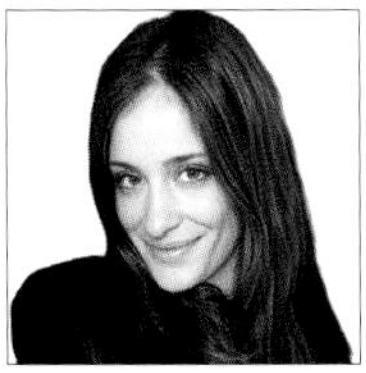

Zoe-Theodora Kolonelos is the Chief Operating Officer of Campisi Clinic Switzerland, where she oversees international communications, research coordination, and expansion initiatives under the direction of Dr. Corrado Campisi. She studied at the University of Detroit Mercy and the University of Windsor, earning degrees in Architectural Design and Visual Arts. Her professional background is distinguished by extensive experience in communications, translation, and consulting across diverse sectors, including architecture, education, entertainment, and hospitality. Since joining Campisi Clinic in 2023, she has collaborated on numerous scientific publications, presentations, and studies. She also co-organizes international congresses, events, and educational courses with Dr. Campisi and actively advocates for greater awareness of lipedema and lymphedema. Her passion for lymphology stems from her close collaboration with Dr. Campisi and her commitment to advancing education and patient advocacy in this evolving field.

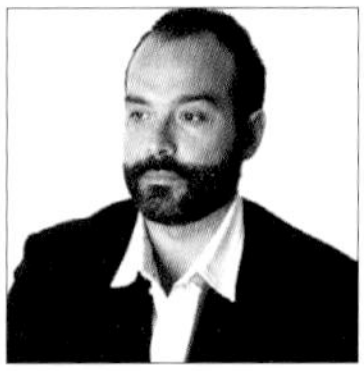

Dr. Michele Maruccia, MD, PhD, is a leading Italian plastic and reconstructive surgeon and Associate Professor at the University of Bari. He specializes in microsurgical treatment of lymphedema and breast reconstruction, with a focus on vascularized lymph node transfers (VLNT). Dr. Maruccia directs the Complex Operations Unit at Bari University Hospital, where he leads advanced surgical programs and research. With over 30 peer-reviewed publications, his work has significantly advanced techniques in lymphedema surgery, improving the quality of life for cancer survivors. A dedicated educator, he trains future surgeons in microsurgery and frequently presents at international conferences.

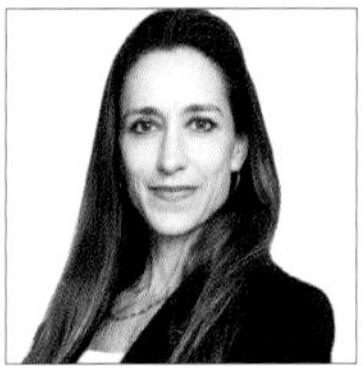

Professor Tracey Lynn McLaughlin, MD, MS, is a Professor of Medicine in Endocrinology at Stanford University School of Medicine. Board-certified in internal medicine and endocrinology, she specializes in diabetes, PCOS, and metabolic diseases. Her research focuses on adipose tissue, insulin resistance, and post-bariatric hypoglycemia, advancing personalized treatment strategies through continuous glucose monitoring. A leader in clinical care and research, she is the co-founder (and former chair) of Stanford Hospital's Diabetes Task Force and an active member of the Endocrine Society and the American Diabetes Association. Professor McLaughlin has had continuous research funding from the American Diabetes Association and the NIH for over 25 years to study the relationship between obesity and metabolic disease. She has been honored with multiple awards, including the NIH K23 Career Development Award.

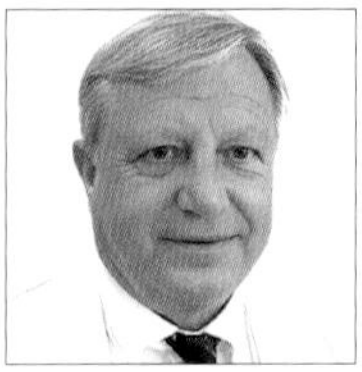

Dr. Sandro Michelini, MD, PhD, is a leading Italian vascular rehabilitation specialist with over 40 years of experience in lymphatic and adipose diseases. He heads the Department of Vascular Rehabilitation at San Giovanni Battista Hospital in Rome and teaches lymphology at multiple Italian universities. A past President of the European Society of Lymphology, Dr. Michelini has published extensively on lipedema, lymphatic dysfunction, and metabolic overlap. He contributes to international guidelines and leads multidisciplinary efforts to advance holistic lymphatic care. Dr. Michelini is also the Founding President of the Lipedema World Alliance (LWA), a global nonprofit dedicated to uniting clinicians, researchers, and advocates to promote greater understanding, recognition, and treatment of lipedema. Under his leadership, the LWA has spearheaded global scientific collaboration, including the

Lipedema World Congress and the development of a consensus-based position paper on the disease. His work bridges clinical excellence, research, and patient advocacy across Europe and beyond.

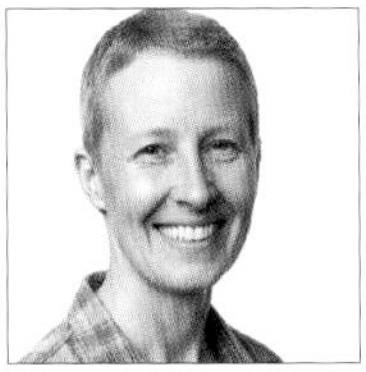

Professor Pia Ostergaard, PhD is a renowned geneticist and Professor of Human Genetics at St George's, University of London. She leads the Lymphovascular Research Group and has identified key genes underlying primary lymphedema, including *EPHB4*, *VEGFC*, and *GATA2*. Her work bridges genetic discovery with clinical application, improving diagnoses and opening doors to targeted therapies for lymphatic diseases. A former Daphne Jackson Fellow, she is also a recipient of the LE&RN-Gordon Research Conference Career Achievement Award. Professor Ostergaard continues to shape the field through cutting-edge research, national service leadership, and mentorship of emerging scientists.

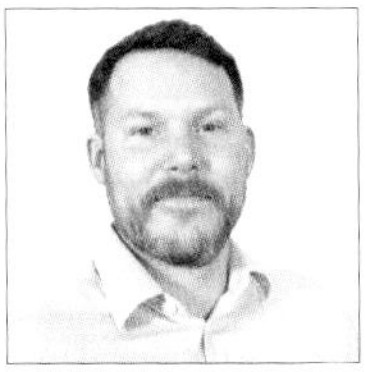

Dr. Alan Michael Pittman, PhD, is a Senior Lecturer in computational genetics at St George's, University of London, specializing in human genomics and rare diseases. With a PhD in neuroscience from University College London, he leads the university's virtual bioinformatics unit and co-investigates a genome-wide association study (GWAS) on lipedema. His work integrates whole-genome sequencing and functional genomics to explore neurological diseases, cancer genetics, and lipid metabolism. Author of over 100 publications, Dr. Pittman plays a pivotal role in advancing genomic education and clinical diagnostics through St George's postgraduate programs in genomic and translational medicine.

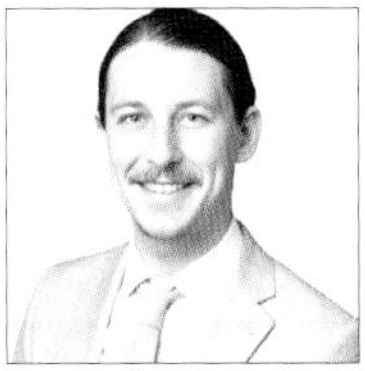

Dr. Michael Pridmore, PhD, is an Assistant Professor in the Department of Radiology & Radiological Sciences at Vanderbilt University and a researcher with the Vanderbilt University Institute of Imaging Science (VUIIS). His expertise spans MRI applications across neuro, cardiac, and peripheral nerve studies. His research includes pioneering the application of diffusion tensor imaging for nerve injury, sodium MRI in conditions such as lipedema, lymphedema, and salt-sensitive hypertension, as well as hippocampal segmentation in mild cognitive impairment. Collaborating with Dr. Crescenzi's SALT Lab, he advances the acquisition and processing of multi-nuclear and proton/sodium MRI.

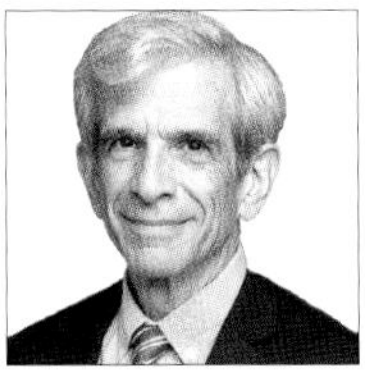

Dr. Stanley G. Rockson, MD, FACP, FACC, is the Allan and Tina Neill Professor of Lymphatic Research and Medicine at Stanford University School of Medicine, where he also serves as Chief of Consultative Cardiology and Director of the Stanford Center for Lymphatic and Venous Diseases. A graduate of Duke University School of Medicine and having completed postgraduate training at Harvard-affiliated institutions, Dr. Rockson has dedicated over four decades to basic and clinical research in lymphatic disease and cardiovascular medicine. He has authored more than 200 peer-reviewed papers, book chapters, and reviews, focused on lymphatic pathophysiology, biomarkers, and innovative therapeutics, and his leadership extends to major roles such as Editor-in-Chief of *Lymphatic Research and Biology*, founding

Chair of the Lymphatic Education & Research Network (LE&RN), and contributions to multiple NIH advisory panels. Dr. Rockson leads clinical trials on lymphedema pathogenesis and treatment, aiming to translate scientific insights into real-world therapies, and has been recognized with awards including Stanford's Dean's Award for Excellence in Teaching and the Lymphatic Research Leadership Award. His dynamic career combines patient care, mentorship, and cutting-edge research, reflecting his enduring commitment to improving outcomes for individuals with lymphatic and vascular diseases.

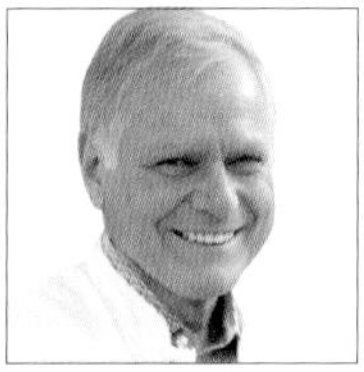

Dr. Franz-Josef Schingale, MD, is a leading expert in phlebology and lymphology, and the Medical Director of the Lympho-Opt Clinic in Pommelsbrunn, Germany, which he founded in 1982. With nearly 50 years of experience, he has authored over 30 publications on compression therapy, lymphatic imaging, and the management of edema. A recognized leader in the field, he is a member of major lymphology societies and a co-founder of the International Council of Lymphology (ICL) and the International Council of Lymphology Research (ICLR). Dr. Schingale is known internationally for pioneering lymphatic rehabilitation techniques and remains a dedicated clinician, researcher, and mentor in advancing lymphatic care.

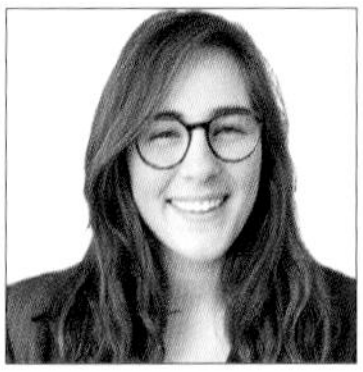

Allison O'Brien Scott, MSc, is a Research Scientist specializing in qualitative data and public health approaches in the University of Virginia Department of Radiology and Medical Imaging. As a key member of Dr. Crescenzi's SALT Lab, Allison supports the development and implementation of cutting-edge imaging protocols, qualitative data assessments, data analysis pipelines, and cross-disciplinary collaborations aimed at translating novel MRI methodologies into clinical and scientific impact. She is conducting independent research to shed light on quality of life impacted by lipedema and address barriers to care for patients with lipedema.

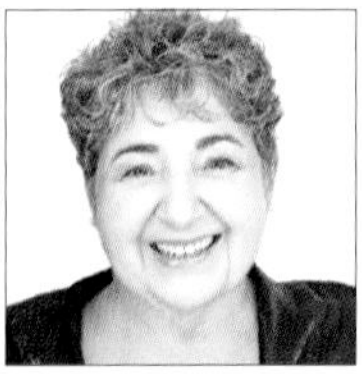

Dr. Catherine Seo, PhD, is a researcher, educator, and advocate recognized internationally for her leadership in the field of lipedema. She is the founder and CEO of Lipedema Simplified and The Lipedema Project initiatives dedicated to advancing awareness, diagnosis, and treatment of lipedema. Her media psychology doctorate centers on the psychosocial impact of hidden illnesses. Dr. Seo directed the documentary *Lipedema: The Disease They Call FAT* and is co-author of the monograph *Lipedema – The Disease They Call FAT: An Overview for Clinicians.* She has co-authored numerous journal articles furthering the understanding and awareness of lipedema in the medical community. Through education, research, and community engagement, she works to transform care and empower those living with lipedema worldwide.

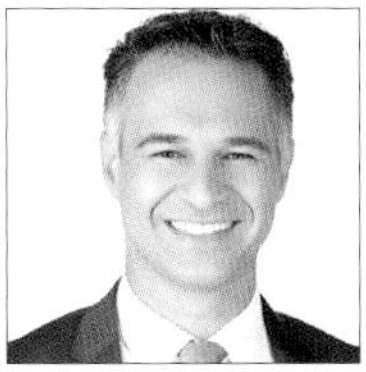

Dr. Ramin Shayan, MBBS, PhD, FRACS (Plastics), is a leading Australian plastic and reconstructive surgeon and Associate Professor at the University of Melbourne, Australia. He directs the O'Brien Institute at St Vincent's Institute for Medical Research and is internationally recognized for his work in lymphatic surgery and reconstructive microsurgery. With over 70 publications and a PhD in cancer metastasis and lymphedema, Dr. Shayan's research bridges the fields of molecular biology and surgical innovation. He also leads advanced projects on lipedema and lymphatic imaging and is a highly regarded educator, mentor, and recipient of numerous clinical and academic honors.

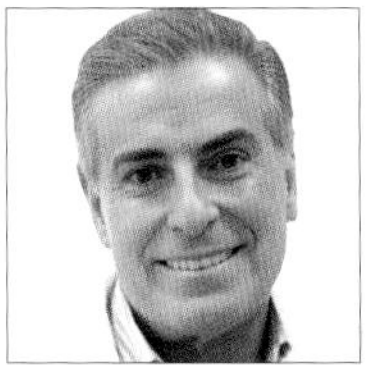

Dr. José Luis Simarro, MD, is a pioneering Spanish physician and the Medical Director of the Instituto del Lipedema in Madrid, which he founded in 2007 as the first medical center in Spain exclusively dedicated to the diagnosis and treatment of lipedema. He earned his medical degree from the Complutense University of Madrid and holds certification in aesthetic medicine from the Official College of Physicians of Madrid. Today, he is widely recognized for his contributions to advancing lipedema care through surgical techniques such as Water-Assisted Liposuction (WAL), as well as innovative non-surgical protocols. Dr. Simarro is also a respected academic and international speaker. He has lectured at the Autonomous University of Barcelona and the University of Barcelona in postgraduate programs on lipedema and regularly presents at national and global conferences. He is known for his work on the pathogenetic theory of lipedema, including his hypothesis around subclinical compartment syndrome as a contributing factor. Committed to evidence-based, patient-centered care, Dr. Simarro continues to lead clinical research and actively participates in scientific societies related to aesthetic medicine, lipedema, and the human microbiota.

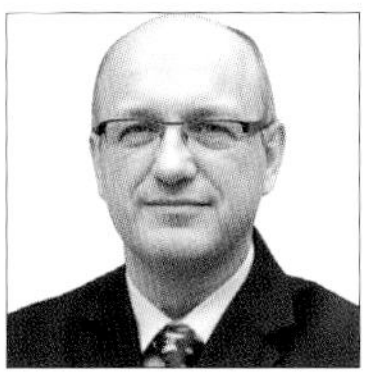

Professor Andrzej Szuba, MD, PhD, is Professor of Medicine and Head of Angiology and Internal Medicine at Wroclaw Medical University in Poland. A leading expert in vascular and lymphatic medicine, he has authored over 240 publications and served as past President of the International Society of Lymphology. Professor Szuba holds editorial roles in major journals and ranks among the top global scholars in lymphology. He also leads Poland's Lymphological Chapter and is a founding member of the International Lipoedema Association, widely recognized for his contributions to advancing lymphatic disease care and research.

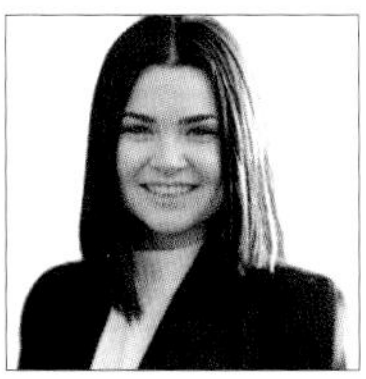

Shannon Taylor, is a Ph.D. candidate in Biomedical Engineering at Vanderbilt University, affiliated with the Vanderbilt Institute for Surgery and Engineering (VISE) and the Vanderbilt University Institute of Imaging Science (VUIIS). Her research focuses on image-guided surgery, sodium (^{23}Na) MRI, and computational tools for disease characterization. She holds a BS in Bioengineering from Lehigh University and has co-authored several publications, including studies on imaging in lipedema. Shannon is a Dean's Graduate Fellow and Russell G. Hamilton Scholar, dedicated to advancing imaging innovations in clinical care.

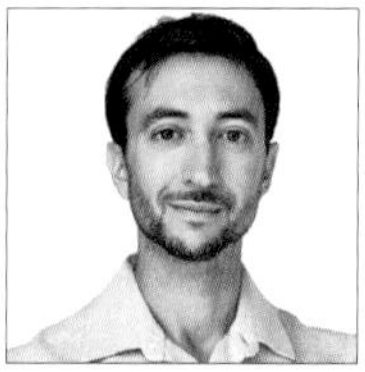

Dr. Juan Vázquez Díez, MD, is a Spanish physician specializing in the rehabilitation of lymphedema and lipedema. Based in Castellón de la Plana in Spain, he earned his medical degree from the University of Valencia and has since contributed to research and clinical practice through the Spanish Group for Lymphology. His work includes studies on joint hypermobility in lipedema and trials on compression therapy. A frequent presenter at international conferences, including the Lipedema World Congress, Dr. Vázquez Díez champions a multidisciplinary, evidence-based approach to lymphatic care that integrates research, clinical innovation, and patient advocacy.

Foreword

William Repicci
President & CEO, Lymphatic Education & Research Network (LE&RN)

When I first began hearing the stories of those living with lipedema, I was struck by a common thread – pain, not just from the disease itself but from being unseen. Women shared how they'd spent years seeking answers, only to be dismissed, misdiagnosed, or told it was their fault. As President & CEO of the Lymphatic Education & Research Network (LE&RN), I've made it our mission to change that. We are now on the brink of a paradigm shift, and this book is a landmark in that transformation.

This volume serves as the most comprehensive, multidisciplinary reference on lipedema to date. Its scope is both broad and deep, featuring 20 chapters that cover the biology, diagnosis, treatment, and lived experiences of this complex disease. The authors include some of the world's foremost clinicians, researchers, and advocates, creating a blueprint for the future of lipedema care – one built on evidence, collaboration, and compassion.

This book brings lipedema out of the shadows and into the heart of clinical understanding. It is the bridge between patient experience and provider action.

The opening chapters lay the groundwork. Drs. Sandro Michelini and José Luis Simarro clarify the elusive definition of lipedema, while Dr. Matthew Carmody tackles a foundational challenge: the role of the primary care physician. He reminds us that early recognition starts in the exam room, and that education must begin where patients first seek help.

The genetics section represents a milestone. What was once speculative is now becoming a scientific reality. Genome-wide association studies and gene signaling analyses – led by researchers such as Professor Pia Ostergaard and her team, along with Drs. Ramin Shayan and Tara Karnezis – are revealing a biological basis for lipedema. These findings offer promise for precision diagnostics and, one day, targeted treatments.

The differential diagnosis section is equally critical. Lipedema is often mistaken for obesity, lymphedema, or other common co-morbidities that frequently accompany this disease. Chapters by Professors Kristiana Gordon and Tracey McLaughlin, Dr. Angelika Chachaj, and Professor Andrzej Szuba provide vital distinctions. Dr. Joanna Dudek's work on weight stigma challenges us to confront systemic bias in the healthcare system.

The imaging section brings innovation to the forefront. While conventional tools like ultrasound and lymphoscintigraphy still serve an essential role as delineated by Dr. Isabel Forner Cordero and her team, new imaging techniques – particularly high-resolution MRI – are reshaping how we view the disease internally. These advances, led by Dr. Rachelle Crescenzi and her team, elevate diagnosis from subjective pattern recognition to objective visualization.

Treatment is presented through a holistic lens. From manual lymphatic drainage and compression (Dr. Franz-Josef Schingale) to anti-inflammatory nutrition (Dr. Gabriele Faerber) and complementary therapies (Professor Pınar Borman and Dr. Ayça Utkan Karasu), this book promotes a whole-body, patient-centered approach. Notably, the work of Dr. Carmody and Siobhan Huggins bridges clinical care with lifestyle interventions, demonstrating how truly integrated treatment can support long-term well-being.

Surgical options, once considered controversial, are presented here with depth and responsibility. Dr. Ramin Shayan and Dr. Corrado Campisi offer a measured, evidence-informed approach to lipedema surgery. Their chapters address risk, outcomes, and ethical standards – a must-read for any clinician contemplating operative care for patients with lipedema.

Perhaps most moving is the chapter on self-care. Kate Forster's contribution reminds us that many people with lipedema have had to become their own care coordinators, educators, and advocates. Her chapter elevates self-care not just as a coping mechanism but as a form of resilience and empowerment.

The final sections direct our focus toward the future. Dr. Catherine Seo and Dr. Leslyn Keith provide an actionable roadmap for finding support, seeking treatment, and fostering community. In the closing chapter, Dr. Stanley Rockson's vision for the next steps in lipedema research and care is bold and clear: we need systemic integration of lipedema into the broader field of lymphatic diseases, supported by funding, training and policy reform.

This volume is not just a medical text. It is a declaration: that lipedema is real, that it is treatable, and that the time to act is now.

For those of us in the lymphatic field, this book serves as a call to action. It affirms the importance of interdisciplinary collaboration. It encourages clinicians to learn. Most importantly, it addresses the needs of patients who have waited far too long for the medical world to take them seriously.

To every provider, researcher, and student who reads these pages: thank you for choosing to learn. Thank you for standing by your patients. And thank you for being part of the change.

William Repicci
President and CEO, Lymphatic Education
and Research Network (LE&RN)

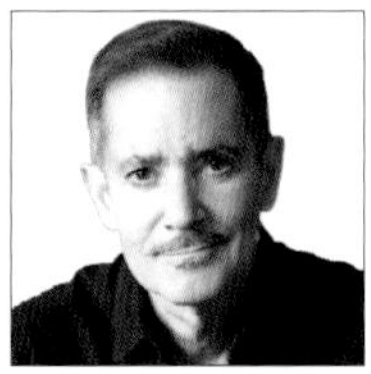

I
Lipedema definition and diagnosis

Please note: Within the medical literature, the disease focus of this volume is variously referred to as **lipedema** (US spelling) or **lipoedema** (British/European/Australian spelling). We have titled the book with the American version; within the text of the individual chapters, we have left the decision to the discretion of the authors and their respective countries of origin.

Chapter One
What is lipedema? Moving towards a widely accepted definition

Sandro Michelini and José Luis Simarro

Introduction

Is it possible that a disease as old as humankind, first identified only in 1940 by two researchers of exceptional clinical insight and diagnostic ability, was only officially recognized by the World Health Organization (WHO) in 2022 with the publication of the 11th edition of the *International Classification of Diseases*?[1, 2] We are referring to lipedema (also spelled 'lipoedema' in some countries), a disease of adipose tissue that, at last, has been assigned its diagnostic code. The answer is, yes.

Lipedema, first described by Drs. Allen and Hines of the Mayo Clinic in the United States, is characterized by the abnormal accumulation of adipose tissue in the lower and upper limbs, notably sparing the distal extremities. This pathological fat exhibits behavior distinct from adipose tissue in unaffected areas of the body. Specifically, lipedema tissue responds poorly to conventional low-calorie diets, shows minimal reduction with physical activity, and remains unresponsive primarily to bariatric surgery techniques, even in patients undergoing procedures for overt obesity.[3, 4]

Lipedema is a disease that affects almost exclusively women and has a hereditary basis, as it is often possible to identify other affected individuals within both the maternal and paternal lines of a family. In many pedigrees, transmission appears to occur through a male who, although genetically carrying the predisposition, does not exhibit the phenotypic features of the disease.[5, 6, 7, 8] In one case we observed, lipedema was inherited from the maternal side; however, the patient's mother, who accompanied her at the time of diagnosis, reported that she had inherited it from her paternal grandmother. Given that lipedema often went undiagnosed in previous generations, it is plausible that the genetic predisposition may be more widespread than currently recognized.

Some aspects of the disease are now known and accepted by the entire international scientific community; others, on the other hand, remain the subject of much ongoing discussion and await more consistent and reliable studies and clinical trials before they can be fully understood and accepted. However, let's try to distinguish the information that does not raise doubts about its reliability regarding the disease from the other information whose validity still awaits definitive confirmation.

Epidemiology and etiopathogenesis

As with other diseases, it is appropriate to

begin by considering the epidemiology and etiopathogenesis of the disease. At one time, it was thought that lipedema could be regarded as a rare disease.[7] Today, according to various authors, the incidence appears to be around 10% of the population, with more than 95% of cases being female.[5, 6, 7, 8] This aspect is undoubtedly related to the age of onset, which, in the vast majority of cases, coincides with female sexual maturation (puberty), specifically at the time when hormone production becomes most pronounced, and will accompany the woman throughout her fertile years.

It is precisely during times of hormonal balance transition (especially during the menopausal and climacteric periods) that further transformations of the affected body areas can occur. The same association with polycystic ovary syndrome (PCOS), or endometriosis, which is present in more than 25% of cases, testifies to the close interrelation between the effects of hormones and clinical pictures. According to some, there is a 'prepubertal' form of the disease that would essentially affect the leg and then extend to the thighs and buttocks at the time of puberty. This is in contrast to a 'pubertal' presentation, which co-occurs in all affected areas.

It has been shown that lipedema can begin before puberty.[9] Preliminary results from a study soon to be published by the authors of this chapter indicate that it could be related to connective tissue pathologies present since childhood and that they could be the cause of prepubertal lipedema that is not associated with female hormones.[10]

Considerable speculation has focused on the role of estrogens, acting through their estrogen receptor α (ERα) and estrogen receptor β (ERβ) receptors, in promoting adipocyte hyperplasia in lipedema. However, during the second phase of the menstrual cycle, the effects of estrogen are typically counteracted by progesterone. If this regulatory mechanism is impaired, potentially due to resistance at the progesterone receptors (PRα and PRβ), it may contribute to the development of adipocyte hypertrophy.[5, 11] Nonetheless, in our clinical experience, the use of progestins, whether administered orally or via intrauterine devices (IUDs), does not appear to exacerbate lipedema symptoms.

The influence of female sex hormones has more than one explanation: it is no coincidence that the few cases affecting men develop in particular clinical conditions characterized by a lack of action of male sex hormones, such as during cirrhosis of the liver or anti-androgen treatment in cases of prostate cancer.[11] An estrogenic influx or the action of estrogenic or pseudo-estrogenic interferents, such as nickel or bisphenol, may cause male breasts to delvelop during male puberty. Similarly, they can also induce the transformation of mesenchymal stem cells from adipose tissue into adipocytes, in larger quantities than usual at male puberty, since male mesenchymal stem cells also have receptors for estrogen. Once developed, these adipocytes would give rise to lipedema in males. We see this in transgender individuals receiving female hormones.

The first gene identified as potentially related to the development of lipedema, *AKR1C1*, is also involved in the metabolism of progesterone. (See Section II of this textbook for more on the genetics of lipedema.) Mutations in this gene appear to impair the body's ability to catabolize progesterone, allowing the hormone to continue exerting its effects even when plasma concentrations remain within normal limits.[7, 8] This mechanism will be explored in greater detail in a later chapter.

More specifically, progesterone is known to play a role in activating the calcium pump. In lipedema, tissue samples of adipocytes have been found to contain abnormally high levels of intracellular calcium ions, which inhibit cytoplasmic phospholipases.[12] This inhibition leads to the intracellular accumulation of phospholipids, resulting in cytotoxic effects. Importantly, the relationship between lipedema and obesity is not axiomatic; it is inconsistent and certainly not pathognomonic. In contrast, features such as systemic lymphostasis (distinct from lymphedema), frequent association with lower limb varicose syndrome, and vascular meiopragia (manifested by spontaneous hematomas following minor trauma) are more consistently observed in affected individuals.

From a biochemical perspective, a recent study[13] demonstrated that pathological tissue samples from individuals with lipedema contain a highly biologically active microRNA that is exclusively present in the affected tissue, when compared to healthy tissue from the same individuals. Ongoing research aims to characterize this finding further, as it holds promise as a potential biomarker for the disease.

Clinical diagnosis

Clinically, lipedema presents itself, as already mentioned, with a volumetric increase in the lower limbs, sometimes associated with similar deposits in the upper limbs, with consistent sparing of the extremities of the limbs themselves (feet and hands).[11, 12] Depending on the predominant location of fat deposits, the disease is typically classified into the following five types, as illustrated in Figure 1.1.

As far as the clinical evolution is concerned, it is usually divided into the following three stages, with the third split into moderate and severe (see Figure 1.2):

- **Stage 1:** the skin surface is normal, and the subcutaneous tissue has a soft consistency but with multiple nodules that can be appreciated on palpation.

- **Stage 2:** the skin surface becomes irregular and hard, related to the nodular structure (large nodules) of the subcutaneous fatty tissue (liposclerosis).

- **Stage 3 moderate:** characterized by a lobular deformation of the skin surface in relation to increased adipose tissue. The nodules vary in size and are distinguishable from the surrounding tissue on

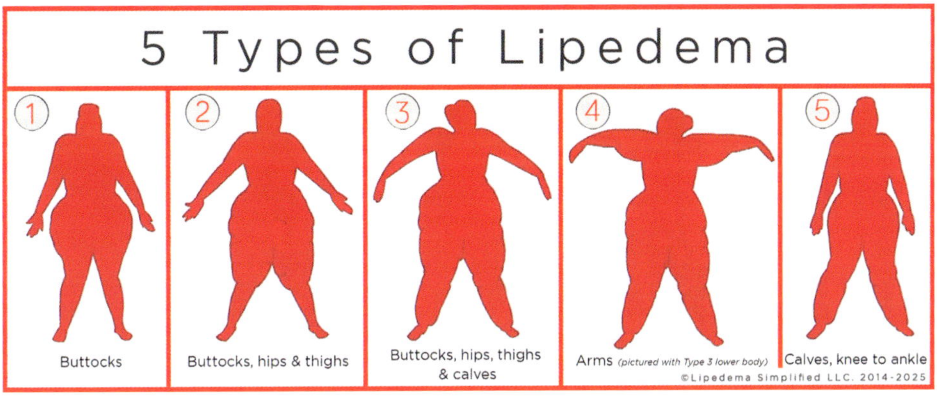

Figure 1.1: Five types of lipedema dependent on the location of excessive adipose tissue including: Type 1 (buttocks); Type 2 (buttocks, hips, and thighs); Type 3 (buttocks, hips, thighs, and calves); Type 4 (arms are affected and generally co-occurs with another type); and Type 5 (calves are the most affected, knee to the ankle). Used with permission from Lipedema Simplified LLC.

palpation. The orange peel phenomenon is appreciated on skin compression.

- **Stage 3 severe:** characterized by severe limb deformity and major functional problems.

Clinical examination of symptoms

Currently, the diagnosis of lipedema is based primarily on clinical examination. Therefore, the physical examination should carefully assess the following signs and characteristics. Refer to Chapter 2 for further discussion on the clinical examination process.

Pain

Pain remains a controversial feature of lipedema. However, it is reported by more than 80% of affected individuals and is typically localized to the areas involved by the disease. Pain is often exacerbated by local pressure during physical examination. Although inherently subjective, pain intensity can be quantified by patients using the numerical rating scale (NRS), with reported values ranging from 0 to 10.[14, 15, 16, 17, 18, 19]

The pain associated with lipedema is generally less intense in the early hours of the day. It tends to worsen progressively, particularly in the afternoon and evening, sometimes reaching maximum intensity (10/10 on the NRS), especially following periods of increased physical activity. When this occurs, it is often accompanied by swelling in the peri-malleolar region, further intensifying the pain. In some cases, a whole night of rest is required for the local swelling to subside and the pain to diminish. The release of inflammatory chemical mediators within the pathological adipose septa leads to vasodilation, which simultaneously increases the volume of the affected anatomical compartment and exacerbates the associated pain. Although the causes of pain in lipedema are multifactorial, it is essential to note that, contrary to its classification by the WHO as a non-inflammatory adipose tissue disease, lipedema is, by definition, an inflammatory disease of adipose tissue.

Although inflammation is a consistent finding in lipedematous tissue and contributes significantly to the disease process, other factors also play a role in the development of pain. For example, mechanical compression of peripheral sensory receptors and nerve fibers can independently evoke pain. Additionally, GABAA

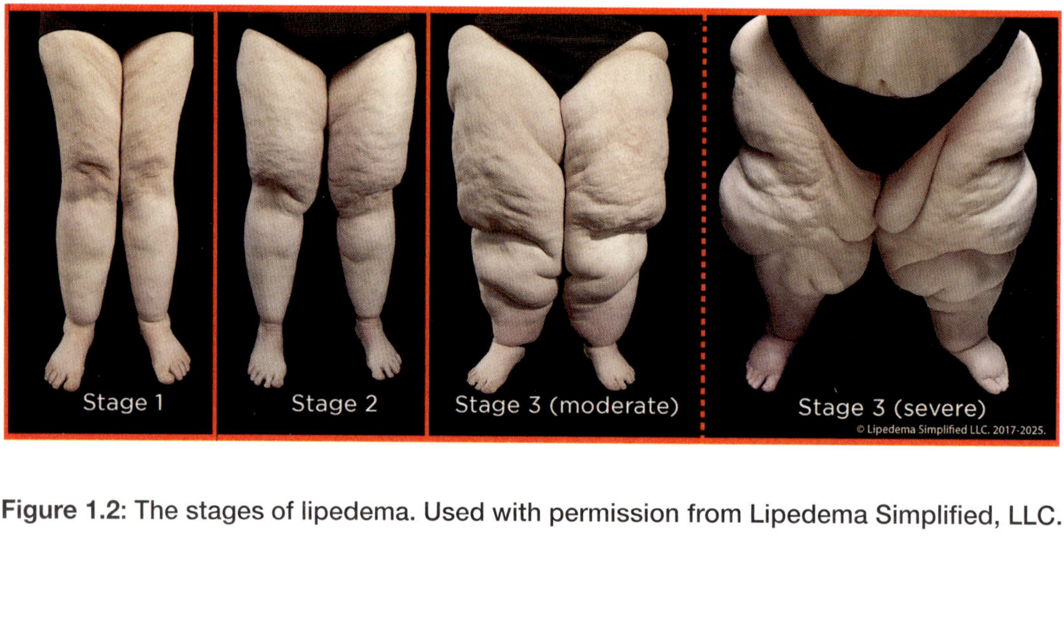

Figure 1.2: The stages of lipedema. Used with permission from Lipedema Simplified, LLC.

channels, which are involved in the pain transmission pathway* and are inhibited by pregnenolone,† also contribute to pain modulation. Clinically, it is often observed that patients with lower plasma concentrations of pregnenolone, frequently below the lower limit of the reference range, report higher levels of perceived pain compared to those whose pregnenolone levels are higher but still within the normal range.

The guidelines of some countries differ significantly in the requirement for pain to diagnose lipedema. The US document *Standard of Care for Lipedema*, for example, reports pain as a persistent and disabling symptom, but not pathognomonic for the diagnosis of the disease.[3] The new German guidelines on the disease, on the other hand, start from the statement that 'all manifestations of fatty tissue changes affecting the limbs in the absence of pain are not covered by these guidelines'.[19] Recognizing that pain perception varies widely among individuals, the US consensus document aligns more closely with common clinical experience.

Assessment of pain is accomplished using external pressure on the affected tissue by the examiner, in particular with the 'pinching' of the tissue constituting the greater and lesser saphenous vein compartments in the lower extremity, and the posterior brachial compartment of the arm. This will generally evoke significant pain in the affected areas in the patient with lipedema to such a degree that, in the absence of a pain response, one could practically exclude the existence of lipedema.‡

Skin and tissue changes

Another clinical manifestation is vascular fragility expressed by the presence of hematomas, mainly located in the limbs themselves. The clinical sign of fovea, at least in the initial stages, is absent, just as Stemmer's sign is negative in the lower limb (and this alone would be sufficient to distinguish it from lymphedema). Skin temperature sign itself is negative; that is, there are no significant changes in skin temperature in lipedema.[3]

Edema

Regarding the issue of edema, there is an ongoing debate about whether the term lipedema should be revised, as fluid stagnation in the interstitial matrix is not always present in uncomplicated cases of lipedema. Some have proposed alternative names, such as painful lipohypertrophy, lipalgia, or lipodystrophy with pain. However, it seems more appropriate to retain the term lipedema, both because the WHO has formally recognized it and because, when considering the etymology, 'edema' simply refers to an increase in tissue volume, regardless of the underlying cause.

Evaluation of co-morbidities during the examination process

In addition to the clinical examination, however, one must also consider the possible association with other aspects, as this disease manifests similarly to others. The prognosis is variable and depends on the possible co-morbidities present in each individual. See Chapters 6, 7, and 9 in this

*The pain transmission chain is a series of neurons and other cells that transmit pain signals from the body to the brain and includes the peripheral receptor, followed by the first sensory neuron, the second neuron of the spinothalamic bundle, the thalamus, and finally the sensory cerebral cortex.

† Pregnenolone is produced by the adrenal gland and is synthesized from the cholesterol molecule. It is a precursor to testosterone, progesterone, cortisol, estrogen, and other hormones.

‡ 1. Deep pressure on the greater saphenous vein compartment (saphenous nerve) was positive in 98.7% of 1788 patients.
2. Pressure on the lesser saphenous vein compartment (sural nerve) is particularly painful and was positive in 98.5% of 1783 patients.

Table 1.1: Differential diagnosis of lymphedema and lipedema.

Lymphedema	Clinical variable	Lipedema
Possible	**Family history**	Certain
Male/female	**Gender**	Female
Uni/bilateral	**Limb Involvement**	Bilateral
Always present in the primary forms, late in the secondary ones	**Involvement of the distal extremities (hands and feet)**	Absent
Congenital, praecox, tarda	**Age of onset**	Puberty (may appear before puberty)
Absent	**Articular hypermobility**	Often present
Present	**Pitting test**	Absent
Always present in the primary forms, late in the secondary ones	**Stemmer sign**	Absent
Usually absent	**Pain**	Present
Good	**Response to the physical therapy**	Varies
Varies	**Response to the surgical therapy**	Good
Flat texture made-to-measure II-III-IV class	**Final garment**	Flat texture made-to-measure I-II-III class – leggings
Regularly	**Clinical follow-up**	When needed

text for a more extensive discussion of common co-morbidities of lipedema.

Indeed, a complete laboratory and instrumental study, complementary to the clinical examination, allows one to cover any conditions that favor the progression of the disease (insulin resistance, thyroiditis, etc.). The involvement of the patient in their therapeutic plan is significant and must necessarily include guidance for daily activities including physical exercise of medium-low intensity, appropriate and personalized nutritional regimens, daily use of proper compression garments, performance of conservative care treatments, and periodic clinical and instrumental monitoring. Refer to Section V of this textbook (Summary of conservative treatment methodologies) for a more comprehensive discussion of these topics.

Lymphedema

Lymphedema presents with various clinical forms, some of which are influenced by specific genetic mutations that determine the individual presentation. A similar genetic basis may be hypothesized for lipedema. Depending on the complexity of the case, specific diagnostic imaging or instrumental examinations should be included as part of the assessment. Lymphedema is discussed further in Chapter 6. Table 1.1 can be used in the differential diagnosis process.

Obesity

Obesity is frequently associated with lipedema but is not caused by it; the two conditions are independent. One of the most commonly discussed topics in the scientific community is the distinction between body mass index (BMI) and waist-to-height ratio (WHtR) when evaluating patients with lipedema. Relying solely on BMI often leads to the misclassification of patients with lipedema as obese, whereas WHtR tends to identify far fewer of these individuals as obese.[20] This distinction is critical, as many patients with undiagnosed lipedema are still being inappropriately referred for bariatric surgery. This intervention can lead to a further decline in their quality of life. Visual differences between lipedema and obesity are shown in Figure 1.3. See Chapter 7 for an in-depth discussion on obesity.

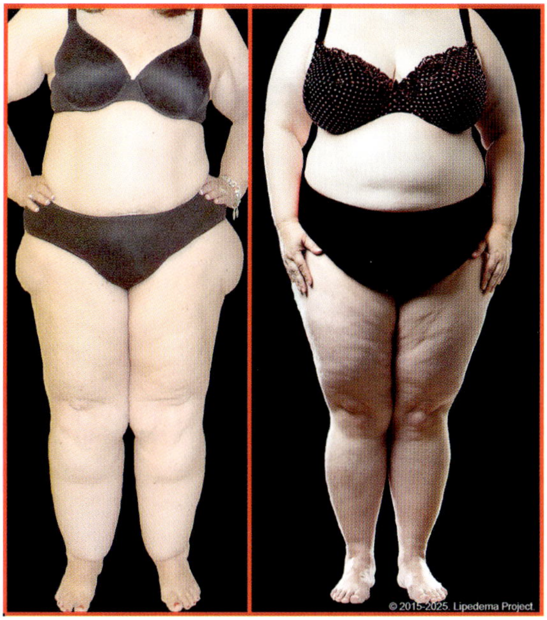

Figure 1.3: Lipedema (left) vs. obesity (right). Photo used with permission from the Lipedema Project.

Polycystic ovary syndrome

Polycystic ovary syndrome (PCOS) and endometriosis can be assessed by clinical, laboratory, and imaging (ultrasound) examinations. Patients with lipedema were asked the following four questions about their menstruation pattern between the ages of 12 and 20 years:[10]

- Was menstruation so painful that you required the use of painkillers?
- Were you forced to miss work or commitments on the first day of menstruation?
- Were your periods heavy?
- Did your menstrual cycle typically not last 28 days?

Because 76% of the 1376 patients queried responded positively to two or more of these questions, this suggests that in lipedema, there may be an ovarian-uterine inflammatory disease, termed ovarian inflammatory dysfunction, likely related to endometriosis and estrogen dominance syndrome (EDS).[11] Given that a very significant number of these patients were prescribed oral contraceptives with estrogen and progestin, the most common treatment for EDS, and were between the ages of 18 and 25, in our clinical experience and agreed by other authors, they are unlikely to experience an improvement in symptoms. On the contrary, these symptoms seem to worsen or even trigger the symptoms of lipedema. This can only be because, in this case, EDS is due to an alteration or resistance of progesterone receptors, caused by the sub-chronic inflammation accompanying lipedema. In extreme cases, this estrogen dominance would lead to PCOS or endometriosis.

Joint hypermobility/Ehlers-Danlos syndrome

Ehlers-Danlos Syndrome (EDS), hypermobility type, can be a co-morbidity of lipedema. EDS is a group of inherited diseases that affect connective tissues, resulting in issues with skin, joints, and blood vessels. These diseases are caused by mutations in genes that affect the structure and function of collagen and related proteins.

Joint hypermobility can be assessed through a comprehensive analysis using the Beighton Scale.[21] In one study, 96.9% of 1750 patients diagnosed with lipedema tested positive on the Beighton Scale.[10] It is not uncommon, in this regard, to formulate a suspicion spectrum of hypermobile Ehlers-Danlos syndrome during an examination for suspected lipedema (see Figure 1.4).

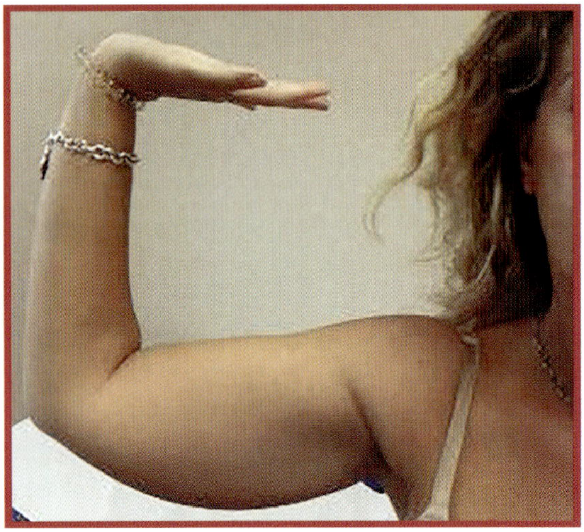

Figure 1.4: Joint hypermobility and EDS can be a co-morbidity of lipedema (demonstrated here in the wrist joint). Courtesy of Dr. Sandro Michelini.

Hypothyroidism

Latent or manifest hypothyroidism is often dependent on autoimmune Hashimoto's thyroiditis.[3, 19] Thyroid nodules are also common in lipedema, with 88.6% of 474 patients diagnosed with lipedema having thyroid nodules using ultrasound imaging.[10]

Insulin resistance

Insulin resistance is frequently found during investigations for lipedema and is often present in subjects with a clear family history of diabetes mellitus.[3, 19]

Hypovitaminosis D

Vitamin D is fat-soluble, and it is not uncommon for individuals with affected conditions to have low plasma concentrations of this vitamin, necessitating supplementation.[22]

Allergies

Allergies to various substances have been noted, first and foremost, nickel.[23] One study showed 67.7% of the 88 patients diagnosed with lipedema had a clinical history of nickel allergy.[10]

Phlebolymphatic insufficiency

Phlebolymphatic insufficiency must always be ruled out as a possible association and contributory cause of local edema.

Instrumental diagnosis

The following methods are possible and practical for instrumental diagnosis. See Chapters 10 and 11 for a more in-depth examination of these tools for instrumental diagnosis.

Bioimpedance testing

Bioimpedance is a non-invasive technique used to assess body composition, including fat, muscle, water, and bone, by measuring electrical impedance – the resistance of body tissues to a small, safe electrical current. Tissues with higher water content, such as muscle, conduct electricity more easily, whereas fat and bone have lower conductivity and therefore greater resistance.[24, 25]

In lipedema, it is found that the percentage of fat mass is much higher in the lower and upper limbs than in the trunk. Bioimpedance measurement of extracellular and intracellular water typically reveals a higher accumulation of fluid in the extracellular matrix compared to the general population.

High-resolution ultrasound

Ultrasonography can also help in diagnosing lipedema, revealing various signs indicating extracellular fluid retention and partial lymphatic system dysfunction. However, we agree with other works that B-mode ultrasound alone is not diagnostic,[26] although it is indicative when accompanied by other signs and symptoms of lipedema.

Magnetic resonance imaging

Magnetic resonance imaging (MRI) enables us to assess the depth of the fat layer in the scanned area.[27] It is a diagnostic tool that allows us to differentiate lipedema from other pathologies, such as lymphedema, venous insufficiency, and obesity, by providing detailed images of the soft tissue. MRI can show diffuse fat hypertrophy in patients with lipedema, but it can also demonstrate this feature in patients with lipohypertrophy. High cost, low spatial resolution, and sensitivity are limitations of MRI.[28, 29]

Lymphoscintigraphy

Lymphoscintigraphy enables the assessment of damage to the lymphatic system, allowing for the differentiation between lipedema and lymphedema, or when the two diseases co-occur. However, its use in lipedema is limited for the following reasons:

1. In initial cases of lipedema, the damage to the lymphatic system is minor and generally undetectable with this test. Only experienced operators detect the slowing of the radiotracer transit.[30]
2. Although the radiation dose is low, there is some exposure, which may be a risk for some patients.
3. Lymphoscintigraphy is expensive and, therefore, not a simple means of screening. Furthermore, evaluation and anatomical correlation are difficult to interpret.
4. Typically, the injection of the radiolabel is performed subcutaneously in the second interdigital space. Not only does this prevent us from seeing the deep lymphatic system, but only a portion of the superficial lymphatic system is viewed.[31, 32]
5. According to some authors, lymphatic damage may be due to causes other than lipedema, limiting the diagnostic applicability of this imaging technique.[33]

Therapeutic approach

Decongestive therapy

Comprehensive decongestive therapy (CDT) consists of the use of manual lymphatic drainage (MLD), compression therapy, skin care, and patient education.[15,34] CDT shows an improvement in the patient's general condition and a decrease in pain; its effects disappear when treatment ceases, and they do not reduce the amount of adipose tissue.[14, 35, 36, 37, 38, 39, 40, 41, 42]

MLD is a manual therapy that stimulates the drainage of the lymphatic system, facilitating the removal of excess fluid and waste products from the interstitial spaces (see Figure 1.5). In the case of lipedema, it is efficacious in improving the sensation of swelling, although its effectiveness is short-lived and does not address the underlying fat in the lipedema. Compression therapy is the application of controlled pressure using elastic garments or multi-layer bandages. Skin care and patient education focus on hygiene and skin hydration, avoidance of infections and irritants, and protecting the skin from trauma. Intermittent pneumatic compression devices, often used in conjunction with CDT, improve lymphatic and venous return when applied correctly and with specific pressures and programs for lipedema. Please see Chapter 12 for a more in-depth discussion of CDT and MLD.

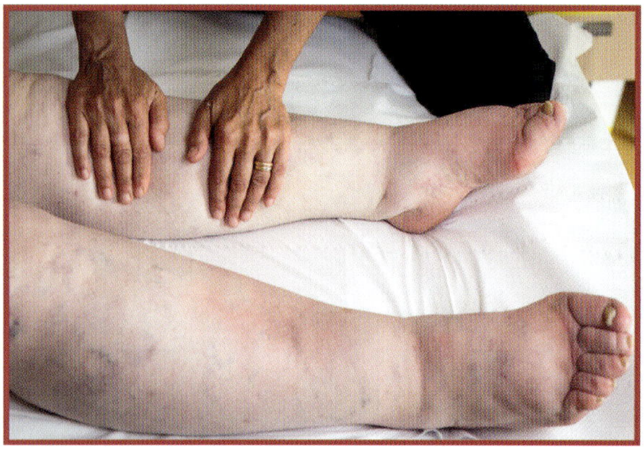

Figure 1.5: Manual lymphatic drainage (MLD) for a patient with lipedema and secondary lymphedema.

Exercise programs

Exercise programs can include water activities, flexibility and balance exercises, strength training, and low-impact aerobic exercises. Postural and gait training is also valuable, as it reduces joint stress, optimizes gait mechanics, increases functional independence, improves mobility and stability, and enhances alignment. Exercise is discussed further in Chapters 12 and 18.

Medical therapy

There is no medical therapy that has been shown scientifically to be effective for lipedema.

Surgical therapy

Surgical treatment for the removal of pathological adipose tissue (also sometimes called 'liposuction') constitutes an important therapeutic solution, especially in the more advanced clinical stages and in the presence of significant painful symptoms. Different techniques are known, although water-assisted liposuction (WAL),[43] power-assisted liposuction (PAL),[44] and Vaser[45] appear to be more effective in maintaining long-term clinical results. Surgical procedures for lipedema are discussed further in Chapters 16 and 17.

Bariatric surgery does not solve the problem of lipedema. It is known that a patient undergoing one of the known bariatric surgical techniques has weight and volume loss in the same body areas that respond to standard low-calorie diets or exercise, but not in those body areas affected by lipedema.[4]

Nutrition

There are various nutritional approaches to treating lipedema, which may depend on the patient's overall condition and any co-existing conditions. In general, an anti-inflammatory diet substantially improves pain associated with the disease and stops the clinical progression of the disease. In many cases, the patient seems to respond better to a ketogenic diet, with many symptoms of lipedema reducing or resolving.[46, 47] See Chapter 14 for a more extensive discussion of ketogenic diets used for lipedema.

Elastic garments

In the absence of venous and/or lymphatic insufficiency in the limbs affected by lipedema, some international compression garment companies have developed 'leggings' for the lower limbs and a 'bolero' for the upper limbs, which come in compression classes I and II. These products help reduce the growth of pathological fatty tissue, alleviate painful symptoms, and improve the personal, relational, and social functioning of individuals affected by the disease. For more information on this topic, see Chapters 12 and 18.

Conclusion

The disease of lipedema requires further epidemiological, etiopathogenic, clinical, and instrumental investigations that will allow a better understanding of the mechanisms leading to the pathological picture. Research focuses on the various emergent theories, including macroscopic and microscopic anatomy, biochemistry, proteomics, metabolomics, genetics, somatics, and germ cells, as well as the well-accepted therapeutic directions. Closely dependent on the scientific achievements that are gradually being gathered, they aim at increasingly targeted objectives and toward constant and lasting results.

References

1. Allen EV, Hines EA. Lipedema of the legs: a syndrome characterized by fat legs and orthostatic edema. *Proc Staff Meet Mayo Clin* 1940;15(15):184–7. Available from: https://klosetraining.com/wp-content/uploads/2021/03/1940-Lipedema-of-the-Legs.pdf
2. WHO. *International Statistical Classification of Diseases and Related Health Problems.* 11th ed. Geneva, Switzerland: World Health Organization (WHO); 2022. Available from: https://www.who.int/standards/classifications/classification-of-diseases
3. Herbst KL, Kahn LA, Iker E, Ehrlich C, Wright T, McHutchison L, et al. Standard of care for lipedema in the United States. *Phlebology* 2021 Dec 1;36(10):779–96. DOI: https://doi.org/10.1177/02683555211015887
4. Bast JH, Ahmed L, Engdahl R. Lipedema in patients after bariatric surgery. *Surg Obes Relat Dis* 2016 Jun;12(5):1131–2. DOI: https://doi.org/10.1016/j.soard.2016.04.013
5. Michelini S, Chiurazzi P, Marino V, Dell'Orco D, Manara E, Baglivo M, et al. Aldo-keto reductase 1C1 (AKR1C1) as the first mutated gene in a family with nonsyndromic primary lipedema. *Int J Mol Sci* 2020 Jan;21(17):6264. DOI: https://doi.org/10.3390/ijms21176264
6. Paolacci S, Precone V, Acquaviva F, Chiurazzi P, Fulcheri E, Pinelli M, et al. Genetics of lipedema: new perspectives on genetic research and molecular diagnoses. *Eur Rev Med Pharmacol Sci* 2019 Jul;23(13):5581–94. DOI: https://doi.org/10.26355/eurrev_201907_18292
7. Child AH, Gordon KD, Sharpe P, Brice G, Ostergaard P, Jeffery S, et al. Lipedema: an inherited condition. *Am J Med Genet A* 2010;152A(4):970–6. DOI: https://doi.org/10.1002/ajmg.a.33313
8. Michelini S, Herbst KL, Precone V, Manara E, Marceddu G, Dautaj A, et al. A multi-gene panel to identify lipedema-predisposing genetic variants by a next-generation sequencing strategy. *J Pers Med* 2022 Feb 11;12(2):268. DOI: https://doi.org/10.3390/jpm12020268
9. Schook CC, Mulliken JB, Fishman SJ, Alomari AI, Grant FD, Greene AK. Differential diagnosis of lower extremity enlargement in pediatric patients referred with a diagnosis of lymphedema. *Plast Reconstr Surg* 2011 Apr;127(4):1571. DOI: https://doi.org/10.1097/PRS.0b013e31820a64f3
10. Simarro JL, Michelini S, Andres-Gasco M, et al. Clinical signs at diagnosis and comorbidities in a large cohort of patients with lipedema in Spain. *Biomedicines MDPI* 2026 (accepted for publication: www.preprints.org/manuscript/202510.1397/v1)
11. Katzer K, Hill JL, McIver KB. Lipedema and the potential role of estrogen in excessive adipose tissue accumulation. *Int J Mol Sci* 2021;22(21):11720. DOI: https://doi.org/10.3390/ijms222111720
12. Barbagallo M, Dominguez LJ, Licata G, Shan J, Bing L, Karpinski E, et al. Vascular effects of progesterone. *Hypertension.* 2001 Jan;37(1):142–7. DOI: https://doi.org/10.1161/01.HYP.37.1.142
13. Cione E, Michelini S, Abrego-Guandique DM, Vaia N, Michelini S, Puleo V, et al. Identification of specific microRNAs in adipose tissue affected by lipedema. *Curr Issues Mol Biol* 2024 Nov;46(11):11957–74. DOI: https://doi.org/10.3390/cimb46110710
14. Szolnoky G, Varga E, Varga M, Tuczai M, Dosa-Racz E, Kemeny L. Lymphedema treatment decreases pain intensity in lipedema. *Lymphology* 2011 Aug 20;44(4):178–82. Available from: https://journals.uair.arizona.edu/index.php/lymph/article/view/17067
15. Kruppa P, Georgiou I, Biermann N, Prantl L, Klein-Weigel P, Ghods M. Lipedema – pathogenesis, diagnosis, and treatment options. *Dtsch Ärztebl Int* 2020 Jun;117(22–23):396. DOI: https://doi.org/10.3238/arztebl.2020.0396
16. Nair AS, Diwan S. Allopregnanolone: a

neurosteroid for managing acute and chronic pain conditions. *Saudi J Anaesth* 2019;13(3):264–6. DOI: https://doi.org/10.4103/sja.SJA_830_18
17. Cornely ME, Hasenberg T, Cornely OA, Ure C, Hettenhausen C, Schmidt J. Persistent lipedema pain in patients after bariatric surgery: a case series of 13 patients. *Surg Obes Relat Dis* 2022 May 1;18(5):628–33. DOI: https://doi.org/10.1016/j.soard.2021.12.027
18. Aksoy H, Karadag AS, Wollina U. Cause and management of lipedema-associated pain. *Dermatol Ther.* 2021 Jan;34(1):e14364. DOI: https://doi.org/10.1111/dth.14364
19. Faerber G, Cornely M, Daubert C, Erbacher G, Fink J, Hirsch T, et al. S2k guideline lipedema. *JDDG J Dtsch Dermatol Ges* 2024;22(9):1303–15. DOI: https://doi.org/10.1111/ddg.15513
20. Pereira de Godoy LM, Pereira de Godoy HJ, Pereira de Godoy Capeletto P, Guerreiro Godoy M de F, Pereira de Godoy JM. Lipedema and the evolution to lymphedema with the progression of obesity. *Cureus* 2020;12(12):e11854. DOI: https://doi.org/10.7759/cureus.11854
21. Hakim AJ, Grahame R. A simple questionnaire to detect hypermobility: an adjunct to the assessment of patients with diffuse musculoskeletal pain. *Int J Clin Pract* 2003 Apr;57(3):163–6. DOI: https://doi.org/10.1111/j.1742-1241.2003.tb10455.x
22. Pereira-Santos M, Costa PRF, Assis AMO, Santos C.A. ST, Santos DB. Obesity and vitamin D deficiency: a systematic review and meta-analysis. *Obes Rev Off J Int Assoc Study Obes* 2015 Apr;16(4):341–9. DOI: https://doi.org/10.1111/obr.12239
23. Ehrlich C, Iker E, Herbst KL. *Lymphedema and lipedema nutrition guide: foods, vitamins, minerals, and supplements.* San Francisco, CA: Lymph Notes; 2017. Available from: https://www.lymphnotes.com/nutrition-guide-introduction
24. Stellmaker R, Thompson B, Mackie H, Koelmeyer L. Comparison of fluid and body composition measures in women with lipoedema, lymphoedema, and control participants. *Clin Obes* 2024 Aug;14(4):e12658. DOI: https://doi.org/10.1111/cob.12658
25. Ward LC, Thompson B, Gaitatzis K, Koelmeyer LA. Comparison of volume measurements and bioimpedance spectroscopy using a stand-on device for assessment of unilateral breast cancer-related lymphedema. *Eur J Breast Health* 2024 Apr;20(2):141–8. DOI: https://doi.org/10.4274/ejbh.galenos.2024.2023-12-8
26. Hirsch T, Schleinitz J, Marshall M, Faerber G. Is differential diagnosis of lipedema possible using high-resolution sonography? *Phlebologie* 2018 Aug 22;47:182–7. DOI: https://doi.org/10.12687/phleb2431-4-2018
27. Taylor SL, Donahue PMC, Pridmore MD, Garza ME, Patel NJ, Custer CA, et al. Semiautomated segmentation of lower extremity MRI reveals distinctive subcutaneous adipose tissue in lipedema: a pilot study. *J Med Imaging* 2023 May;10(3):036001. DOI: https://doi.org/10.1117/1.JMI.10.3.036001
28. Markarian B, Toro C, Moreira K, Polam S, Mathew N, Mayrovitz HN. Assessment modalities for lower extremity edema, lymphedema, and lipedema: a scoping review. *Cureus* 2024 Mar;16(3):e55906. DOI: https://doi.org/10.7759/cureus.55906
29. Munn LL, Padera TP. Imaging the lymphatic system. *Microvasc Res* 2014 Nov;96:55–63. DOI: https://doi.org/10.1016/j.mvr.2014.06.006
30. Forner-Cordero I, Oliván-Sasot P, Ruiz-Llorca C, Muñoz-Langa J. Lymphoscintigraphic findings in patients with lipedema. *Rev Esp Med Nucl E Imagen Mol Engl Ed* 2018 Nov 1;37(6):341–8. DOI: https://doi.org/10.1016/j.remnie.2018.10.013
31. Shinaoka A. A new lymphography protocol and interpretation principles based on functional lymphatic anatomy in lower limb lymphedema. *Anat Sci Int* 2024 Mar 1;99(2):153–8. DOI: https://doi.org/10.1007/s12565-023-00754-2
32. Bräutigam P, Földi E, Schaiper I, Krause T, Vanscheidt W, Moser E. Analysis of lymphatic drainage in various forms of leg edema using two compartment lymphoscintigraphy. *Lymphology* 1998 Jun;31(2):43–55. Available from: https://journals.librarypublishing.arizona.edu/lymph/article/id/3343/
33. Chachaj A, Dudka I, Jeziorek M, Sowicz M, Adaszyńska A, Szuba A. Lymphoscintigraphic alterations in lower limbs in women with lipedema in comparison to women with overweight/

obesity. *Front Physiol* 2023 Apr 10;14. Available from: https://www.frontiersin.org/journals/physiology/articles/10.3389/fphys.2023.1099555/full

34. Reich-Schupke S, Schmeller W, Brauer WJ, Cornely ME, Faerber G, Ludwig M, et al. S1 guidelines: lipedema. *J Dtsch Dermatol Ges* 2017;15(7):758–67. DOI: https://doi.org/10.1111/ddg.13036
35. Donahue PMC, Crescenzi R, Petersen KJ, Garza M, Patel N, Lee C, et al. Physical therapy in women with early stage lipedema: potential impact of multimodal manual therapy, compression, exercise, and education interventions. *Lymphat Res Biol* 2022 Aug;20(4):382–90. DOI: https://doi.org/10.1089/lrb.2021.0039
36. Czerwińska M, Teodorczyk J, Spychała D, Hansdorfer-Korzon R. The usefulness of the application of compression therapy among lipedema patients – pilot study. *Int J Environ Res Public Health* 2023 Jan 4;20(2):914. DOI: https://doi.org/10.3390/ijerph20020914
37. Atan T, Bahar-Özdemir Y. The effects of complete decongestive therapy or intermittent pneumatic compression therapy or exercise only in the treatment of severe lipedema: a randomized controlled trial. *Lymphat Res Biol* 2021 Feb;19(1):86–95. DOI: https://doi.org/10.1089/lrb.2020.0019
38. Volkan-Yazici M, Esmer M. Reducing circumference and volume in upper extremity lipedema: the role of complex decongestive physiotherapy. *Lymphat Res Biol* 2022 Feb;20(1):71–5. DOI: https://doi.org/10.1089/lrb.2020.0128
39. Herbst KL, Ussery C, Eekema A. Pilot study: whole body manual subcutaneous adipose tissue (SAT) therapy improved pain and SAT structure in women with lipedema. *Horm Mol Biol Clin Investig* 2017 Sep 20;33(2). DOI: https://doi.org/10.1515/hmbci-2017-0035
40. Esmer M, Schingale FJ, Unal D, Yazıcı MV, Güzel NA. Physiotherapy and rehabilitation applications in lipedema management: a literature review. *Lymphology* 2020;53(2):88–95. Available from: https://journals.librarypublishing.arizona.edu/lymph/article/id/4659/
41. Schneider R. Low-frequency vibrotherapy considerably improves the effectiveness of manual lymphatic drainage (MLD) in patients with lipedema: a two-armed, randomized, controlled pragmatic trial. *Physiother Theory Pract* 2020 Jan;36(1):63–70. DOI: https://doi.org/10.1080/09593985.2018.1479474
42. Michelini S, Musa F, Vetrano M, Santoboni F, Nusca SM, Latini E, et al. Defocused and radial shock wave therapy, mesotherapy, and kinesio taping effects in patients with lipedema: a pilot study. *Lymphology* 2023;56(1):13–26. DOI: https://doi.org/10.2458/lymph.5872
43. Witte T, Dadras M, Heck FC, Heck M, Habermalz B, Welss S, et al. Water-jet-assisted liposuction for the treatment of lipedema: standardized treatment protocol and results of 63 patients. *J Plast Reconstr Aesthet Surg* 2020 Sep 1;73(9):1637–44. DOI: https://doi.org/10.1016/j.bjps.2020.03.002
44. Abboud MH, Dibo SA, Abboud NM. Power-assisted liposuction and lipofilling: techniques and experience in large-volume fat grafting. *Aesthet Surg J* 2020 Jan 29;40(2):180–90. DOI: https://doi.org/10.1093/asj/sjz019
45. de Souza Pinto EB, Abdala PC de SP, Maciel CM, dos Santos F de PT, de Souza RPM. Liposuction and VASER. *Clin Plast Surg* 2006 Jan;33(1):107–15, vii. DOI: https://doi.org/10.1016/j.cps.2005.09.001
46. Cannataro R, Michelini S, Ricolfi L, Caroleo MC, Gallelli L, De Sarro G, et al. Management of lipedema with ketogenic diet: 22-month follow-up. *Life* 2021 Dec;11(12):1402. DOI: https://doi.org/10.3390/life11121402
47. Keith L, Seo CA, Rowsemitt C, Pfeffer M, Wahi M, Staggs M, et al. Ketogenic diet as a potential intervention for lipedema. *Med Hypotheses* 2021 Jan 1;146:110435.d DOI: https://doi.org/10.1016/j.mehy.2020.110435

Chapter Two
Addressing lipedema: challenges to the primary care physician

Matthew Carmody

Introduction

Drs. Allen and Hines spoke to the staff of the Mayo Clinic 85 years ago, describing lipedema with these words (see Figure 2.1):[1] 'a clinical syndrome, lipedema of the legs…which was frequently very distressing…present for many years in some since girlhood. Enlargement of the limbs has always been generalized and symmetrical…associated with a gradual increase in body weight…aching distress in the legs is common. There is a history of a similar in other members of the family.' They continued: 'Such patients are sensitive about the appearance of their limbs…occasionally a patient feels that her large legs have 'ruined her life'…deposition of the fat beneath the skin of the buttocks and legs only, is not easy to explain, although in many instances it is a hereditary trait.'

An astute patient in my practice, with long-standing central obesity, controlled with exercise and variable dietary management, presented complaining of painful proximal legs and arms, recently increased in size without pitting edema, erythema, or signs of vascular compromise. She was recently menopausal. Droopy fatty tissue had increased in her proximal arms, which she remarked was 'just hanging there…loose!'

Multiple consultations in Boston medical systems (Harvard, Tufts, Boston University) ensued, during which most consultants believed it was obesity (of some kind) or lymphedema. She already had years of well-managed obesity and mild lymphedema. This most recent incidence of swelling was 'quite painful'. With her careful research, she emerged from the Foeldi Clinic for Lymphology in Germany with a diagnosis of lipedema, a disease that is well known in Europe but generally less so in the United States, except for some institutions involved in in-depth research.

At last, I learned my patient had lipedema. Thereafter, I recognized seven other 'obese' patients with painful arms, legs, and sometimes buttocks as having lipedema that I had previously diagnosed as obesity alone. This made the diagnosis challenging, but it was still achievable with a thorough examination and careful consideration of the patient's personal and family history, as well as distinct physical exam findings. My lipedema practice gradually grew to hundreds of patients referred to me by other recently diagnosed patients, as well as providers who were wondering if some of their patients with obesity also had lipedema.

I wish to emphasize the importance of the Sulkowitch test in determining the excretion of calcium. It is of importance in determining the efficacy of treatment of parathyroid insufficiency with calcium and vitamin C. It is of greater importance, as emphasized by Albright and his group, in the diagnosis of hyperparathyroidism. This easily performed diagnostic test should be used for every patient suspected of having this disease and every patient who has renal stones. The earlier we can diagnose hyperparathyroidism, the less damage will have been done to the patient.

VASCULAR CLINICS. X.
LIPEDEMA OF THE LEGS: A SYNDROME CHARACTERIZED BY FAT LEGS AND ORTHOSTATIC EDEMA

E. V. Allen, M. D., and E. A. Hines, Jr., M. D., Division of Medicine: We wish to describe a clinical syndrome, lipedema of the legs, which is frequently very distressing. In our experience it affects solely women. The chief complaint is of swelling of the legs and feet which has been present for many years; in some instances, first noted in girlhood. On questioning, the physician may elicit that enlargement of the limbs has always been generalized and symmetrical. Usually, it is associated with gradual increase in body weight. There is never a history of recurrent episodes of acute cellulitis such as may occur in the course of lymphedema. The swelling below the knees is accentuated when patients are on their feet much and in warm weather. Aching distress in the legs is common. In many instances, there is a history of a similar condition in other members of the family. Ordinarily, such patients are very sensitive about the appearance of their limbs; they wear long skirts and stand behind chairs when in the presence of strangers. They avoid swimming. Evidence of neurosis is likely to be found. Occasionally, a patient feels that her large legs have "ruined her life." Many are "ashamed" of their legs.

ANATOMIC AND PHYSIOLOGIC BASIS

The basic difficulty in lipedema is the deposition of an unusual amount of fat beneath the skin. An intake of food exceeding the caloric requirements of the body is the obvious cause in cases of generalized obesity. The deposition of fat beneath the skin of the buttocks and legs only, is not easily explained although in many instances it is a hereditary trait. Whatever the basis for increased subcutaneous fat may be, it offers abnormally poor resistance to the passage of fluid into the tissue from the blood and thus permits edema to occur.

Edema is a manifestation of disturbed exchange between the fluid of the blood and that of the tissue. If more fluid than usual leaves blood vessels or if the removal of fluid from the limb is hindered, edema results. Although the transfer of fluid from blood to tissue is primarily controlled by capillary and colloid osmotic pressure, it is greatly influenced by a number of secondary factors, particularly by posture. There is a great tendency toward edema of the feet of well people when they are in the erect posture because the venous pressures rise to as much as 120 cm. of water. Edema is prevented in the erect posture in normal persons as a

result of an increase in colloid osmotic pressure in the blood of the veins of the feet, as a result of a decrease in volume and velocity of circulation of blood in the legs and as a result of an increase in tissue pressure due to filtration of fluid from blood vessels into extravascular spaces. In the erect posture, this increase in tissue pressure seems to be three to five times as important in limiting loss of fluid from the blood as is the increase in colloid osmotic pressure.[1,2] More simply stated, a very important mechanism in preventing edema in the erect posture is that by which fluid which leaves the blood vessels and enters the extravascular spaces thereby increases the tissue pressure; this condition in turn hinders the further filtration of the fluid of the blood into tissue spaces. When a person first

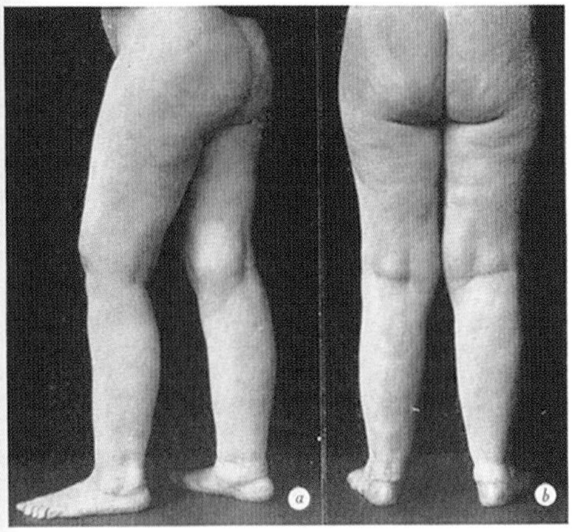

Fig. 1. Lipedema of the lower extremities of a woman aged forty-six years; a, left lateral aspect; b, posterior aspect.

stands, the filtering pressure exceeds the antifiltering pressure but equilibrium occurs in about thirty minutes. If edema occurs as a result of standing, equilibrium is reached only after more than the ordinary amount of fluid has passed from the blood into extravascular spaces.

An obviously very important extravascular factor in determining when tissue pressure will become great enough to prevent further loss of fluid

1. Youmans, J. B., Wells, H. S., Donley, Dorothy, and Miller, D. G.: The effect of posture (standing) on the serum protein concentration and colloid osmotic pressure of blood from the foot in relation to the formation of edema. J. Clin. Investigation 13: 447-459 (May) 1934.
2. Youmans, J. B., Akeroyd, J. H., Jr., and Frank, Helen: Changes in the blood and circulation with changes in posture: the effect of exercise and vasodilatation. J. Clin. Investigation 14: 739-753 (Nov.) 1935.

Figure 2.1: Original publication regarding lipedema from the Mayo Clinic Staff Meetings, March 20, 1940.

Lipedema practice challenges

Over the last 18 years, I have become aware of multiple challenges a primary care provider faces when taking on this fascinating patient population with lipedema. This chapter aims to address the challenges of lipedema practice, mitigate difficulties, and provide a foundation for compassionate care by discussing the seven most significant challenges to lipedema care.

Challenge #1. Lipedema and differential diagnosis: treating multiple co-occurring diseases

We will explore the co-occurring diseases, namely obesity and lymphedema, that may have hidden lipedema right in front of us for years. However, all complicating conditions need to be determined, appreciated, and addressed.

Key health issues in a lipedema practice:

1. Lipedema often co-occurs with obesity

and/or lymphedema.

2. Obesity is co-incident to lipedema in as many as 80% of cases (of which 50% is morbid obesity or BMI ≥40).[2]
3. Lipedema does not cause obesity or lymphedema.[2]
4. Obesity can cause lymphedema.[3]
5. Obesity is an aggravating factor for lipedema.[2, 4]
6. Obesity can cause/induce other chronic diseases, such as diabetes mellitus (type 2), cardiovascular disease (stroke/MI), renal failure, liver disease (cirrhosis, cancer, and liver failure), ovarian and uterine cancer; sleep apnea, osteoarthritis of weight-bearing joints, depression, and internalized anti-fat bias.[5]
7. Identifying associated complications involves a thorough physical examination, careful mental health screening, including assessment for internalized weight bias, as well as laboratory tests and EKG evaluation.

Diagnosing co-morbidities enables more targeted and effective interventions. Chapter 9 addresses how to distinguish between lipedema, lymphedema, and obesity. Here, the focus of the first challenge in a lipedema practice is on determining which of these diseases, or what combination of them, may be present in your patient. The diagnostic frameworks outlined below can support this evaluation.

Diagnostic formulations

Lipedema is diagnosed based on the certainty gained by applying the proposed framework for a case definition of lipedema, as defined by Keith et al.,[6] to the patient's history and physical examination. Reaching the diagnosis using combinations of agreed upon characteristics (female, pain, disproportionate distribution of adipose tissue to limbs, skin and tissue changes, and unresponsive to diet) and, if necessary, additional evidence (wrist/ankle cuffing, non-pitting edema with negative Kaposi-Stemmer sign, onset/exacerbation with hormone flux, family history, and easy bruising without trauma) achieves confirmation.[6]

Obesity is diagnosed using a waist-to-height ratio (WHtR) and by examining the patient to appreciate adipose tissue in the trunk. In this way, we can assess the significant metabolic health risk(s) of central obesity and estimate the severity of that risk. A WHtR of greater than 0.5 is indicative of obesity, while less than or equal to 0.5 is normal.[7]

When obesity is diagnosed, body mass index (BMI) is calculated to determine the severity. BMI calculators are available online. The patient with lipedema typically has a gynoid shape, with the most prominent fat deposition below the waist, and will have a normal waist-to-height ratio (WHtR). A patient with both lipedema and obesity will have symptoms of lipedema and WHtR greater than 0.5, along with truncal adipose tissue.

Obesity-induced lymphedema is a secondary lymphedema that occurs when BMI is ≥30 and is almost universally present when the BMI is 60. Obesity has a negative impact on lymphatic density in subcutaneous tissue, lymphatic endothelial cell proliferation, macromolecule clearance, integrity and function of the lymphatic vessels, and the collecting vessel pump capacity, which, in the end, induces more adipose tissue deposition and worsens obesity and lymphedema. If the patient is non-ambulatory, obesity-induced lymphedema can occur at a lower weight and BMI.[3]

Chronic venous disease

Beyond obesity-induced lymphedema, there are many other etiologies of lymphedema categorized into functional and venous hypertension. Diagnosing these specifically allows a more targeted intervention. Table 2.1 shows various diagnoses that can cause functional venous insufficiency.

Table 2.1: Diagnoses associated with functional venous insufficiency leading to lymphatic overload/failure and the development of lymphedema.

Functional venous insufficiency etiology	**Causal diagnoses**
Elevated central pressure	Obesity, obstructive sleep apnea, right heart failure, pulmonary artery vasoconstriction, pulmonary hypertension
Lymphatic dysfunction	Dependent edema, lymphedema, obesity-induced lymphedema
Decreased forward momentum of venous flow	Poor calf and foot pump function, muscle weakness, increased abdominal pressure
Lymphatic dysfunction	Dependent edema lymphedema
Obesity-induced lymphedema	
Decreased forward momentum of venous flow	Poor calf and foot pump function
Muscle weakness	
Increased abdominal pressure	

The CEAP classification system – an acronym for 'clinical signs, etiology, anatomical distribution, and pathophysiology' – is a standardized framework used to classify chronic venous disorders.[8, 9] It provides a consistent method for diagnosing, documenting, and guiding the management of venous diseases by categorizing the condition based on its clinical presentation, underlying cause, affected anatomy, and functional abnormalities. This tool is available at: https://www.sciencedirect.com/science/article/pii/S2213333X20300639.

Venous symptoms worsen in hot environments, with prolonged standing, at the end of the day, and during peri-menstrual periods. Physical exams are done with the patient standing to observe the effect of gravity and body weight. Skin is closely observed for hyperpigmentation (hemosiderin staining), erythema (cellulitis), and skin breakdown.[8]

Discussing co-morbidities

Having a discussion with your patient about their co-existing diseases, particularly obesity if present, can be a challenge. It is important to help improve your patient's understanding of the nature of their various diseases without judgment and with respect. The following is an example of how I discuss obesity with my patients.

Your disease is, in large part, inherited.

Obesity is a complex metabolic disease involving billions of fat cells having a diameter equal to the width of a human hair. These adipocytes are talking to the hypothalamus, a control region at the base of the brain. The fat cell produces a precise amount of the hormone leptin. The amount of leptin tells the brain precisely how much energy is stored in that fat cell. Without you being aware, the brain decides what to do based on this signaling and communicates to other parts of the brain to take action.

This all happens beyond your awareness! Sensor cells in your gut wall tell the brain what you are eating, at the time you eat it, through hormones and nerve signaling. So, the brain and other hormone systems take action! This symphony creates hunger and satiety…your conscious mind is NOT in the decision loop.

Obesity has a significant effect on multiple systems, causing various diseases.

Obesity is a metabolic disorder that increases the risk of other diseases.

We measure the degree of obesity by BMI and note that some low levels of increased BMI (30–35) are sometimes protective. We know that a BMI >40, or a BMI >35 with a co-occurring metabolic disease (such as diabetes), is a severely damaging disease that needs urgent intervention.

We know that every person has a difficult-to-determine weight set point, and they tend toward this set point, despite their efforts to change their weight. This fat regain can occur as much as 3 years after successful weight loss, even when the same weight loss measures are still employed. That means you may have inherited a higher weight, but it is unlikely to be in the obesity range.

Sixty per cent of obesity is genetically determined.[5]

Obesity is worsened by the type of food we eat (but helped by avoiding ultra-high processed food and high carbohydrates); the neighborhood we live in (but helped by a safe neighborhood that allows walking); the regular exercise we achieve (where 20 minutes of walking daily is a significantly positive effect); the number of hours we sleep (we all need ≥7 hrs each night; less sleep is associated with weight increase); the circadian rhythm we establish and refuse to disrupt (we need a regular sleep onset time/pattern) to mention only a few factors. The positive actions, cited in parentheses, are known to help patients maintain a better weight.

These interventions are known to drive the weight toward health! Be clear to your patient that they will improve their obesity and help their lipedema if they start and maintain for the rest of their lives. If there is future cessation, the weight will drift back to the previous weight (also understood as the person's metabolic set point).

Managing co-morbid obesity may require a referral to an obesity medicine specialist, but many primary care physicians are willing and able to collaborate with their patients to develop treatment strategies. Table 2.2 can help practitioners decide which strategies may be used based on the patient's BMI. It is important to remember that if the patient's WHtR does not indicate the presence of obesity, these strategies are not necessarily warranted.

Table 2.2: Weight management strategies based on the World Health Organization (WHO) classification of weight status.[9]

Weight status	Body mass index (kg/m2)	Treatment
Overweight	25.0–29.9	Diet and lifestyle
Obese	>30	Diet and lifestyle
Class I obesity	30.0–34.9	Diet and lifestyle
Class II obesity	35.0–39.9	With one co-existing metabolic disease (e.g. DM2, CVD, HTN), requires intense intervention using those for Class III
Class III obesity	>40	Immediate weight reduction by intense intervention: surgery or using GLP-1 receptor agonists

DM2 = diabetes mellitus, type 2; CVD = cardiovascular disease; HTN = hypertension; GLP-1 = glucogen-like peptide-1.

Challenge #2. Understanding the patient's lived experience

It is important to explore the patient's experience of living with lipedema. A study conducted by Dudek et al.[10] gives insight into the association between lipedema symptom severity and quality of life. For instance, almost 93% of participants reported both fatigue and leg heaviness as moderate to severe, and just under 73% of participants reported moderate to severe pain in their fat tissue. Higher symptom severity correlated with a lower quality of life. As providers, knowing which lipedema symptoms have the highest impact on a patient's quality of life and which symptoms are the most severe allows us to assess the patient's status and be more effective with intervention.

People with lipedema often demonstrate remarkable resilience and inner strength, particularly in managing chronic pain. Over time, many develop coping strategies that allow them to tolerate or minimize their symptoms, which may lead them to underreport the extent of their discomfort. It is essential to examine the patient's understanding of their pain and how they have adjusted to it in their daily life. Many individuals may not even recognize their experience as 'pain' or associate their symptoms with a specific medical condition. For a more detailed discussion of the fluctuating and complex nature of lipedema-related pain, refer to Chapter 1.

Some patients know and understand this summary statement, which is my understanding of what the patient may be experiencing:

Lipedema is a chronic, proliferative, symmetrical fat disease that affects the legs (proximal and/or distal), hips, buttocks, and sometimes the arms (especially proximal). The adipose tissue in these areas is experienced as painful by the patient, 2–3 years after the onset of lipedema…The moderate to severe pain is only present in the lipedema tissue and is likely not present in other fatty areas (e.g. torso, abdomen)…Sometimes the patient describes 'pain' as 'heavy, tight, uncomfortably burning, sharp or congested'. The pain can be induced by a light touch. Lipedema impacts the patient's life, making movement more difficult and painful, limiting social life, disrupting sleep, and subjecting the patient to anti-fat bias.

Through my work with patients, I've learned the importance of letting their stories guide me. I begin by asking them to share what a typical day is like:

'Tell me the story of a day in your life. Help me understand what you're experiencing. How do you adapt to your disease in your daily routines?'

This approach provides valuable insight into their lived experience and helps shape more empathetic, effective care.

Only one person fully experiences all aspects of living with lipedema: the person who has it. Their unique, multidimensional experiential knowledge grants them a form of wisdom not accessible to those without the disease. This inner understanding enables individuals with lipedema to make informed and sensible decisions about their care and treatment. When primary care practitioners support and expand this patient knowledge, it encourages patients to explore beneficial treatments, skills, and insights from other healthcare providers and specialists, provided both the patient and practitioner believe the experience may be valuable. Furthermore, when patients with lipedema connect with others facing the same disease, a powerful multiplier effect can emerge. These collaborative relationships often lead to remarkable innovation and shared wisdom, amplifying individual insights through the strength of community.

Challenge #3. Defining and describing the pathophysiology of lipedema for both patients and colleagues

The pathophysiology of lipedema can be understood by the patient, which helps direct self-care as they can better see and imagine what a treatment intervention is accomplishing. Providing the patient with an understandable pathology may help them take action. A pathophysiology statement for patients (brief and to the point) is:

In lipedema, fat cells enlarge, but their nutrient

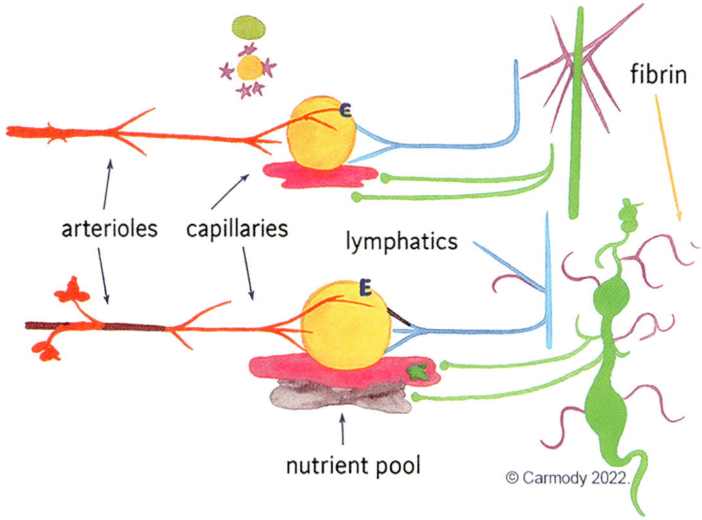

Figure 2.2: Capillary bed for fat cells (E): a capillary (red) brings nutrients to the cell; a vein (blue) takes blood back to the heart; and a lymph vessel (green) returns waste from the fat cell back to the heart.

blood vessels, which should also increase, don't!! The underfed fat cells starve and can't breathe enough oxygen. The distressed fat cells become angry with inflammation and pain. To add more trouble, lymphatic vessels under your skin that should be taking 'used' fluids away to make room for incoming, new nutrient and oxygen-rich fluids are not able to fully accomplish their job. Not taking the waste fluid away causes congestion (backup) and tight, painful tissue (see Figure 2.2).

Here is a more detailed description that can be used with colleagues and other healthcare providers:

Lipedema is a disease of the fat cells (there are 22 billion fat cells that comprise 20% of our weight) in the subcutaneous (under the skin) adipose tissue:

1. Adipocytes (fat cells) increase in size and, eventually, in number of fat cells.
2. But in the disease of lipedema, the number of nutrient-supplying blood vessels (which bring oxygen and nutrients) doesn't increase in number and size sufficiently, and this leads to inadequate circulation to the fat mass. This eventually starves the fat cells of oxygen and nutrients. The fat tissue signals its distress by starting a painful inflammation.
3. To make matters worse, the lymphatic system, which should be getting rid of fat cell waste, is unable to adequately get rid of old oxygen and nutrient-depleted fluid. The fresh supply of incoming oxygen and nutrients is impeded and becomes backed up (congested) from the pathologically slow-moving lymphatic circulation. As tissue fluid builds up and fat tissue becomes more congested, there is further inflammation, which increases pain and heaviness and inflammation.

Fact sheets about lipedema for internal medicine providers

Providing succinct, one-page handouts for colleagues who will likely see patients with lipedema in their practice can raise awareness and recruit more providers for multidisciplinary care. For providers new to diagnosing lipedema, an easy-to-follow fact sheet on diagnostic principles condensed from the *Proposed Framework for Research Case Definitions of Lipedema*[6] can be helpful (see the *Simplified Roadmap for Diagnosing Lipedema* in Chapter 19). Similarly, I developed a handout (see Table 2.3) that summarizes the treatment strategies suggested by the recently published S2k guidelines by the German Society of Phlebology and Lymphology.[6] Both of these papers are highly recommended for further reading.

Challenge #4. Transforming your practice from a traditional care model into one of patient–provider collaboration

After a decade in practice, I realized that there was an expert in the room, and it wasn't me. The wisdom is in the patient. As I reflect on collaborative relationships with patients with lipedema, I realize the patient has a broad appreciation and wisdom about their disease, despite being unaware of the specific diagnosis. Bringing out the brilliance in the patient by asking them about their experience fosters a conversation between co-collaborators, each with different expertise and perspectives, that, when combined, is more effective and inclusive of multiple perspectives, leading to the best path and the best commitment.

Establishing a collaborative relationship begins with trust and respect, and it requires time to develop. The first step is a willingness to truly listen to the patient. Through listening, we begin to understand the specific ways lipedema affects their daily life. When invited, patients often share deeper insights, including the interventions they've tried, the challenges they face, and the strategies that have helped them succeed. In my experience, partnering with patients by

Table 2.3: Fact sheet of practical strategies for the management of lipedema.

Strategy	Purpose	Notes
Psychological factors assessment	Address mental health impact	• Psychological disorders may affect lipedema symptoms • Diagnosis and prescription should be considered for eating disorders, depression, and PTSD after violence and abuse • An interdisciplinary approach can be used
Nutrition	Pain and inflammation management	• Both Mediterranean (especially very low carbohydrates) and ketogenic diets are recommended • Eating habits can have a favorable effect of lowering blood sugar (very low sugar diet) and decreasing pain, inflammation, and excess adipose tissue. Eating between meals is not healthy • For obesity (and lipedema), short-term diets are to be avoided. Sustained change to eating habits using an individually adjusted dietary plan • Leg volume is reduced by weight reduction with a healthy diet

Diagnosis	Allows for timely and appropriate treatment	• Lipedema is usually not regarded as a progressive disease. For instance, Stage 1 does not always eventually become Stage 2 • Co-occurring obesity should be diagnosed and addressed
Compression garments	Pain relief management	• Custom, flat-knit garments may be optimal • Compression garments are targeting pain relief and not necessarily decongestion. Close consultation is needed between the patient, physician, and therapist. The lowest effective compression class avoids complications
Intermittent pneumatic compression	Pain relief management	• These devices can be effective for lipedema pain relief
Medications		• None recommended for lipedema specifically
Manual lymphatic drainage (MLD)	Improve lymphatic flow and reduce fluid buildup	• It can be used to reduce pain based on its effect on C-fiber nerves. Unless there is documented swelling, MLD is not used for its volume reduction effect
Complete decongestive therapy (CDT)	Pain and swelling management	• CDT with a 'training program' was the best for complex patients
Water exercise	Pain and swelling management	• Water exercise, such as aqua cycling, is considered a good addition to CDT (complete decongestive therapy)
Vibration plates	Pain and swelling management	• Vibration plates can increase the pressure pain threshold
Surgery	Remove lipedema fat and alleviate pain	• Surgery for lipedema is considered for documented refractory pain, impaired mobility due to skin or orthopedic problems (joint deterioration), BMI >40, or WHtR >0.55

recognizing the intelligent, lived wisdom they bring to their disease is especially powerful, particularly when the patient is actively engaged in their care. This holds true even when the disease is complex and challenging. Such a respectful and dynamic relationship is truly invaluable.

Initial visit examination

Mutual trust and respect begin with the initial visit. Even if a patient has been previously diagnosed, the practitioner and the patient will significantly benefit from repeating the diagnostic exam and discussing the findings together. A checklist for the physical exam can be found in Table 2.4. The initial assessment and discussion became much more comfortable for me after I had performed it several times. The complexity of an examination for lipedema requires more time, especially as it presents an opportunity for the patient to hear the findings and discuss them with you.

An interview precedes the exam, while they are fully clothed, to establish rapport and calm before performing the physical exam. This interview could include a discussion of their medical and social history, current symptoms and co-morbidities, and the outcome of any interventions they have attempted. Confirming other diagnoses or investigating other complaints the patient may have is an integral part of both the initial interview and the physical examination. After the interview, I would leave the room while they changed for the physical exam. I suggest to the patient (almost all are females) that they wear a bra and underwear with a gown open in the back. During the physical exam, I would continually ask how they would adjust the exam to make it more comfortable for them. I would inform them of what I was finding and what it meant and also invite them to ask me questions.

After the physical exam, the patient and I would review the findings, especially the more unusual parts. Allow valuable moments, both during and after the exam, to be punctuated by conversation and questions. Ask the patient if there is anything they have noticed that they would like checked, or if they have any questions about your current assessment. Elicit the wisdom of your patient by asking if they have a theory about what is happening in their body.

In anticipation of the next visit's conversation, both the patient and the physician should consider the following questions:

1. What needs to be discussed at the next visit?
2. What worked? Which were the successful interventions?
3. What was the attained outcome versus the desired outcome?
4. Are there any new symptoms or needs not previously known or addressed?
5. Assess the support the patient has received from the primary care practice and each of the consulted services.

Second visit and beyond

Here are some general guidelines to keep in mind as the patient-physician collaborative relationship grows and develops:

- Initiate and allow to evolve an agreed-upon description of the patient's current symptoms and the associated methods of addressing those symptoms. Other specialists will be invited to join a multidisciplinary team for the patient's care. See Table 2.7 for suggested specialist strategies.
- Elicit the patient's deep concerns and explore the challenges they face by understanding their support systems and identifying barriers or life burdens. This provides essential context for care and can include learning about the patient's home environment, such as who currently supports them or has supported them in the past, their financial stability, their ability to access planned interventions, the presence of significant pain, and issues such as food insecurity.
- Document all agreed-upon concerns,

Table 2.4: Physical examination checklist for lipedema.

Lipedema WITHOUT obesity	❑ If lipedema is present without obesity, adipose tissue is affected on the arms (usually proximal), and stops at the wrist if the entire arm is affected
	❑ A normal waistline just below the ribs with large hips, buttocks, upper legs, and sometimes lower legs where the adipose tissue stops at the ankle
Lipedema WITH obesity	❑ If there is obesity with the lipedema, a large fat mass at the waist and chest is observed
Lipedema WITH lymphedema	❑ In cases of lymphedema with lipedema, asymmetry is observed with a loss of ankle definition and a swollen foot
Examination areas	
With the exam gown in place, two important regions are examined:	
Proximal upper arm adipose tissue	❑ The arm is held 90 degrees to the side of the body. Feel the hanging adipose tissue between the elbow and armpit
Medial posterior knee adipose tissue	❑ The medial legs. On the inside starting along the course of the saphenous vein, ten inches above and below the knee medially
Identifying the lipedema stage	
Stage 1 lipedema	❑ Two sacks of adipose tissue are examined with the palmar surface of the fingers and then, grasping the fat sack between the thumb on one side and the index and middle finger on the other, rolling the fat between the fingers, feeling the soft bouncy fat (normal fat) or the nodular fat that can feel like lentils/chickpeas embedded in thick yogurt
Stage 2 lipedema	❑ Pain is induced with palpation of fat and/or larger lentils/chickpeas/grape-size nodules are felt embedded in thick fibrous tissue
Stage 3 lipedema	❑ In Stage 3 lipedema, painful, variable nodular deformation of the skin surface itself is observed with the skin, tough, with an orange peel appearance

especially those that were collaboratively addressed, and identify the next steps.

- Explore anti-fat bias or any mental health issues.
- Reassess after intervention attempts by listening to the patient's particular story again afterwards and then identify successes and shortcomings.
- Request updated perspectives from the patient by regularly asking for more details, for example by saying 'Maybe you can help me understand the most important parts better now that we have been working together for a while.'

Goals for lipedema treatment

Setting goals is a meaningful and empowering collaborative process between the primary care practitioner and the patient. It helps the patient identify and prioritize what they hope to achieve, while also giving the physician valuable insight into the patient's values, needs, and motivations. The goals listed below are common among patients with lipedema but should be personalized and adapted to reflect each individual's unique circumstances and aspirations.

1. Reduce pain, tenderness, or heightened sensitivity.
2. Reduce congestion or swelling, including decreasing the sensation of congestion, heaviness, and inflammation.
3. Increase functional mobility by reducing lower limb volume and increasing muscle strength and joint range of motion.
4. Enhance self-management of lipedema by:
   - recognizing lipedema-induced emotional burden
   - appreciating the effect of anti-fat bias and possible internalization of anti-fat bias
   - increasing the patient's knowledge and plan for treatment.
5. Use weight gain stabilization as an indication of successful lipedema intervention.
6. Consider lipedema surgery (tumescent liposuction) if pain and/or weight gain cannot be controlled.
7. Bariatric surgery for BMI >40 or BMI >35 with an obesity comorbidity.

Challenge #5. Accommodating and caring for patients with lipedema in a primary care practice

Effectively serving patients with lipedema requires that all members of the practice have a foundational understanding of the disease, as the entire team is typically involved in the patient's care directly or indirectly. The complexity of the management poses special challenges. Providing office staff and patients with educational materials, establishing clear procedures for specialist referrals and follow-up, and designating communication channels can help ensure that both patients and staff are informed about what is happening, when it will occur, and where it should take place.

Practice office staff as part of the team

Although office staff are not expected to be experts, some knowledge about lipedema will allow them to be more supportive and understanding of patients with lipedema, who may have many questions. Figure 2.3 is a sample fact sheet about lipedema to give to the primary care practice office manager and other staff.

Description of the office organization

A generic process map for a medical practice illustrates the patient journey from initial contact through to discharge, highlighting key touchpoints and decision points along the way. It visually outlines each step, beginning with scheduling the first appointment, navigating referrals, accessing essential services and supplies, and continuing through follow-up care. This general workflow can be adapted for patients with lipedema to ensure appropriate follow-up and track the progress of typical referrals and interventions tailored to their specific needs.

The process map ensures that all team members are aware of the procedures for making and tracking referrals and requests for equipment, garments, and other supplies. The patient, as the key person on this team, also knows what they are supposed to accomplish and who to call. A staff member should be designated as the point person to monitor the patient, ensuring timely referrals, answering questions, and addressing any potential barriers that may arise. See Table 2.5.

Office organization/set up

Clearly defined roles and responsibilities among office staff in a medical practice are essential for ensuring efficient operations, minimizing errors, and delivering high-quality patient care. When each team member understands their specific

Understanding the Pathophysiology and Intervention for Lipedema

PATHOPHYSIOLOGY

We remember that in lipedema:

Excessive Subcutaneous Adipose Tissue (SAT)
Fat cells (adipocytes) are starved and signal by starting inflammation, which causes pain.

↓

Insufficient Arterial Capillaries
The arterial capillaries are not numerous enough to bring the needed oxygen and nutrients to the adipocytes.

↓

Defective Lymphatic Drainage
The defective lymphatics do not remove enough inflammatory cell metabolism waste.

↓

As a result,
The subcutaneous adipose tissue (SAT) is **painful** and **congested.**

INTERVENTION

Compression Methods for Pain Relief

Suggested by U.S. and German lipedema experts.

- Medical compression stockings
- Compression bandages
- Medical adaptive compression systems, *e.g. Velcro products.*
- Intermittent pneumatic compression (IPC) devices

These require **evaluation** and **measurement** by a **compression specialist** for custom garments and medical devices.

Key Notes:
Referral to a certified lymphedema therapist (CLT) trained in complete decongestive therapy (CDT) may be requested.

CDT may include:
- Manual lymph drainage (MLD)
- Compression therapy
- Gentle movement/exercise, and
- Skincare (infection prevention)

Figure 2.3: Sample informational handout about pathophysiology and interventions for lipedema for office staff. Used with permission from Lipedema Simplified LLC.

Table 2.5: Building the office treatment care team. Process map example for a lipedema practice.

Step	Key team member(s)	Description
1. First contact	Clinical secretary	Patient initiates contact or is referred
2. Appointment setting	Clinical secretary	First appointment is scheduled
3. Intake and check-in	Clinical secretary	Patient checked in, messages relayed to clinical team
4. Clinical evaluation	Clinical provider	Medical history, physical exam, initial diagnosis
5. Referral planning	Clinical provider + clinical secretary	Identify necessary referrals (e.g. therapist, surgeon)
6. Supply/equip-ment requests	Clinical secretary to coordinate	Compression garments, IPC devices, etc.
7. Monitoring follow-ups	Assigned point person on staff	Track referrals, answer patient questions
8. Ongoing care	Clinical provider + clinical assistant	Continued management, evaluations, lab work
9. Patient follow-through	**Patient** (central team member)	Patient completes referrals, uses supplies
10. Discharge or transition	Clinical provider	Transition to long-term care or maintenance
Note: A **dedicated point person** should monitor referral progress, address delays, and ensure the patient has clear instructions		

duties and scope of authority, it reduces confusion, prevents duplication of efforts, and promotes accountability. Clear delineation of roles also streamlines workflow, enhances communication between administrative and clinical teams, and facilitates timely task completion. Additionally, it supports staff training, performance evaluation, and professional development by setting expectations and identifying areas for improvement. Ultimately, role clarity fosters a more organized, collaborative, and patient-centered healthcare environment. The suggested roles are outlined in Table 2.6.

Planning the next steps

See Tables 2.5 and 2.6 and the discussion of referrals to specialists under Challenge #7 below for more detail, but in general, here are some basic guidelines for the next steps after the initial visit and physical exam has been performed:

1. Understand the plethora of possible interventions.
2. Choose several interventions based on the patient's immediate needs for relief of symptoms.
3. Discuss the initial treatment referrals that will be made.

Table 2.6: Roles and responsibilities of office staff in a clinical practice.

Role	Responsibilities
Office manager	• Organizes and checks the efficiency and reliability of the practice teams • Organizes meetings with the staff • Communicates with the larger organization
Lead physician	• Organizes the provider team • Checks the provider team's performance • Holds the practice to a high standard of care
Office clinical providers	• Physician • Physician assistant • Nurse practitioner • Others who are primarily involved in ongoing care
Clinical secretary	• Checks patients in for appointments • Answers phone calls from patients • Transmits messages to and from the clinical providers • Schedules office and specialty appointments
Clinical assistant	• Escorts patients to treatment rooms • Takes vital signs • Helps with in-office care and procedures, such as blood draws

4. List tests that need to be done in the near future and the questions those tests are being used to answer.
5. Discuss who from the office should be called if additional help is needed. Discuss who might also be part of the care team and who may be the primary provider for the patient, such as a nurse practitioner or physician assistant.

Challenge #6. Providing support for psychological impacts and biases associated with lipedema

The psychological impacts of lipedema can be significant. Multiple studies have shown that individuals with lipedema experience higher rates of depression, anxiety, and eating disorders compared to the general population.[10,11] Additionally, patients with lipedema often report a lower quality of life and are more likely to encounter stigma and bias related to their weight or body shape.

Many patients will arrive at the primary care setting having endured repeated experiences of weight bias, often from healthcare providers themselves.[12] This chronic exposure can lead to the internalization of harmful stereotypes, contributing to negative self-perception. Internalized weight bias has been linked to further weight gain and a decline in mental health, physical well-being, and self-efficacy related to diet and exercise.[13]

Because weight bias can increase healthcare avoidance, it is essential for providers to actively acknowledge the reality of lipedema as a medical disease and recognize the unique challenges it presents. While evidence-based strategies to reduce internalized weight bias are still emerging, it is clear that weight stigma is both scientifically unfounded and professionally irresponsible.[14] For a deeper exploration of this issue, see Chapter 8: The challenge of weight stigma in recognizing lipedema.

Psychological issues may be brought forward as the patient attempts various interventions and learns to cope with a chronic disease. The primary care physician may note signs of depression in their patient and needs to be ready with proper referrals if their practice is not equipped to manage this diagnosis. A case-finding instrument with a sensitivity of 96% and a specificity of 57%[15] can be applied that requires the interviewer to ask two questions:

1. During the past month, have you often been bothered by feeling down, depressed, or hopeless?
2. During the past month, have you often been bothered by little interest or pleasure in doing things?

The primary care physician will need to be prepared with specialist referrals, support groups, and other online and community resources that can be made available for their patients when these issues arise. It is recommended that the patient be allowed space to create their own language to direct their care so that the discovery of optimal support measures is performed in collaboration between the patient and physician.

Challenge #7. Coordinating care: the primary care provider's role in the coordination of care, providing resources, and making referrals

Lipedema is a multi-faceted and complex disease that may require multiple specialists for optimal management. The primary care physician is uniquely positioned to help patients find appropriate referrals and coordinate their care. Therefore, very early in the collaborative relationship with the patient, the question is asked: *Which specialists are needed to intervene with what therapy that will provide what health effect?* In this way, the initial steps can be taken to identify and recruit specialist team members.

Following the initial visit and physical exam, the primary care physician will begin to understand not only the severity of lipedema symptoms but also begin to identify co-morbid conditions, such as cardiovascular disease, venous disease, obesity, lymphedema, hypothyroidism, depression, and anxiety. Together, the patient and physician will determine which diseases and/or issues should be prioritized and if a specialist referral is required. Table 2.7 provides a list of common interventions available for patients with lipedema, along with specialists who can be consulted for treatment or assistance.

Determining the proper referral may depend on whether the patient has lymphedema and/or obesity along with a lipedema diagnosis. Table 2.8 lists possible interventions and specialists depending on the patient's diagnosis.

Communicating general lifestyle recommendations

Forming healthy lifestyle habits may warrant a referral to a specialist, such as a dietitian, nutritionist, physical therapist, or others, but the patient may also expect some guidance from their primary care provider. Table 2.9 is a sample handout for patients with lifestyle suggestions that the primary care physician can discuss with their patients. Regarding dietary recommendations, see Chapter 14 for a more in-depth discussion.

Table 2.7: Referral to a specialist for lipedema management.

Area of care	**Description**	**Specialist(s)**
Complete decongestive therapy (CDT)	See Chapter 12 for details. Combines MLD, compression, exercise, and skincare	• Certified lymphedema therapist (CLT)
Compression garments	Provides compression to affected areas, typically lower body	• Durable medical equipment (DME) provider (measuring, ordering, donning/doffing instruction) • Certified lymphedema therapist (CLT) (fit verification and effectiveness)
Manual lymph drainage (MLD)	Gentle, manual technique to stimulate lymphatic flow	• Certified lymphedema therapist (CLT)
Daily exercise/ movement	Begin with 20 minutes of activity (e.g. slow walking)	• Certified lymphedema therapist (CLT) • Exercise specialist • Physical therapist • Personal trainer (in collaboration with patient and care team)
Skincare and hygiene	Reduces risk of fungal/ bacterial infections, erysipelas, and cellulitis	• Certified lymphedema therapist (CLT) • Dermatologist • Vascular specialist
Diet and lifestyle	Anti-inflammatory strategies including low-carb or ketogenic diets	• Dietitian/nutritionist/health-and-wellness coach
Weight management	For co-occurring obesity or metabolic concerns	• Obesity medicine specialist (certified by OMA) • Dietitian/nutritionist

Table 2.8: Referrals for diagnosis-specific interventions.

Intervention	Lipedema	Lymphedema	Obesity	Specialist(s)
Specialized techniques	CDT	CDT	Obestiry medicine specialist	CLT
Nutrition	Carb restriction	Carb restriction	Nutrition therapy	Dietitian, nutritionist, keto health coach
Physical activity	(Part of CDT)	(Part of CDT)	Physical activity	CLT, physical therapist, personal trainer
Compression garments	(Part of CDT)	(Part of CDT)	Compression garments	DME provider, CLT
Psychological support	Psychological support	Psychological support	Behavioral modification	Psychologist, psychia-trist, MFT
Medications	Pain management	Investigation for anti-inflammatory meds	Weight-loss medications	PCP, pain specialist, obesity medicine specialist
Surgical procedures	Lymph-sparing liposuction surgery	Lymph-sparing liposuction sur-gery, lymphatic microsurgery	Bariatric procedures	Lymphatic, plastic, or bariatric surgeon

CDT = complete decongestive therapy; CLT = certified lymphedema therapist; MFT = marriage and family therapist; PCP = primary care physician.

Conclusion

We have navigated a series of challenges – beginning with the realization that lipedema is not only real, but often coexists with obesity and, less commonly, with lymphedema. Many of us may not have recognized lipedema as a distinct disease when evaluating patients with obesity. Now, we understand that two separate diseases may be present, distinguishable by clinical examination, touch, and underlying pathophysiology.

Perhaps the most valuable co-expert in this journey has been the patient. I vividly recall how clarity and precision in management began when I approached the patient as a true partner. Together, we uncovered insights that accelerated my learning and revealed just how much there was still to understand about this underrecognized disease.

Introducing these patients to the rest of the care team meant creating a new care map – tailored, yet grounded in the kind of multidisciplinary complexity we had encountered in other disease models. At first, lipedema experts were few and far between – but we found them. They became essential allies on the path to better management.

We also discovered that the lipedema community was already all around us – sometimes virtually – made up of knowledgeable therapists, committed clinicians, and, most inspiring of all, dedicated patients. These individuals understood both the profound toll of the disease and the practical realities of its treatment. They became not only our collaborators but also our inspiration.

Table 2.9: Communicating general lifestyle recommendations for patients with lipedema.

Lifestyle change checklist
Patients should begin with **one strategy at a time** and build steadily toward sustainable lifestyle change. Providers may also consider referrals to specialists (e.g. dietitian, nutritionist, physical therapist).

Lifestyle area	Recommendation	Rationale
Diet	Reduce carbohydrate intake (low sugar and starch)	Supports weight reduction and lipedema symptom management. If treating obesity and lipedema, a ketogenic or low-carb diet is advised
	Commit to staying on the diet long-term	Diet must be sustainable to maintain benefits
	Eliminate highly processed foods	Reduces inflammation and excess caloric intake
Sleep	Get at least 7 hours of sleep per night (no less!)	Improves weight control and overall health
	Go to bed at the same time each night	Stabilizes circadian cycle, which supports better mental health, emotional balance, and weight control
Movement	Movement for 20 minutes or more each day...and more if you are able	Walking, swimming, water-walking, water aerobics, yoga and gentle movement, stretching and exercise enhances lymphatic flow, mobility, and weight control. Increase duration if tolerated

Note: The combination of eliminating processed foods, improving sleep duration and regularity, and walking daily will make a potent addition to a dietary intervention.

References

1. Allen EV, Hines EA. Lipedema of the legs: a syndrome characterized by fat legs and orthostatic edema. *Proc Staff Meet Mayo Clin*. 1940;15(15):184–7. Available from: https://klosetraining.com/wp-content/uploads/2021/03/1940-Lipedema-of-the-Legs.pdf
2. Faerber G, Cornely M, Daubert C, Erbacher G, Fink J, Hirsch T, et al. S2k guideline lipedema. *JDDG J Dtsch Dermatol Ges*. 2024;22(9):1303–15. DOI: https://doi.org/10.1111/ddg.15513
3. Sudduth CL, Greene AK. Lymphedema and obesity. *Cold Spring Harb Perspect Med*. 2022 May 27;12(5):a041176. DOI: https://doi.org/10.1101/cshperspect.a041176
4. Herbst KL, Kahn LA, Iker E, Ehrlich C, Wright T, McHutchison L, et al. Standard of care for lipedema in the United States. *Phlebology*. 2021 Dec 1;36(10):779–96. DOI: https://doi.org/10.1177/02683555211015887
5. Kloock S, Ziegler CG, Dischinger U. Obesity and its comorbidities, current treatment options and future perspectives: challenging bariatric surgery? *Pharmacol Ther*. 2023 Nov 1;251:108549. DOI: https://doi.org/10.1016/j.pharmthera.2023.108549
6. Keith L, Seo C, Wahi MM, Huggins S, Carmody

M, Faerber G, et al. Proposed framework for research case definitions of lipedema. *Lymphat Res Biol*. 2024 Apr;22(2):93–105. DOI: https://doi.org/10.1089/lrb.2023.0062
7. Rubino F, Cummings DE, Eckel RH, Cohen RV, Wilding JPH, Brown WA, et al. Definition and diagnostic criteria of clinical obesity. *Lancet Diabetes Endocrinol*. 2025 Mar;13(3):221–62. DOI: https://doi.org/10.1016/S2213-8587(24)00316-4
8. Fukaya E, Kolluri R. Nonsurgical management of chronic venous insufficiency. *N Engl J Med*. 2024 Dec 19;391(24):2350–9. DOI: https://doi.org/10.1056/NEJMcp2310224
9. Purnell JQ. Definitions, classification, and epidemiology of obesity. In: Feingold KR, Ahmed SF, Anawalt B, Blackman MR, Boyce A, Chrousos G, et al., eds. *Endotext*. South Dartmouth (MA): MDText.com, Inc.; 2000. Available from: http://www.ncbi.nlm.nih.gov/books/NBK279167/
10. Dudek JE, Białaszek W, Gabriel M. Quality of life, its factors, and sociodemographic characteristics of Polish women with lipedema. *BMC Womens Health*. 2021 Jan 15;21(1):27. DOI: https://doi.org/10.1186/s12905-021-01174-y
11. Bauer AT, von Lukowicz D, Lossagk K, Aitzetmueller M, Moog P, Cerny M, et al. New insights on lipedema: the enigmatic disease of the peripheral fat. *Plast Reconstr Surg*. 2019 Dec;144(6):1475–84. DOI: https://doi.org/10.1097/PRS.0000000000006280
12. Dudek JE, Białaszek W, Ostaszewski P, Smidt T. Depression and appearance-related distress in functioning with lipedema. *Psychol Health Med*. 2018 Aug 9;23(7):846–53. DOI: https://doi.org/10.1080/13548506.2018.1459750
13. Puhl R, Suh Y. Health consequences of weight stigma: implications for obesity prevention and treatment. *Curr Obes Rep*. 2015 Jun;4(2):182–90. DOI: https://doi.org/10.1007/s13679-015-0153-z
14. Pearl RL, Puhl RM, Lessard LM, Himmelstein MS, Foster GD. Prevalence and correlates of weight bias internalization in weight management: a multinational study. *SSM – Popul Health*. 2021 Mar 1;13:100755. DOI: https://doi.org/10.1016/j.ssmph.2021.100755
15. Whooley MA, Avins AL, Miranda J, Browner WS. Case-finding instruments for depression. Two questions are as good as many. *J Gen Intern Med*. 1997 Jul;12(7):439–45. DOI: https://doi.org/10.1046/j.1525-1497.1997.00076.x

Recommended reading

Bindlish, S, Ng, J, Ghusn, W, Fitch, A, Bays, HE. Obesity, thrombosis, venous disease, lymphatic disease, and lipedema: an obesity medicine association (OMA) clinical practice statement (CPS). *Obesity Pillars*. 2023; 8:100092. Available from: https://www.sciencedirect.com/science/article/pii/S2667368123000384

Keith, L, Seo, C, Wahi, MM, Huggins, S, Carmody, M, Faerber, G, ... & Rockson, SG. Proposed framework for research case definitions of lipedema. *Lymphatic Research and Biology*. 2024; 22(2), 93–105. DOI: https://doi.org/10.1089/lrb.2023.0062

II
Genetics of lipedema

Chapter Three
Genome-wide association studies of the lipedema phenotype

Sara Dobbins, Pia Ostergaard and Alan Pittman

Introduction

Is there a genetic basis for lipedema? Recent research has provided strong positive evidence, with family history studies playing a crucial role in understanding the hereditary nature of this disease. Clinical observations have noted that individuals with lipedema often report a positive family history, with recent estimates ranging from 40% to 89%.[1, 2, 3] This high prevalence of familial occurrence strongly supports the hypothesis that genetic factors contribute to the development of lipedema.

The genetic architecture of lipedema is most likely complex, involving multiple genes, intricate interactions between genetic variants, and potential environmental influences, which collectively contribute to the development and progression of this disease. Variants, rare in the general population and which play a major role in determining risk, may be inherited in families with multiple affected individuals, as seen in monogenic Mendelian diseases. Common risk variants, with small impact on risk, may act in concert to increase the likelihood of an individual developing the disease (Figure 3.1). Furthermore, common variation may influence the expression of those monogenic variants, and, together with environmental and lifestyle risk factors, contribute to an individual's risk of disease development.

Exploring the underlying genetic basis, or genetic architecture, of an understudied disease such as lipedema requires a range of experimental approaches. Family studies can be used to identify high-penetrant risk variants in specific genes through genome or exome sequencing of multiple individuals from large families. Alternatively, an association study-based approach can be undertaken using cohorts of unrelated individuals with lipedema and unaffected controls. Rare variant association studies (RVAS) typically use exome or genome sequencing data to identify rare variants with increased frequency in cases compared to controls.[4] Gene burden tests, also known as collapsing methods, are used to identify genes that carry a higher frequency of rare variants in cases compared to controls, typically focusing on rare variants that are likely to be pathogenic. At the other end of the spectrum, a genome-wide association study (GWAS) utilizes single nucleotide polymorphism (SNP) array data to identify common disease risk variants, typically of lower penetrance and smaller effect, observed at a significantly higher frequency in cases compared to controls. This approach is most likely to identify low-risk, non-coding genetic variants associated with the disease or trait. The success of these varied approaches in identifying risk variants depends on the number of samples studied (family

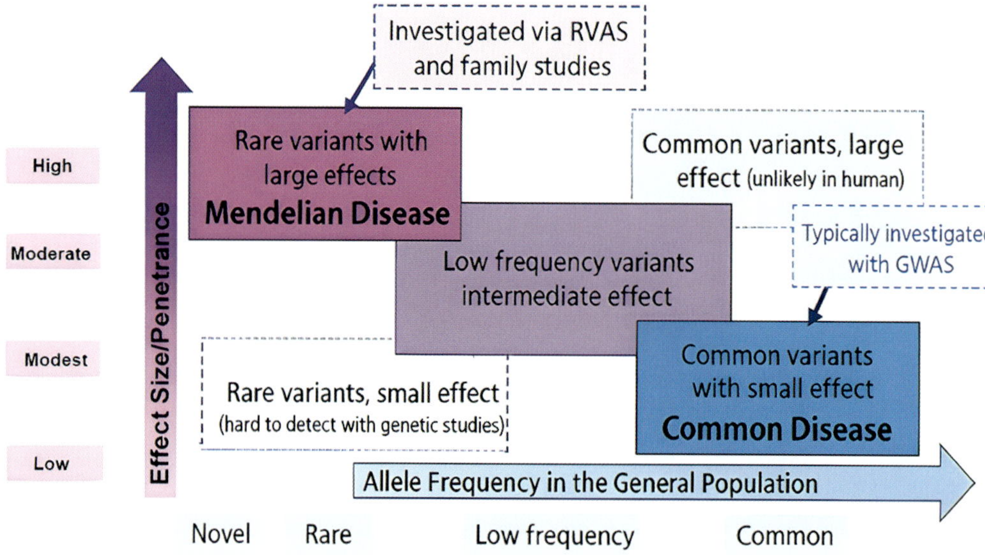

Figure 3.1: Exploring the genetic architecture of human disease. Depending on how frequent a variant is in the general, unselected population (x-axis) and the strength of the genetic effect in producing the disease phenotype (y-axis), different approaches must be taken to identify those variants that contribute to the disease. High penetrance, rare genetic variants are the hallmarks of Mendelian disease, while genetic variants of low penetrance and smaller effect typically contribute to the susceptibility of developing a common disease. It should be noted that while *penetrance* (the proportion of individuals with a particular genotype who express the associated phenotype) and *effect size* (the magnitude of the impact a variant has on a trait) are correlated, the relationship is complex and exceptions exist (Image 'Genetic Architecture' by City St. George's, University of London is licensed under CC BY-SA-4.0.).

or cohort size) and, of course, the underlying genetic architecture of the disease.

This chapter will focus on current efforts to identify common, low-penetrance risk variants for lipedema utilizing GWAS approaches. We will explore how these studies are performed and reveal how they are beginning to uncover the genetic basis of lipedema.

Genome-wide association studies (GWAS)

A GWAS is a powerful genetic research approach, widely adopted in the late 2000s, used to identify common genetic variants, or regions of the genome, that are associated with specific traits or diseases. It is a method that scans genetic variants across the whole genome and compares if they occur more frequently in people with a disease or trait (*cases*) than in people without it (*controls*). Any statistically significant differences are highlighted and may suggest that the variant is associated with the particular trait or disease under investigation.

The development of single-nucleotide variant DNA microarray technology (also known as DNA chips) facilitates the economic interrogation of millions of common genetic variants in thousands of unrelated individuals to agnostically identify associations between these common variants and disease. These variants are most often single-nucleotide polymorphisms (SNPs), characterized by a defined major and minor allele, which represent the nucleotides that occur at a specific position in the genome. A common variant would typically be defined as one with a minor allele frequency (MAF) of greater than five per cent in the population being studied.

Modern GWAS chips can capture approximately 70–90% of common genetic variation (MAF >5%) in the human genome, depending on the chip design. This high level of coverage is achieved through the strategic selection of SNPs that are in strong linkage disequilibrium with nearby variants, so-called tag SNPs. However, the exact coverage can vary significantly depending on the specific chip design, the population being studied, and the genomic region in question.

A typical GWAS approach is outlined in Figure 3.2. Case and control subjects are enrolled in a GWAS study, and researchers isolate DNA, typically extracted from a blood sample. The DNA samples are then genotyped using the high-throughput microarray technology platform to identify the alleles present at several hundred

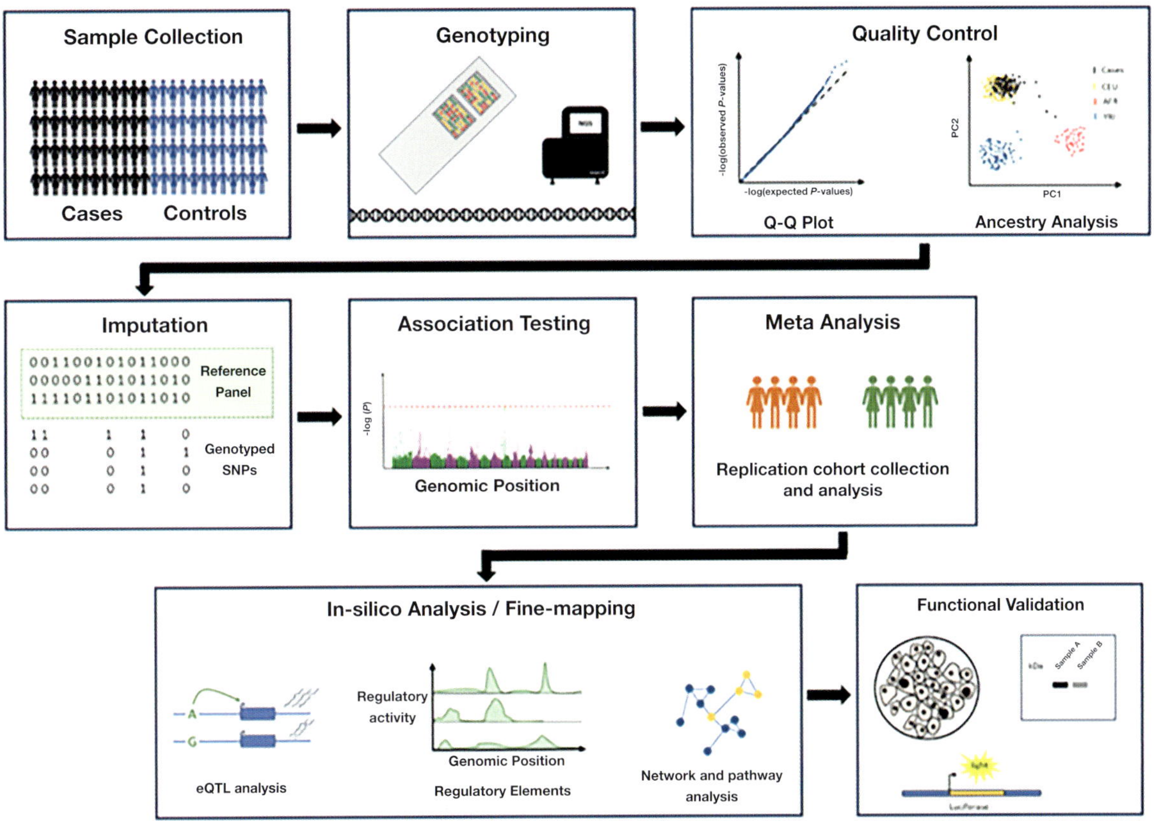

Figure 3.2: Overview of typical GWAS methodology. (Image 'GWAS methodology overview' by City St. George's, University of London is licensed under CC BY-SA-4.0.)

thousand to millions of sites across the entire genome in all subjects. Alternatively, SNP genotypes can be extracted from whole-genome or exome sequencing data. Researchers often use publicly available genotype data to form control cohorts that are matched for sex and ancestry. Even case cohorts may be established from public resources, such as the UK Biobank,[5] where the phenotype is sufficiently represented.

Stringent quality control protocols are implemented to limit potential bias, including removing poorly genotyped SNPs or individuals, checking and adjusting for well-matched ancestry between case and control cohorts, and checking for any sex discrepancies or unexpected relatedness between individuals. Any systematic bias can be assessed using a Q-Q plot, which is especially important when cases and controls have not been genotyped together. Large reference datasets, such as the Haplotype Reference Consortium (HRC), can serve as the basis for genotype imputation to infer the status of ungenotyped SNPs in individuals, thereby increasing the number of SNPs available for study.[6] This powerful technique leverages the extensive genetic information contained in these reference panels to enhance the resolution of the analysis.

Each SNP is then statistically tested for association with the disease or trait, and it is determined if a particular allele is significantly more common in the case group compared to the control group. Due to the large number of statistical tests being performed, a very stringent significance threshold ($5x10^{-8}$) is typically used to reduce the likelihood of false positives.[7, 8] Therefore, depending on the genetic architecture of the trait or disease, large case and control sample sizes are often required to identify genetic variants that are 'genome-wide significant'.

Replication cohorts are also beneficial to confirm that associations are robust to any uncontrolled bias and provide more accurate estimates of effect sizes.[9] Comprehensive studies will often include multiple replication cohorts and

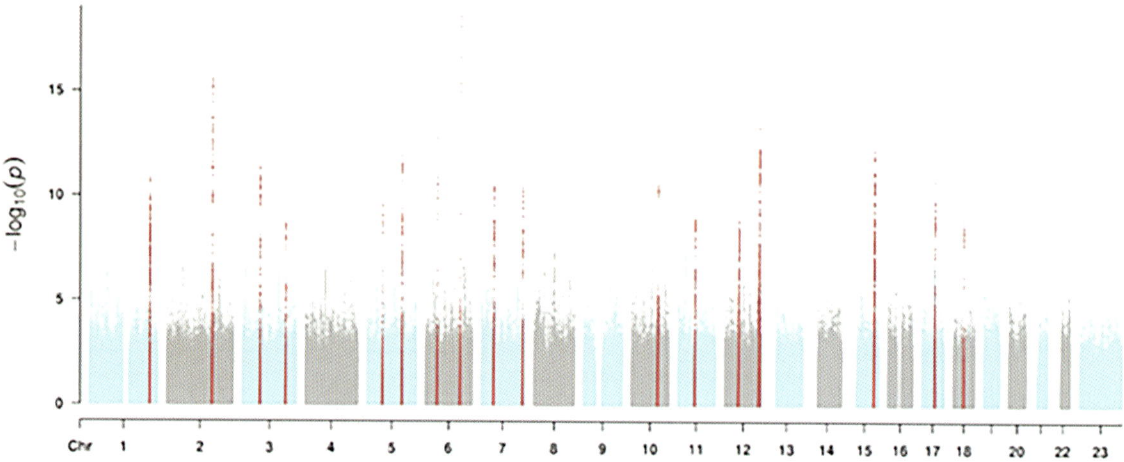

Figure 3.3: Manhattan plot of lipedema GWAS. A Manhattan plot is a graphical summary of the results from a GWAS, where the x-axis displays the genomic location of SNPs across all chromosomes, and the y-axis shows the negative logarithm of the association p-value for each SNP, with significant associations appearing as prominent peaks resembling a city skyline. In this figure, genome-wide significant loci are highlighted in red. Original image provided courtesy of the authors.

meta-analyses. Accounting for any systematic differences in ancestry between cases and controls is a distinct challenge, involving careful study design and the appropriate statistical treatment of ancestry as a covariate in the analysis.[10]

SNPs that are identified and show a genome-wide significant association with the disease or trait highlight regions of the genome that can harbor genes that play a role in the development of the disease or trait, providing new insights into the underlying biology. However, many variants identified through GWAS are themselves non-causal, and the association is driven by linkage disequilibrium between this variant and the true causal variant. Thus, GWAS typically identify risk loci with clusters of statistically significant SNPs, and the next step in the analysis is to perform in-silico fine-mapping to characterize the region, and functional interpretation to identify the most plausible gene impacted either by a coding change, or more likely, by a change in regulation. This 'fine-mapping' can integrate multiple sources of information, such as gene expression data, chromatin accessibility, and histone modifications. For example, expression quantitative trait loci (eQTL) analysis can identify any genetic variants that influence nearby gene expression levels. This can be extended to colocalization analysis, which uses statistical methods to assess the probability that the same causal variant underlies both the GWAS and eQTL signal. Incorporating tissue-specific information and identifying correlations between genetic variants and gene expression can provide insights into the cell types and biological mechanisms underlying disease associations.

The final step may involve performing experiments to functionally validate the findings and demonstrate the measurable impact of variants on gene function or regulation. For example, in luciferase assays, the genomic region containing the variant of interest is cloned into a reporter construct upstream of a luciferase gene. The construct is transfected into cells, and the luciferase activity is measured to quantify the impact of the variant on gene expression. Other approaches, such as Hi-C (chromatin capture), western blots, quantitative polymerase chain reaction (qPCR), electrophoretic mobility shift assays (EMSA), and CRISPR-Cas9, may be useful in exploring the relationship between variant associations and the underlying biological mechanisms leading to the trait or disease.

GWAS can identify genetic risk factors for disease, which can lead not only to a better understanding of how diseases develop but also help identify individuals in the population who are at a higher risk. GWAS are applicable in a wide range of fields, from common complex diseases like hypertension and diabetes to traits such as height, body mass index (BMI), and body fat distribution. Since the first GWAS in 2005,[11] over three thousand GWAS have been published for over a thousand different traits and diseases,[12] with some cohorts exceeding a million participants.[13,14] Tens of thousands of genetic risk variants have been identified, and these results have greatly increased our understanding of the genetic architecture of these traits and diseases.[15] Occasionally, these findings have led to further insight into disease mechanisms and even the development of new therapies through the identification of new druggable targets.[16]

Genome-wide association studies of body fat distribution

To date, there have been several GWAS studies that have been conducted on body fat distribution,[17]a highly heritable trait. These studies have identified genetic variants associated with how and where the body stores fat and have been crucial in understanding the genetic architecture of fat and metabolic diseases. Since lipedema may be considered an extreme phenotype of body fat distribution, genetic variants uncovered by such studies may play a role in understanding the etiology of this disease.

Early studies performed meta-analyses of GWAS data with relevant anthropometric measures of central obesity and fat distribution.[18] These studies identified several genetic loci associated specifically with waist-to-hip ratio (WtHR), a common measure of body fat distribution, often measured in individuals with lipedema, independent of body mass index (BMI). Intriguingly, Heid et. al.[18] revealed sexual dimorphism, highlighting differences in genetic effects between men and women. These findings have been consistently replicated in larger studies[19] and have also identified distinct sex-specific signatures associated with different patterns of body fat distribution.[20] Another GWAS identified genetic loci linking adipose and insulin biology to body fat distribution,[21] identifying 49 loci associated with WtHR adjusted for BMI ($WtHR_{adjBMI}$). Age-dependent genetic effects on BMI, but not $WtHR_{adjBMI}$, have also been reported in a large-scale meta-analysis.[22] The development of techniques for measuring body fat distribution, such as CT scans, has provided additional insights, allowing differentiation between subcutaneous and visceral fat deposition,

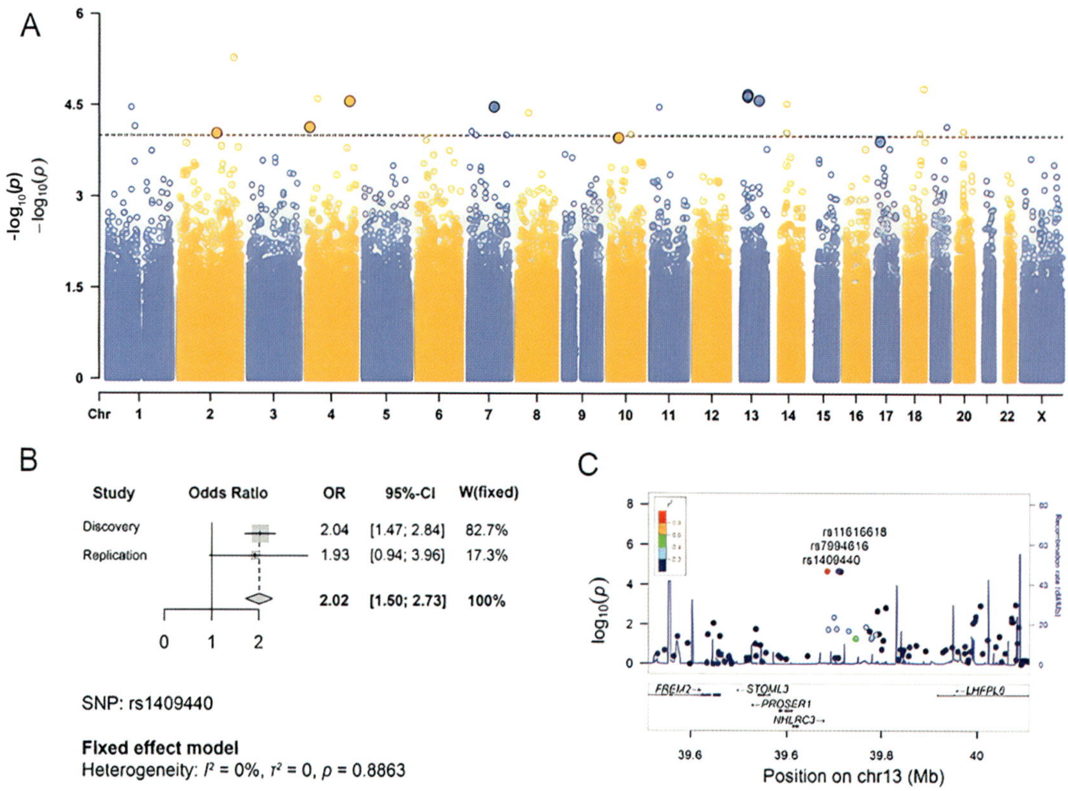

Figure 3.4: Results from the UK genome-wide association study (GWAS): (A) Manhattan plot of the P-values ($-\log_{10}$ scale) for each variant association with lipedema in the discovery cohort. The highlighted SNPs (dots with black outline) were tested in the replication cohort and have $p_{meta} < 1\times10^{-4}$ and the same direction of effect in both studies; (B) Forest plot of chromosome 13 rs1409440 SNP meta-analysis pooled odds ratio and 95% confidence intervals; (C) Regional association plot of chr13q13.3 showing the top three SNPs (rs1409440, rs7994616, rs11616618) from the meta-analysis. Images reproduced from Grigoriadis et al.[31] under CC BY license.

and highlighting the benefits of utilizing metrics from imaging over anthropometric measures[23, 24] for use in GWAS.

A recent GWAS identified new loci associated with BMI and fat distribution in diverse populations, demonstrating that including individuals from a broader range of ethnic ancestries can improve discovery for complex traits.[25] Lipedema is a disease that affects women worldwide, and it will be important to study the genetic basis of the disease in as many diverse populations as possible. The relationship between genetic variation and body fat distribution in relation to lipedema is not entirely clear, but it is entirely plausible that lipedema may be a distinct clinical entity heavily influenced by genetic determinants of body fat distribution.

Genome-wide association studies of the lipedema phenotype

In 2023, Klimentidis and colleagues published a landmark GWAS on the lipedema phenotype using data from the UK Biobank, a prospective cohort of approximately half a million UK adults aged 41 to 72.[26] The resource includes a wealth of data, including lifestyle and health information, imaging, and biological samples (including DNA for sequencing), with the possibility of linking to the individual's national health records. It is therefore currently one of the most powerful resources to study the genetic basis of common, complex diseases and traits.[27] Because assembling a large prospective cohort of individuals with lipedema is difficult, partly due to its low diagnosis rate, this study's use of existing population-scale data represents a practical and informative approach.

In their study, Klimentidis and colleagues[26] used body fat percentage and anthropometric measurements in the UK Biobank to classify women who appear to have a lipedema phenotype. Women were deemed to be lipedema cases if they fell within the >65th percentile of leg fat percentage residual and <51.3rd percentile of the waist circumference residual (to achieve a prevalence of 10%). Control subjects, also from the UK Biobank, were defined as those women with ≤45th leg fat percentile residual and ≥71.3rd waist circumference residual percentile, and a lack of a positive response to the recruitment question: 'Do you get pain in either leg on walking?' The GWAS was performed on this proxy lipedema cohort by testing the association between each of the 1.8 million SNPs that were available for analysis using linear regression, identifying 18 regions of the genome significantly associated with the lipedema phenotype (Figure 3.3). The genetic loci identified with the lipedema phenotype also associate with other anthropomorphic features such as body fat and leptin levels, and at nominal significance levels with hip circumference, primary biliary cirrhosis, BMI, WtHR, age at first birth, birth weight, and age at menopause. Several of the identified loci have previously been found to be associated with WtHR, exhibit more potent effects in women than in men,[21] and are associated with leg fat percentage independent of hip circumference.

This important study has highlighted that susceptibility to lipedema is influenced by common genetic factors and provides a starting point in understanding the genetic architecture and physiological basis of the disease. One caveat of this study is that these samples have not been clinically ascertained, and we must ask how closely the genetic architecture observed here will resemble that of clinically defined lipedema. However, in a replication cohort of clinically ascertained individuals with lipedema from the UK lipoedema cohort (discussed in more detail in the next section) two statistically significant associations (the *VEGFA* and *GRB14-COBLL1* loci) were identified, suggesting this study approach provides a means to detect clinically relevant lipedema genetic loci, capitalizing on the power of large-scale population-based genetic datasets.

The genes identified from this study are

interesting and provide insight into the underlying biology of lipedema, informing future avenues of research. For example, there has been an established link between *VEGFA*, angiogenesis, and adipogenesis, and there is also some evidence in the literature suggesting a link between lymphangiogenesis and adipose cells.[28, 29] *COBLL1* plays a role in the regulation of the actin cytoskeleton in adipocytes,[30] and following *COBLL1* knockdown, stress fibers in subcutaneous adipocytes failed to degrade, preventing cells from remodeling the cytoskeleton and becoming metabolically active.[30]

Genome-wide association studies in clinical lipedema subjects

In parallel to the UK Biobank study, Grigoriadis and colleagues[31] investigated phenotypic characteristics and genome-wide associations in the UK lipoedema cohort. Two hundred women were recruited from two UK-based clinics, with review from specialist clinicians, according to strict diagnostic criteria including bilateral excess adipose deposition from the hips to the ankles, age of onset <35 years, BMI ≤40 kg/m^2 without excess upper body fat, WtHR ≤0.85, soft and 'doughy' tissues, and sparing of the feet. Women with proximal upper limb lipedema were also included in the study. The average age of reported onset was 16.8 (SD±9.0), with an average BMI of 33.4 (SD±7.2) but WtHR of 0.76 (SD±<0.07), indicating minimal central obesity. A family history of lipedema was reported in 58.2% of participants, with data on other clinical features of bruising, edema, venous abnormalities, hypermobility, pain, and dieting recorded.

Of the recruited cases, 130 were included in the GWAS cohort, and a control cohort was constructed with genotype data from women recruited to the *Understanding Society* UK study.[32] A small replication cohort was identified from individuals recruited to the 100,000 Genomes Project Rare Diseases Program v11 with lipedema.[33] Due to the modest size of both the discovery and replication cohorts, no loci were identified as statistically significant after adjustment for multiple testing ($p<5x10^{-8}$).

However, multiple genomic loci were associated with lipedema at a nominal significance level of $P<2x10^{-4}$ (Figure 3.4). The top SNP from the analysis maps to chr13q13.3 with a risk allele frequency of 0.17 in cases versus 0.09 in controls (p meta=3.98x10^{-6}). Defining a 40kb region based on linkage disequilibrium and interrogation of expression and regulation datasets identifies regulation of *LHFPL6* as a potential candidate for the association signal (Figure 3.4). Women carrying this variant were more likely to report a direct maternal relative with lipedema. *LHFPL6* is a member of the lipoma HMGIC (high mobility group protein isoform C) fusion partner (*LHFP*) gene family. Interestingly, *LHFP* has previously been implicated in polyunsaturated fat levels in adipose tissue in chicken thighs.[34] Furthermore, structural variation at chr13q13 has been identified in lipomas, including a gene fusion of *LHFP* with HMGIC,[35] with haploinsufficiency of *LHFP* postured as a mechanism for lipoma formation.[36] Lipomas are common benign soft tissue tumors of mature adipocytes and have been reported in association with lipedema.[37, 38] Indeed, the occurrence of lipomas in Dercum's disease,[39] which shares some clinical similarities with lipedema, is well-documented. The frequently observed fatty tissue around the knees in women with lipedema may represent lipoma-like adipose tissue.[40, 41]

While these observations are intriguing, it is important to note that the specific relationship between lipoma and lipedema etiology remains unclear. Furthermore, the association is unsupported by the analysis of the UK Biobank proxy lipoedema cohort, which, although not clinically ascertained, is much larger. Further research is needed to confirm these findings and establish a definitive link between the two diseases. Additional genetic studies involving diverse groups of clinically diagnosed lipedema participants would be valuable in elucidating the potential relationship between lipedema and lipoma-like tissue formations.

The analysis of well-phenotyped, clinically ascertained samples was central to the study design of this GWAS, facilitating the identification of association signals with a clear lipedema phenotype. This is in contrast to biobank-based strategies, which offer large cohort sizes and increased statistical power, at the potential cost of a clinically robust definition of lipedema cases. Given the small sample size of the UK lipoedema cohort, it was only powered to identify common variants with large effects, and its failure to do so only provides us with indications about the likely architecture of the disease. Therefore, while the results of this GWAS are promising, the study implies larger sample sizes will be required to robustly identify common genetic variants underlying lipedema.

Conclusion

A combined approach of pragmatically utilizing data from large-scale biobanks to define lipedema cohorts in conjunction with analysis of smaller, but precisely phenotyped, clinically ascertained cohorts is likely the way forward to further investigate the genetic architecture of lipedema. A concerted worldwide effort to produce large-scale lipedema cohorts of well-defined, clinically ascertained cases will be necessary, including a marked effort to diversify collection from European samples to capture underlying variation across all ancestries.

Sample numbers will also be bolstered by the impressive efforts of the international community to provide easy access to population-scale databanks,[42] such as All of Us[43] and FinnGen.[44] These, in conjunction with the UK Biobank (as discussed above), will provide additional cohorts in which to validate findings and explore differences between variants. This will facilitate defining lipedema susceptibility versus standard body fat distribution metrics such as the waist-to-hip ratio.

As these datasets grow, we will be able to utilize additional approaches in statistical genetics to explore our understanding of lipedema. These include polygenic risk scoring,[45] which creates a scoring model by aggregating the effects of multiple genetic markers across the genome to provide an individualized risk score. This could be used to define a risk score for lipedema, as well as to explore the risk profile of individuals with lipedema in relation to other related phenotypes, such as waist-hip ratio and obesity. Another technique, Mendelian randomization,[46] uses genetic variants as instrumental variables to examine the causal effect of an exposure on outcomes. This could be used to explore the relationship between lipedema and other health outcomes such as diabetes or heart disease.

We have discussed in detail here the basics of genome-wide association studies, with reference to the identification of common variants with small effect sizes. These same cohorts, when sequenced, can also be utilized to undertake genome-wide rare variant association studies (RVAS), where, if sample size is sufficient, rare variants can also be identified. An alternative approach is gene burden testing, where genes enriched for rare variation in cases compared to controls are identified. These will likely be fruitful once sufficient sample sizes have been collected. These types of analyses will complement the analysis of large, multi-generational families, where rare variants with larger effect sizes are most easily identified.

References

1. Forner-Cordero I, Szolnoky G, Forner-Cordero A, Kemény L. Lipedema: an overview of its clinical manifestations, diagnosis and treatment of the disproportional fatty deposition syndrome – systematic review. *Clin*

Obes. 2012;2(3–4):86–95. DOI: https://doi.org/10.1111/j.1758-8111.2012.00045.x
2. Harwood CA, Bull RH, Evans J, Mortimer PS. Lymphatic and venous function in lipoedema. *Br J Dermatol*. 1996 Jan;134(1):1–6. DOI: https://doi.org/10.1046/j.1365-2133.1996.d01-741.x
3. Rudkin GH, Miller TA. Lipedema: a clinical entity distinct from lymphedema. *Plast Reconstr Surg*. 1994 Nov;94(6):841. Available from: https://journals.lww.com/plasreconsurg/abstract/1994/11000/lipedema__a_clinical_entity_distinct_from.14.aspx
4. Lee S, Abecasis GR, Boehnke M, Lin X. Rare-variant association analysis: study designs and statistical tests. *Am J Hum Genet*. 2014 Jul 3;95(1):5–23. DOI: https://doi.org/10.1016/j.ajhg.2014.06.009
5. Manolio TA. UK Biobank debuts as a powerful resource for genomic research. *Nat Med*. 2018 Dec;24(12):1792–4. DOI: https://doi.org/10.1038/s41591-018-0276-3
6. McCarthy S, Das S, Kretzschmar W, Delaneau O, Wood AR, Teumer A, et al. A reference panel of 64,976 haplotypes for genotype imputation. *Nat Genet*. 2016 Oct;48(10):1279–83. DOI: https://doi.org/10.1038/ng.3643
7. Chen Z, Boehnke M, Wen X, Mukherjee B. Revisiting the genome-wide significance threshold for common variant GWAS. *G3 GenesGenomesGenetics*. 2021 Feb 1;11(2):jkaa056. DOI: https://doi.org/10.1093/g3journal/jkaa056
8. Risch N, Merikangas K. The future of genetic studies of complex human diseases. *Science*. 1996 Sep 13;273(5281):1516–7. DOI: https://doi.org/10.1126/science.273.5281.1516
9. Kraft P, Zeggini E, Ioannidis JPA. Replication in genome-wide association studies. *Stat Sci Rev J Inst Math Stat*. 2009 Nov 1;24(4):561–73. DOI: https://doi.org/10.1214/09-STS290
10. Uffelmann E, Huang QQ, Munung NS, de Vries J, Okada Y, Martin AR, et al. Genome-wide association studies. *Nat Rev Methods Primer*. 2021 Aug 26;1(1):1–21. DOI: https://doi.org/10.1038/s43586-021-00056-9
11. Klein RJ, Zeiss C, Chew EY, Tsai JY, Sackler RS, Haynes C, et al. Complement factor H polymorphism in age-related macular degeneration. *Science*. 2005 Apr 15;308(5720):385–9. DOI: https://doi.org/10.1126/science.1109557
12. Buniello A, MacArthur JAL, Cerezo M, Harris LW, Hayhurst J, Malangone C, et al. The NHGRI-EBI GWAS catalog of published genome-wide association studies, targeted arrays and summary statistics 2019. *Nucleic Acids Res*. 2019 Jan 8;47(D1):D1005–12. DOI: https://doi.org/10.1093/nar/gky1120
13. Jansen PR, Watanabe K, Stringer S, Skene N, Bryois J, Hammerschlag AR, et al. Genome-wide analysis of insomnia in 1,331,010 individuals identifies new risk loci and functional pathways. *Nat Genet*. 2019 Mar;51(3):394–403. DOI: https://doi.org/10.1038/s41588-018-0333-3
14. Lee JJ, Wedow R, Okbay A, Kong E, Maghzian O, Zacher M, et al. Gene discovery and polygenic prediction from a genome-wide association study of educational attainment in 1.1 million individuals. *Nat Genet*. 2018 Aug;50(8):1112–21. DOI: https://doi.org/10.1038/s41588-018-0147-3
15. Loos RJF. 15 years of genome-wide association studies and no signs of slowing down. *Nat Commun*. 2020 Nov 19;11(1):5900. DOI: https://doi.org/10.1038/s41467-020-19653-5
16. Stankey CT, Bourges C, Haag LM, Turner-Stokes T, Piedade AP, Palmer-Jones C, et al. A disease-associated gene desert directs macrophage inflammation through ETS2. *Nature*. 2024 Jun;630(8016):447–56. DOI: https://doi.org/10.1038/s41586-024-07501-1
17. Saini S, Walia GK, Sachdeva MP, Gupta V. Genomics of body fat distribution. *J Genet*. 2021 May 24;100(2):32. DOI: https://doi.org/10.1007/s12041-021-01281-7
18. Heid IM, Jackson AU, Randall JC, Winkler TW, Qi L, Steinthorsdottir V, et al. Meta-analysis identifies 13 new loci associated with waist-hip ratio and reveals sexual dimorphism in the genetic basis of fat distribution. *Nat Genet*. 2010 Nov;42(11):949–60. DOI: https://doi.org/10.1038/ng.685
19. Pulit SL, Stoneman C, Morris AP, Wood AR, Glastonbury CA, Tyrrell J, et al. Meta-analysis of genome-wide association studies for body fat distribution in 694 649 individuals of European ancestry. *Hum Mol Genet*. 2019 Jan 1;28(1):166–74. DOI: https://doi.org/10.1093/hmg/ddy327
20. Rask-Andersen M, Karlsson T, Ek WE, Johansson

Å. Genome-wide association study of body fat distribution identifies adiposity loci and sex-specific genetic effects. *Nat Commun*. 2019 Jan 21;10(1):339.
DOI: https://doi.org/10.1038/s41467-018-08000-4

21. Shungin D, Winkler TW, Croteau-Chonka DC, Ferreira T, Locke AE, Mägi R, et al. New genetic loci link adipose and insulin biology to body fat distribution. *Nature*. 2015 Feb;518(7538):187–96. DOI: https://doi.org/10.1038/nature14132
22. Winkler TW, Justice AE, Graff M, Barata L, Feitosa MF, Chu S, et al. The influence of age and sex on genetic associations with adult body size and shape: a large-scale genome-wide interaction study. *PloS Genet*. 2015 Oct 1;11(10):e1005378. DOI: https://doi.org/10.1371/journal.pgen.1005378
23. Fox CS, Liu Y, White CC, Feitosa M, Smith AV, Heard-Costa N, et al. Genome-wide association for abdominal subcutaneous and visceral adipose reveals a novel locus for visceral fat in women. *PloS Genet*. 2012 May 10;8(5):e1002695. DOI: https://doi.org/10.1371/journal.pgen.1002695
24. Plourde M, Vohl MC, Bellis C, Carless M, Dyer T, Dolley G, et al. A variant in the LRRFIP1 gene is associated with adiposity and inflammation. *Obesity*. 2013;21(1):185–92.
DOI: https://doi.org/10.1002/oby.20242
25. Wojcik GL, Graff M, Nishimura KK, Tao R, Haessler J, Gignoux CR, et al. Genetic analyses of diverse populations improves discovery for complex traits. *Nature*. 2019 Jun;570(7762):514–8.
DOI: https://doi.org/10.1038/s41586-019-1310-4
26. Klimentidis YC, Chen Z, Gonzalez-Garay ML, Grigoriadis D, Sackey E, Pittman A, et al. Genome-wide association study of a lipedema phenotype among women in the UK Biobank identifies multiple genetic risk factors. *Eur J Hum Genet*. 2023 Mar;31(3):338–44.
DOI: https://doi.org/10.1038/s41431-022-01231-6
27. Bycroft C, Freeman C, Petkova D, Band G, Elliott LT, Sharp K, et al. The UK Biobank resource with deep phenotyping and genomic data. *Nature*. 2018 Oct;562(7726):203–9.
DOI: https://doi.org/10.1038/s41586-018-0579-z
28. Ahmadzadeh N, Robering JW, Kengelbach-Weigand A, Al-Abboodi M, Beier JP, Horch RE, et al. Human adipose-derived stem cells support lymphangiogenesis *in vitro* by secretion of lymphangiogenic factors. Exp Cell Res. 2020 Mar 15;388(2):111816.
DOI: https://doi.org/10.1016/j.yexcr.2020.111816
29. Phan TT, Chakraborty A, Tatum MA, Lima-Orellana A, Reyna AJ, Rutkowski JM. Increased adipose tissue lymphatic vessel density inhibits thermogenesis through elevated neurotensin levels. *Front Cell Dev Biol* . 2023 Jan 27;11. Available from: https://www.frontiersin.org/journals/cell-and-developmental-biology/articles/10.3389/fcell.2023.1100788/full
30. Glunk V, Laber S, Sinnott-Armstrong N, Sobreira DR, Strobel SM, Batista TM, et al. A non-coding variant linked to metabolic obesity with normal weight affects actin remodelling in subcutaneous adipocytes. *Nat Metab*. 2023 May;5(5):861–79. DOI: https://doi.org/10.1038/s42255-023-00807-w
31. Grigoriadis D, Sackey E, Riches K, Zanten M van, Brice G, England R, et al. Investigation of clinical characteristics and genome associations in the 'UK lipoedema' cohort. *PloS ONE*. 2022 Oct 13;17(10):e0274867. DOI: https://doi.org/10.1371/journal.pone.0274867
32. Reynolds C, Thompson J, Hawthorne I, Turner W. Understanding society: a longitudinal study of social and economic dynamics in the UK. *Int J Soc Sci Res*. 2023;2(1):1–7.
DOI: https://doi.org/10.58531/ijssr/1/2/1
33. The 100,000 Genome Project Investigators. 100,000 genomes pilot on rare-disease diagnosis in health care – preliminary report. *N Engl J Med*. 2021 Nov 10;385(20):1868–80.
DOI: https://doi.org/10.1056/NEJMoa2035790
34. Yang S, Wang Y, Wang L, Shi Z, Ou X, Wu D, et al. RNA-Seq reveals differentially expressed genes affecting polyunsaturated fatty acids percentage in the Huangshan Black chicken population. *PloS ONE*. 2018 Apr 19;13(4):e0195132. DOI: https://doi.org/10.1371/journal.pone.0195132
35. Petit MMR, Schoenmakers EFPM, Huysmans C, Geurts JMW, Mandahl N, Van de Ven WJM. *LHFP*, a novel translocation partner gene of *HMGIC* in a lipoma, is a member of a new family of *LHFP*-like genes. *Genomics*. 1999 May 1;57(3):438–41.
DOI: https://doi.org/10.1006/geno.1999.5778

36. Dahlén A, Debiec-Rychter M, Pedeutour F, Domanski HA, Höglund M, Bauer HCF, et al. Clustering of deletions on chromosome 13 in benign and low-malignant lipomatous tumors. *Int J Cancer*. 2003;103(5):616–23. DOI: https://doi.org/10.1002/ijc.10864
37. Fife C, Maus E, Carter M. Lipedema: A frequently misdiagnosed and misunderstood fatty deposition syndrome. *Adv Skin Wound Care*. 2010 Feb;23(2):81–92. DOI: https://doi.org/10.1097/01.ASW.0000363503.92360.91
38. Pascucci A, Lynch PJ. Lipedema with multiple lipomas. *Dermatol Online J*. 2010 Sep 15;16(9):4. Available from: https://pubmed.ncbi.nlm.nih.gov/20875325/
39. Hansson E, Svensson H, Brorson H. Review of Dercum's disease and proposal of diagnostic criteria, diagnostic methods, classification and management. *Orphanet J Rare Dis*. 2012 Apr 30;7(1):23. DOI: https://doi.org/10.1186/1750-1172-7-23
40. Eisman J, Swezey RL. Juxta-articular adiposis dolorosa: what is it? Report of 2 cases. *Ann Rheum Dis*. 1979 Oct 1;38(5):479–82. DOI: https://doi.org/10.1136/ard.38.5.479
41. Herbst KL. Subcutaneous adipose tissue diseases: Dercum disease, lipedema, familial multiple lipomatosis, and Madelung disease. In: Feingold KR, Ahmed SF, Anawalt B, Blackman MR, Boyce A, Chrousos G, et al., editors. *Endotext* . South Dartmouth (MA): MDText.com, Inc.; 2000. Available from: http://www.ncbi.nlm.nih.gov/books/NBK552156/
42. Lieb W, Strathmann EA, Röder C, Jacobs G, Gaede KI, Richter G, et al. Population-based biobanking. *Genes*. 2024 Jan;15(1):66. DOI: https://doi.org/10.3390/genes15010066
43. Bick AG, Metcalf GA, Mayo KR, Lichtenstein L, Rura S, Carroll RJ, et al. Genomic data in the All of Us research program. *Nature*. 2024 Mar;627(8003):340–6. DOI: https://doi.org/10.1038/s41586-023-06957-x
44. Kurki MI, Karjalainen J, Palta P, Sipilä TP, Kristiansson K, Donner KM, et al. FinnGen provides genetic insights from a well-phenotyped isolated population. *Nature*. 2023 Jan;613(7944):508–18. DOI: https://doi.org/10.1038/s41586-022-05473-8
45. Choi SW, Mak TSH, O'Reilly PF. Tutorial: a guide to performing polygenic risk score analyses. *Nat Protoc*. 2020 Sep;15(9):2759–72. DOI: https://doi.org/10.1038/s41596-020-0353-1
46. Sanderson E, Glymour MM, Holmes MV, Kang H, Morrison J, Munafò MR, et al. Mendelian randomization. *Nat Rev Methods Primer*. 2022 Feb 10;2(1):1–21. DOI: https://doi.org/10.1038/s43586-021-00092-5

Chapter Four

Genetic analysis of non-syndromic primary lipedema

Sandro Michelini

Introduction

Lipedema is a chronic, progressive disease characterized by the abnormal, symmetrical accumulation of adipose tissue, primarily affecting the limbs and occurring almost exclusively in women.[1] This disease is notably resistant to conventional weight management strategies, including dietary modifications, physical exercise, and even bariatric surgery. In recognition of its distinct clinical presentation, the World Health Organization recently included lipedema in the *International Classification of Diseases (ICD-11)* under the code EF02.2. [2]

Although lipedema was first described more than half a century ago, standardized diagnostic criteria and management guidelines have only emerged in recent years. Current clinical recommendations have improved awareness and treatment outcomes by outlining clear strategies for diagnosis and care.[3, 4, 5] Advances in imaging modalities, such as lymphoscintigraphy, ultrasound, and MRI, have further enhanced diagnostic precision by revealing characteristic patterns of adipose tissue distribution and structural changes, aiding in differentiation from other fat diseases and lymphedema.[6, 7, 8]

The clinical course of lipedema is closely tied to hormonal changes, often worsening during puberty, pregnancy, and menopause, suggesting a strong hormonal influence. Recent genetic studies have further deepened our understanding of lipedema, uncovering specific mutations and revealing complex hereditary patterns.[9, 10] These findings support the view that lipedema is a multifactorial disease with both genetic and hormonal components.

This chapter explores the emerging role of genetics in lipedema, reviewing current discoveries related to gene mutations and inheritance patterns. It also examines the implications of these findings for improved diagnostics, individualized treatment strategies, and the potential for future gene-targeted therapies.

Syndromic vs. non-syndromic lipedema

Syndromic lipedema involves specific genetic mutations or chromosomal abnormalities that lead to both lipedema and other distinct symptoms and features characteristic of a recognized syndrome, such as Sotos syndrome, Williams-Beuren syndrome, pseudoxanthoma elasticum, and cutis laxa type III.[11] Non-syndromic lipedema, on the other hand, is characterized by the typical features of lipedema as discussed above, without the presence of other associated symptoms or anomalies that define a specific syndrome.[12]

Genetic basis and familial studies

Genetic investigations have consistently identified a hereditary component in lipedema. Early familial studies by Child et al.[9] confirmed an autosomal dominant inheritance with sex limitation, where the genetic susceptibility is transmitted predominantly through asymptomatic males to affected females. Extensive pedigree studies systematically recorded affected family members across several generations, highlighting this inheritance pattern. These studies focused on identifying both symptomatic and asymptomatic carriers and delineating clear genetic transmission pathways, essential for accurate diagnosis and effective genetic counseling.[9,10,13]

Identification of the *AKR1C1* mutation

A significant advancement in understanding the genetic basis of lipedema was the identification of mutations in the *AKR1C1* gene. Michelini et al. [10] detailed a specific mutation characterized by the Leu213Gln substitution, significantly impairing enzyme function critical in progesterone metabolism. This mutation impacts adipogenesis and potentially modifies pain perception through altered metabolism of neurosteroids like allopregnanolone, thus providing insights into possible therapeutic targets.[10]

Additional genetic insights and candidate genes

Research has identified multiple genes potentially associated with lipedema, expanding beyond *AKR1C1* to include *PPARG*, *AKT2*, *LIPE*, *Plin1*, and *MFN2*.[10] This highlights the concept that lipedema is likely polygenic.[13] *PPARG* plays a crucial role in adipocyte differentiation and glucose homeostasis, and mutations have been associated with familial partial lipodystrophy, a disease that shares features with lipedema.[10] *AKT2*, another candidate gene, regulates crucial metabolic pathways, including glucose metabolism and adipocyte function. Mutations in *AKT2* have been linked to severe metabolic disturbances, highlighting its potential relevance in lipedema.[10] *LIPE*, encoding hormone-sensitive lipase, and *Plin1*, involved in lipid droplet regulation within adipocytes, both significantly influence adipocyte metabolism. Mutations in these genes have been identified in other adipose diseases, suggesting their involvement in the abnormal fat distribution observed in lipedema.[10]

MFN2 mutations, associated primarily with Madelung's disease, have highlighted significant clinical overlap with lipedema, suggesting potential shared pathogenic mechanisms and further complicating diagnostic clarity.[10] Additional implicated genes, including *ALDH18A1*, *GHR*, *RB1*, *ABCC6*, *BBS10*, and PITPN1, illustrate the genetic heterogeneity and complexity underlying lipedema. Mutations in these genes have been linked to metabolic, hormonal, and connective tissue diseases, thereby expanding the genetic spectrum associated with lipedema pathology.[10]

Diagnostic challenges and advanced genetic testing

Diagnostic differentiation of lipedema from obesity, lymphedema, and other related diseases remains challenging. Next-generation sequencing (NGS) panels have emerged as critical tools, enabling precise identification of genetic markers that distinguish lipedema from phenotypically overlapping diseases. These genetic panels allow comprehensive screening for known associated genes and mutations, significantly improving diagnostic accuracy and informing personalized management strategies.[14] The frequent coexistence of lipedema with various diseases, including metabolic syndrome, insulin resistance, autoimmune thyroiditis (Hashimoto's thyroiditis), hypermobile Ehlers-Danlos syndrome, polycystic ovary syndrome (PCOS), and endometriosis, highlights the need for genetic tests capable of differentiating among overlapping clinical presentations.[11, 14, 15, 16, 17]

Concerning somatic mutations in a diseased tissue sample, we observed a mutation in the peroxisome proliferator-activated receptor gamma gene (PPARG), a master regulator of adipocyte differentiation.[10] This aspect must be developed and studied. In a study involving tissue samples from both a healthy area and an area affected by lipedema (clinical stage 2) in the same patient, we identified several highly active RNAs.[18] We analyzed 800 microRNAs in tissue samples from both regions and found 13 that showed differential expression. One microRNA, in particular, appears to be a potential biomarker for the disease. This may be particularly relevant as, currently, a diagnosis of lipedema is based solely on clinical criteria.[15, 19, 20]

Implications of genetic research on therapeutic considerations

Current management strategies for lipedema include both surgical and non-surgical interventions. Among surgical options, liposuction has shown effectiveness in reducing symptoms and improving quality of life.[21] However, it is important to note that surgery is not curative. Many patients continue to experience symptoms such as chronic pain following the procedure, underscoring the need for ongoing care and individualized treatment planning.[21, 22]

Noninvasive therapies also play a critical role in lipedema management. Manual subcutaneous adipose tissue (SAT) therapy, for example, has shown promise in reducing pain and improving tissue architecture.[23] These outcomes support the value of integrative, multidisciplinary approaches that address both functional impairment and symptom burden.[20, 21] Genetic profiling may eventually help identify which patients are most likely to benefit from such conservative therapies, including physical treatment modalities and dietary interventions.

As genetic research into lipedema advances, it holds the potential to significantly refine and personalize treatment strategies. For instance, identifying genetic subtypes of lipedema may help clinicians determine which patients are best suited for surgical intervention, and even guide the extent or technique of liposuction to minimize complications and reduce the risk of recurrence. Likewise, insights into a patient's genetic profile may predict responsiveness to conservative treatments, enabling more targeted and effective management.[24]

Importantly, genetic studies have begun to shed light on the mechanisms underlying one of lipedema's most distressing symptoms: chronic pain. Neurosteroids, particularly those derived from progesterone, such as allopregnanolone, have demonstrated analgesic effects and may play a role in modulating lipedema-associated pain.[25] Mutations in genes like *AKR1C1*, which are involved in neurosteroid metabolism, may contribute to increased pain sensitivity in lipedema. These findings open the door to novel therapeutic targets that extend beyond symptom management to address the biological basis of pain in this disease.[26]

Conclusion

As our understanding of lipedema continues to grow, recent genetic discoveries, particularly involving mutations in *AKR1C1* and other emerging candidate genes, offer new hope for uncovering the biological roots of this complex disease. Comprehensive genetic testing, including next-generation sequencing (NGS) panels, holds great promise for improving diagnostic accuracy, guiding individualized treatment, and ultimately enhancing patient care through targeted therapies and genetic counseling. Ongoing research, including segregation studies and investigations into somatic mutations, is essential for identifying additional genetic factors. These advancements bring us closer to earlier diagnosis, more effective treatments, and a better quality of life for those living with lipedema.

References

1. Földi M, Földi E. *Földi's Textbook of Lymphology: for Physicians and Lymphedema Therapists.* 3rd ed. München: Elsevier Urban & Fischer; 2012. Available from: https://search.worldcat.org/title/Foldi's-textbook-of-lymphology-:-for-physicians-and-lymphedema-therapists/oclc/792987093
2. WHO. *International Statistical Classification of Diseases and Related Health Problems.* 11th ed. Geneva, Switzerland: World Health Organization (WHO); 2022. Available from: https://www.who.int/standards/classifications/classification-of-diseases
3. Wold L, Hines EA, Allen EV. Lipedema of the legs: a syndrome characterized by fat legs and edema. *Ann Intern Med.* 1951;34(5):1243–50. Available from: https://klosetraining.com/wp-content/uploads/2021/03/1940-Lipedema-of-the-Legs.pdf
4. Reich-Schupke S, Schmeller W, Brauer WJ, Cornely ME, Faerber G, Ludwig M, et al. S1 guidelines: lipedema. *J Dtsch Dermatol Ges.* 2017;15(7):758–67. DOI: https://doi.org/10.1111/ddg.13036
5. Herbst KL, Kahn LA, Iker E, Ehrlich C, Wright T, McHutchison L, et al. Standard of care for lipedema in the United States. *Phlebology.* 2021 Dec 1;36(10):779–96. DOI: https://doi.org/10.1177/02683555211015887
6. Szolnoky G, Ifeoluwa A, Tuczai M, Varga E, Varga M, Dosa-Racz E, et al. Measurement of capillary fragility: a useful tool to differentiate lipedema from obesity? *Lymphology.* 2017;50(4):203–9. Available from: https://pubmed.ncbi.nlm.nih.gov/30248725/
7. Forner-Cordero I, Oliván-Sasot P, Ruiz-Llorca C, Muñoz-Langa J. Lymphoscintigraphic findings in patients with lipedema. *Rev Esp Med Nucl E Imagen Mol Engl Ed.* 2018 Nov 1;37(6):341–8. DOI: https://doi.org/10.1016/j.remnie.2018.10.013
8. Dimakakos PB, Stefanopoulos T, Antoniades P, Antoniou A, Gouliamos A, Rizos D. MRI and ultrasonographic findings in the investigation of lymphedema and lipedema. *Int Surg.* 1997;82(4):411–6. Available from: https://pubmed.ncbi.nlm.nih.gov/9412843/
9. Child AH, Gordon KD, Sharpe P, Brice G, Ostergaard P, Jeffery S, et al. Lipedema: an inherited condition. *Am J Med Genet A.* 2010;152A(4):970–6. DOI: https://doi.org/10.1002/ajmg.a.33313
10. Michelini S, Chiurazzi P, Marino V, Dell'Orco D, Manara E, Baglivo M, et al. Aldo-keto reductase 1C1 (AKR1C1) as the first mutated gene in a family with nonsyndromic primary lipedema. *Int J Mol Sci.* 2020 Jan;21(17):6264. DOI: https://doi.org/10.3390/ijms21176264
11. Paolacci S, Precone V, Acquaviva F, Chiurazzi P, Fulcheri E, Pinelli M, et al. Genetics of lipedema: new perspectives on genetic research and molecular diagnoses. *Eur Rev Med Pharmacol Sci.* 2019 Jul;23(13):5581–94. DOI: https://doi.org/10.26355/eurrev_201907_18292
12. Forner-Cordero I, Forner-Cordero A, Szolnoky G. Update in the management of lipedema. *Int Angiol J Int Union Angiol.* 2021 Aug;40(4):345–57. DOI: https://doi.org/10.23736/S0392-9590.21.04604-6
13. Morgan S, Reid I, Bendon C, Ishaq M, Shayan R, Pope B, et al. A family-based study of inherited genetic risk in lipedema. *Lymphat Res Biol.* 2024 Apr 1;22(2):106–11. DOI: https://doi.org/10.1089/lrb.2023.0065
14. Michelini S, Herbst KL, Precone V, Manara E, Marceddu G, Dautaj A, et al. A multi-gene panel to identify lipedema-predisposing genetic variants by a next-generation sequencing strategy. *J Pers Med.* 2022 Feb 11;12(2):268. DOI: https://doi.org/10.3390/jpm12020268
15. Forner-Cordero I, Szolnoky G, Forner-Cordero A, Kemény L. Lipedema: an overview of its clinical manifestations, diagnosis and treatment of the disproportional fatty deposition syndrome – systematic review. *Clin Obes.* 2012;2(3–4):86–95. DOI: https://doi.org/10.1111/j.1758-8111.2012.00045.x
16. Herbst KL, Mirkovskaya L, Bharhagava A, Chava Y, Te CH. Lipedema fat and signs and

symptoms of illness, increase with advancing stage. *Archives of Medicine*. 2015;7(4):8. Available from: https://www.semanticscholar.org/paper/Lipedema-Fat-and-Signs-and-Symptoms-of-Illness%2C-Herbst-Mirkovskaya/8b0e0bed68581bc6d602792109f58ca9f745e5ab

17. Herbst KL. Subcutaneous adipose tissue diseases: Dercum disease, lipedema, familial multiple lipomatosis, and Madelung disease. In: Feingold KR, Ahmed SF, Anawalt B, Blackman MR, Boyce A, Chrousos G, et al., editors. *Endotext* . South Dartmouth (MA): MDText.com, Inc.; 2000. Available from: http://www.ncbi.nlm.nih.gov/books/NBK552156/
18. Cione E, Michelini S, Abrego-Guandique DM, Vaia N, Michelini S, Puleo V, et al. Identification of specific microRNAs in adipose tissue affected by lipedema. *Curr Issues Mol Biol*. 2024 Nov;46(11):11957–74. DOI: https://doi.org/10.3390/cimb46110710
19. Wollina U. Lipedema – an update. *Dermatol Ther*. 2019;32(2):e12805. DOI: https://doi.org/10.1111/dth.12805
20. Todd M. Diagnosis and management of lipoedema in the community. *Br J Community Nurs*. 2016 Oct;21(Sup10):S6–12. DOI: https://doi.org/10.12968/bjcn.2016.21.Sup10.S6
21. Ghods M, Kruppa P. [Surgical treatment of lipoedema]. *Handchirurgie Mikrochirurgie Plastische Chirurgie*. 2018 Dec;50(6):400–11. DOI: https://doi.org/10.1055/a-0767-6808
22. Cornely ME, Hasenberg T, Cornely OA, Ure C, Hettenhausen C, Schmidt J. Persistent lipedema pain in patients after bariatric surgery: a case series of 13 patients. *Surg Obes Relat Dis*. 2022 May 1;18(5):628–33. DOI: https://doi.org/10.1016/j.soard.2021.12.027
23. Herbst KL, Ussery C, Eekema A. Pilot study: whole body manual subcutaneous adipose tissue (SAT) therapy improved pain and SAT structure in women with lipedema. *Horm Mol Biol Clin Investig*. 2017 Sep 20;33(2). DOI: https://doi.org/10.1515/hmbci-2017-0035
24. Vettori A, Paolacci S, Maltese PE, Herbst KL, Cestari M, Michelini S, et al. Genetic determinants of the effects of training on muscle and adipose tissue homeostasis in obesity associated with lymphedema. *Lymphat Res Biol*. 2021 Aug;19(4):322–33. DOI: https://doi.org/10.1089/lrb.2020.0057
25. Joksimovic SL, Covey DF, Jevtovic-Todorovic V, Todorovic SM. Neurosteroids in Pain management: a new perspective on an old player. *Front Pharmacol* . 2018 Oct 2;9. Available from: https://www.frontiersin.org/journals/pharmacology/articles/10.3389/fphar.2018.01127/full
26. Xu Y, López M. Central regulation of energy metabolism by estrogens. *Mol Metab*. 2018 Sep 1;15:104–15. DOI: https://doi.org/10.1016/j.molmet.2018.05.012

Chapter Five

Interrogating genes and the gene signaling networks implicated in patients with lipedema:

what we know and where we are headed

Ramin Shayan and Tara Karnezis

Introduction

The unique adipose distribution in the lipedema disease state has been recorded in the classical works of the Dutch master Peter Paul Rubens. For decades, since the 1940s, the recognition of the disease in a minority of medical circles has not necessarily translated into either greater compassion for those suffering in silence with the disease, nor into a greater scientific understanding. Lipedema (also referred to as lipoedema in some jurisdictions) is a chronic and progressive disease characterized by the abnormal, bilateral, and symmetrical accumulation of subcutaneous adipose tissue, primarily in the limbs. Lipedema predominantly affects women and manifests clinically as disproportionate fat distribution, often in the lower extremities, which can lead to significant physical and psychological burdens. Reported symptoms frequently include extreme leg sensitivity with exquisite pain to point touch, hyperadiposity, interstitial fluid swelling (lymphedema), general pain, malaise, easy bruising, and musculoskeletal and joint complications such as hypermobility and subsequent arthritis.

Despite its significant physical and psychological impacts, the underlying mechanisms driving lipedema have remained poorly understood since the description of the disease in the medical literature in the 1940s. Lipedema predominantly affects women, usually commencing and often exacerbated, during phases of life that are characterized by hormonal change, such as during puberty, in vitro fertilization (IVF), pregnancy, and menopause. The overall clinical picture may result in impairment of patient gait and mobility, as well as complex distortion of body image, which is exacerbated by the 'fat-shaming' culture exhibited in many modern Western cultures.[1]

Lipedema is frequently confused and may also be overlaid with obesity, primary or secondary lymphedema, lipodystrophies, and other adipose tissue diseases.[2] Adding to the confusion regarding the degree of overlap of the above-mentioned diseases is the additional fact that the diagnosis of lipedema is still made on clinical grounds. Therefore, one of the major remaining clinical challenges in the lipedema field is the absence of a reliable diagnostic marker. The quest to identify a dedicated, specific, reproducible diagnostic marker, be it genetic or biochemical, is also one of the holy grails of lipedema researchers. While reports continue to differentiate the entities of lipedema and obesity,[2] the exact cellular microenvironment in the tissues that are affected by lipedema has yet to be elucidated.[3]

Familial patterns, hereditary basis and genetic predisposition to lipedema

A pattern of genetic inheritance is suggested by emerging research, as lipedema tends to run in families. A positive family history has been identified in 60%–80% of cases.[3] Although early studies have primarily focused on clinical observations and phenotypic presentations, genetic investigations are beginning to unveil the intricate relationships between gene variants and the development of lipedema. Suggestions of a genetic basis for lipedema have included either X-linked dominant inheritance or, more likely, autosomal dominant inheritance with sex limitation, as suggested by Child et al. in 2010.[4]

This observation of a family history and resulting hypothesis regarding a putative genetic origin to lipedema, as well as an observation that many patients also had lymphedema, and thus that there may be a relationship to lymphatic dysregulation, led the St George's lymphedema group to investigate further the contribution of genetics in lipedema.[5] To address this question, they recruited a tightly phenotyped cohort of 200 UK-based patients with lipedema across two separate clinics and collated clinical and quality-of-life characteristics of the respective cohorts. To better probe the genetic architecture of the disease, a genome-wide association study (GWAS) using genome-wide single-nucleotide polymorphism (SNP) genotype data was performed on 130 of the recruits. The resulting analysis suggested certain genetic loci to be associated with the lipedema phenotype, with validation using a comparison with an independent cohort taken from the 100,000 Genomes Project.

The top SNP was located upstream of *LHFPL6* and implicated in the formation of lipomas. Although the exact way in which these findings relate to lipedema is yet to be fully elucidated, this study was the first GWAS conducted on a lipedema cohort. It identified potentially important genetic regions that were suggestive of an association with the lipedema disease state. However, the group concluded that only further replication of such findings in other independent populations would be required to definitively identify any key genes. An additional GWAS analysis by the same group was performed on a select group of patients from the UK Biobank based on a distinct phenotype: those with a high percentage of fat in the lower limbs and relatively small waist, adjusting for hip circumference.[6] Patients with the characteristic 'lipedema' body shape had gene variants that clustered to two loci (*VEGFA* and *GRB14-COBLL1*), suggesting that there is an enrichment of gene variants in blood vessels and adipose tissue associated with lipedema.

In 2020, the Michelini group studied a family with three family members affected by sex-limited autosomal dominant non-syndromic lipedema.[7] They screened the family with whole-exome sequencing and found that none of the variants found were in genes already associated with syndromes that include lipedema. Instead, some variants were found in genes that regulated steroid hormone signaling and are associated with abdominal obesity or metabolic syndrome. These included the *NGEF* gene (abdominal obesity) and *FBXL7*, which has been described as associated with both metabolic syndrome and an abnormal pharmacological response to corticosteroids.

The authors also identified a missense variant p. (Leu213Gln) in *AKR1C1*, a gene involved in the reduction of progesterone to its inactive form. The analysis was performed by sequencing the exons and intron-exon junctions of all known genes, focusing on heterozygous variants observed in affected patients but not in clinically unaffected family members. Comparative molecular dynamics suggested a partial loss-of-function of the identified variant that could contribute to slower, less efficient processing of progesterone to hydroxyprogesterone and increased subcutaneous fat deposition in carriers.[7]

This discovery of a missense variant in *AKR1C1* in this family of patients with lipedema suggested that *AKR1C1* was one of the first candidate genes associated with non-syndromic lipedema. Sanger sequencing confirmed the presence of this missense variant found to be functionally detrimental to the encoded protein's function, either preventing substrate activation or the cofactor binding in the three affected females but not in nine unaffected family members. Further, eight of 265 *AKR1C1* variants taken from the gnomAD database proved to be detrimental to the function of the protein by the criteria developed in this study.[7] The authors concluded that hormonal influence appears to play a role in the pathogenesis of lipedema. Genetic variants in *AKR1C1* may predispose some patients to the disease, particularly in the context of hormone imbalance. This imbalance could result from altered dietary intake, such as changes in protein, dairy, or vegetable consumption, or exposure to endocrine-disrupting compounds. Therefore, monitoring and controlling steroid hormone levels in patients with lipedema, or those with a family history of the disease, may help prevent disease onset.

To build on these early genetic studies of lipedema, alternative comprehensive approaches were envisaged. In 2022, Michelini et al.[8] conducted a study incorporating a next-generation sequencing (NGS) panel designed to help in the diagnosis of lipedema by identifying genes specific for lipedema, but also genes for overlapping diseases, and potential targets for tailored treatments for these diseases. The NGS gene panel that was utilized consisted of 305 genes potentially associated with lipedema based on extrapolation from existing literature investigating lipedema and putative overlapping diseases with a biological relevance, adjacency, or overlap with lipedema. The genomes of 162 Italian and American patients with lipedema were sequenced using the designed gene panel. Within this tested cohort, twenty-one deleterious variants were detected in 17 patients, according to a score of at least 3 out of 5 predetermined predictors. These genes included *PLIN1, LIPE, ALDH18A1, PPARG, GHR, INSR, RYR1, NPC1, POMC, NR0B2, GCKR, PPARA*. Further work to validate many of these gene candidates is required.

More recent studies utilizing bioinformatics approaches also report a strong familial predisposition but suggest that rather than one 'magic bullet' deleterious pathway being at the root of lipedema phenotypes, multiple genetic factors are more likely to contribute to the risk of developing lipedema. For instance, the Karnezis lab conducted a familial aggregation study, demonstrating that women with a family history of lipedema were indeed significantly more likely to develop the disease themselves.[3] DNA from 31 individuals from 9 lipedema families was analyzed to reveal genetic variants predicted to alter protein function, yielding candidate variants in 469 genes. Of these, 366 genes were predicted to alter protein function based on variant annotation, and genes related to extracellular matrix (ECM) were overrepresented in this candidate gene set.

This was the first exome-wide analysis to identify ECM-related rare genetic variants in families with lipedema. Seven variants were shortlisted for Sanger sequencing based on variant annotation score and previous literature, to be validated. Importantly, the inheritance models identified for the seven validated genetic variants indicated that lipedema has an autosomal dominant inheritance pattern, which allows for male carriers (a point of contention previously). Taken together, these findings point to a 'set of genes' influencing lipedema related to the ECM, rather than one specific gene in all patients. No one gene was found to be mutated in every family, supporting the concept that no single exomic factor is responsible for all lipedema cases. A Gene Ontology (GO) analysis of the filtered variant set also identified overrepresentation of variants related to vasopressin receptor activity, microfibril binding, and patched binding. The connection between microfibril binding and lipedema is of particular interest, as microfibrils are known to play a crucial role in connective tissue function that could be altered in the clinical presentation of lipedema.[3]

Collectively, these genetic studies indicated a heritability but highlighted the fact that lipedema is not caused by a single exomic genetic factor alone, and the study provided more robust support for the hypothesis of genetic heterogeneity in the etiology of lipedema.[3] Importantly, the authors identified two genetic variants associated with ECM, which were also observed in the study by Michelini et al.,[8] conducted in a distinct population. Morgan et al.[3] identified variants in seven of the genes that were also contained in the lipedema panel assembled by Michelini and colleagues, namely, *BBS1, BBS4, POMC, NCOA1, RREB1, STAB1*, and *TNXB*. Both studies identified genetic variants in the *POMC* gene, which is linked to a predisposition to obesity. Morgan et al.[3] identified a missense mutation that was predicted to be deleterious, while Michelini et al.[8] detected a truncating variant. Two of the genes contained in the Michelini et al.[8] lipedema panel and identified in the Morgan et al.[3] analysis were *STAB1* and tenascin-X (TNX)B (*TNXB*), both of which are closely associated with the ECM, and in line with the overrepresentation of microfibril binding from the GO analysis.

TNX is a glycoprotein thought to mediate cell-ECM interactions via direct fibrillary collagen binding through decorin and cell surface integrin.[9] *TNXB* gene variants are linked to classical-like Ehlers-Danlos syndrome type 1 (clEDS1), one of the 13 types of Ehlers-Danlos syndrome (EDS),[9, 10] a rare but heterogeneous group of connective tissue diseases that, while it has not been directly linked to lipedema, has been thought to be closely associated. The evidence of separate studies that identify the *TNXB* association may provide the first link between the two. While haploinsufficiency of *TNXB* is associated with EDS, deficiency of tenascin-X also causes abnormal elastin fiber morphology and reduced collagen levels in the dermis, a feature commonly identified in lipedema.[4] *STAB1*, in contrast, encodes a scavenger receptor that clears collagen-binding proteins in the ECM and has also been associated with waist-to-hip ratio in humans, a key feature in the clinical diagnosis of lipedema.[11]

Both studies also identified genetic variants in the *POMC* gene, which is linked to obesity predisposition,[12] a key co-morbidity and confounding differential diagnosis in lipedema. Congenital deficiency of proopiomelanocortin (POMC) protein results in a syndrome of hypoadrenalism, severe obesity, and altered skin and hair pigmentation, while loss of one copy of the *POMC* gene predisposes to obesity.[12] In the Farooqi et al.[12] study of *POMC* heterozygotes, 11 of 12 heterozygotes were obese or overweight, compared with only 1 of 7 of the wild-type control relatives from his large Turkish cohort. Unfortunately, the presence of lipedema in this cohort was not assessed in the Farooqi et al. cohort, but the presence of this *POMC* in both the Michelini et al.[8] and the Morgan et al.[3] studies indicated that this gene may be important in determining the manifestation of obesity, which is thought to have at least an interrelationship with the clinical manifestation of lipedema. We identified a missense mutation that was predicted to be deleterious,[3] while Michelini et al.[8] detected a truncating variant.

Collectively, while interrogating the genetics underlying lipedema by various groups around the world has proved encouraging, what these genetic studies have revealed is that a single gene that may be targeted as a 'silver bullet' for lipedema is increasingly unlikely. It may be a more plausible hypothesis that there is a spectrum of gene variants or clusters leading to the heterogeneity observed in this disease. Therefore, alternative complementary strategies are likely to be needed.

Understanding what is different about lipedema tissue

While genetics provides a powerful means to interrogate drivers of disease, it is equally important to understand how tissue is affected by the causative gene variant(s). 'OMICs' refer to the collective technologies used to explore the roles, relationships, and actions of biological molecules within cells and tissues. Recent advancements in the field of the so-called 'OMICs' technologies have enabled researchers to conduct comprehensive analyses of transcriptomic, metabolomic, and lipidomic profiles, providing deeper insights into the pathophysiology of lipedema. In the context of lipedema, transcriptomics (the study of gene expression), metabolomics (the study of metabolic profiles), and lipidomics (the analysis of lipid species) collectively provide a multifaceted view of the disease. This section explores these interrelated domains, reflecting on how they contribute to a holistic understanding of the disease.

Transcriptomics

Transcriptomic analysis involves the examination of RNA transcripts to understand gene expression patterns. The analysis of gene expression profiles has been a cornerstone of understanding various diseases, including lipedema. The dysregulation of genes related to lipid metabolism, inflammation, and adipogenesis in lipedema has gained particular attention, as these dysregulations contribute to the biological functions that seem to be altered as a part of the disease's etiology. Studies employing RNA sequencing and microarrays have identified significant alterations in gene expression levels compared to healthy controls (see below), indicating a biological signature peculiar to lipedema. Key gene transcription pathways that are altered in the pathological states in lipedema relate to the expression of genes involved in inflammation, insulin resistance, and adipose tissue development.

1. Inflammatory markers: Numerous studies suggest an inflammatory component in lipedema. Increased expression of pro-inflammatory cytokines such as IL-1β, IL-6, and TNF-α has been observed, implicating systemic inflammation in disease progression.[13, 14, 15] Elevated levels of these cytokines can promote adipocyte hypertrophy and contribute to altered vascular permeability, leading to fluid accumulation.
2. Adipogenesis-related genes: Genes that regulate differentiation and proliferation of adipocytes, such as PPARγ (peroxisome proliferator-activated receptor gamma) and C/EBPα (CCAAT/enhancer-binding protein alpha), show altered expression patterns in lipedema.[16] These findings suggest that the mechanism of adipocyte formation and function may be dysregulated, resulting in the characteristic fat deposition patterns seen in affected individuals.
3. Angiogenesis: Another compelling aspect of transcriptomic analysis in lipedema is the potential involvement of angiogenic pathways. Increased expression of angiogenic factors like VEGF (vascular endothelial growth factor) protein may contribute to the compromised lymphatic function observed in patients with lipedema, indicating that vascular

alterations might exacerbate or cause several symptoms of the disease.[17]

Metabolomics

Metabolomics has emerged as a powerful tool for investigating the biochemical changes associated with lipedema. Metabolomic approaches examine and compare the small-molecule metabolites within different biological samples. These metabolites may be critical in functional metabolic pathways or may be breakdown products that indicate the activity or inactivity of key metabolic processes. In lipedema, alterations in metabolic pathways related to lipid and carbohydrate metabolism are particularly relevant and may manifest as distinctive metabolic phenotypes. Understanding these changes enhances both our knowledge of the disease mechanism and may suggest which metabolic pathways may constitute potential therapeutic targets.

1. Energy metabolism: Alterations in glucose and lipid metabolism have been documented in patients with lipedema.[18] For instance, dysregulated levels of intermediates in glycolysis and the citric acid cycle suggest that energy production may not proceed efficiently. This metabolic inflexibility may lead to the accumulation of lipids, exacerbating the pathogenesis of the disease.
2. Lipid metabolites: Specific lipid metabolites, such as ceramides and sphingolipids, have been implicated in lipedema.[2]These compounds play crucial roles in cell signaling and inflammation. Elevated levels of certain lipid species may serve as markers for inflammation and could be potential therapeutic targets.
3. Hormonal influence: Metabolomic studies also indicate hormonal involvement in lipedema. Altered levels of adipokines such as leptin and adiponectin have been reported, which may contribute to the development of insulin resistance and abnormal lipid accumulation.[18, 19] Insight into these hormonal changes is vital for understanding the syndrome's metabolic dysfunction.

Lipidomics

Given that lipedema is fundamentally characterized by lipid dysregulation, lipidomic analyses are critical in elucidating the exact changes that occur at the lipid level during the disease process. Lipidomic analysis focuses on the vast array of lipids present in different biological systems at the level of fatty acids. Given that lipedema is characterized by abnormal lipid accumulation, lipidomics is crucial in revealing the composition and distribution of lipid species that may be unique to affected individuals. This analysis not only delineates the lipids involved but also uncovers the potential pathways leading to dysregulated lipid storage.

1. Lipid composition: Lipidomic profiling has revealed distinct patterns of lipid species in patients with lipedema compared to controls. These findings include alterations in triglyceride composition, changes in phospholipid levels, and an increase in long-chain fatty acids.[13, 20] Such modifications can affect cellular processes such as membrane fluidity and energy storage.
2. Role of fatty acids: Specific fatty acids might play significant roles in lipedema pathology. For instance, omega-3 and omega-6 fatty acids have well-documented effects on inflammation and metabolism. The balance between these fatty acids can influence tissue integrity and the inflammatory response, highlighting the potential of dietary interventions. Understanding the lipidomic landscape of lipedema can open new avenues for targeted therapies. For example, modulating lipid metabolism through dietary changes

or the use of pharmaceuticals aimed at specific lipid pathways could provide innovative and effective treatment strategies for managing lipedema.

The role of an integrated OMICs platform

The integration of transcriptomic, metabolomic, and lipidomic data provides a comprehensive lens through which to view lipedema. Each OMIC layer contributes distinct information that, when combined, offers a richer understanding of the complex interplay of genetics, metabolism, and lipid dysregulation in the disease. To further expand upon the genetic theories of lipedema development and the interconnection of various pathways outlined above, the Karnezis lab undertook a series of comprehensive, comparative multi-omics analyses of adipose tissue, adipose stem cells, and adipocytes from patients with and without lipedema.[2]

A comprehensive global lipidomic and metabolomic analysis, transcriptional profiling, and validation using complementary functional assays identified signaling events central to the enhanced stem cell proliferation seen in lipedema.[2] The transcriptional profiling study revealed >4,400 significant differences in lipedema tissue, with altered levels of genes expressed that are involved in critical signaling and cell function-regulating pathways (e.g. lipid metabolism and cell-cycle/proliferation). Profiling lipedema adipocytes revealed >900 changes in lipid composition (including cell signaling lipids PA170/141, PC282, LysoPE241, and PEO-160/130) and >600 differentially altered metabolites, implicated in cell growth and expansion. Functional assays demonstrated that dysregulated Bub1 protein signaling drives increased proliferation of lipedema stem cells, suggesting a potential mechanism for enhanced adipogenesis in lipedema. Importantly, by applying a comprehensive OMICs approach to lipedema tissue, the relationships among gene expression, metabolic profiles, and lipid compositions reveal interconnected biological pathways that contribute to lipedema.

There remains significant scope for future research, particularly in longitudinal studies that track these OMIC parameters over time. Investigating the effects of various interventions (such as diet, exercise, and pharmacotherapy, such as the bourgeoning GLP-1 inhibitor class of treatment) across the OMIC domains can elucidate novel and distinct mechanisms of action and tailored therapeutic options for patients with lipedema.

Where we are headed in lipedema research

The role of sex and hormonal influences

Lipedema predominantly affects women, which suggests that sex-specific genetic factors may play a critical role. Hormonal influences, particularly estrogen, have been proposed as modulatory factors in the development of lipedema. A 2021 study by Katzer et al.[21] discussed how estrogen regulation might affect adipose tissue distribution and fatty acid metabolism, implicating dysregulation of estrogens in the pathogenesis of lipedema. This work underscores the need for further investigation into the interplay between genetics, hormones, and environmental factors, and the introduction of newer technologies, as outlined in this chapter, may facilitate the re-examination of the hormonal cues that are at play in lipedema.

Epigenetic factors

In addition to genetic predisposition, epigenetic modifications may also play a crucial role in lipedema. Epigenetics refers to changes in gene expression that do not involve alterations in the DNA sequence itself. Evidence suggests that environmental factors, diet, and trauma can lead to epigenetic modifications that may exacerbate or trigger lipedema.[22] The Karnezis lab is currently investigating chromatin structure and remodeling in stem cells isolated from patients with lipedema. Our research has shown that a key epigenetic regulator of adipose tissue development is overexpressed in lipedema tissue. This overexpression leads to an 'open chromatin' configuration, which exposes a significant number of adipose-specific regions for transcription [Bandara et al., unpublished]. Understanding these mechanisms could help identify new therapeutic targets for managing lipedema.

The fat atlas

The growing complexity of the adipose organ is underscored by recent advances in the study of lipedema. Once considered a biologically uniform and unremarkable tissue, adipose tissue is now recognized for its diversity, distinguished by types such as brown, white, and beige fat, and for its varied stem cell composition, a topic of increasing scientific interest. Additionally, the clinical use of fat grafting in both reconstructive and aesthetic surgery has become well established.

However, a fundamental question in lipedema research remains largely unexplored: how does stem cell composition and function differ between various anatomical fat depots? This question is critical, as regional variation must be understood before it can be ruled out as a contributing factor to the tissue or cellular differences observed between lipedema and control samples. To address this, future studies must first characterize these regional differences and establish standardized anatomical sampling protocols across subject and control groups. Without this standardization, conclusions may be premature, and the applicability of findings to the broader patient population remains uncertain.

Sampling methodology limitations

Similarly, a major limitation in the field lies in the varied methods used to obtain adipose tissue samples. Tissue harvested via liposuction introduces several confounding factors, including tissue trauma, hypoxia, imprecise anatomical origin, and disruption of native architecture. These variables add to an already complex landscape of uncontrollable influences.

Superficial tissue biopsies, while less invasive, are limited by their inability to access deeper fat layers, which may hold the most pathologically relevant information. In contrast, whole tissue samples that preserve anatomical integrity could overcome many of these limitations. However, such samples are rarely obtained from early-stage patients with lipedema, meaning that available specimens often represent only later stages of the disease, potentially skewing findings and limiting their generalizability.

Conclusion

The genetic insights into lipedema have significant implications for clinical practice. As our understanding of the genetic basis of lipedema deepens, the potential for personalized treatment approaches becomes feasible. Genetic screening may eventually lead to the early identification of at-risk individuals, allowing for timely interventions that could mitigate the severity of the disease. The identification of candidate genes and their association with lipedema remains in its infancy. Ongoing research initiatives, including collaborative genome-wide association studies (GWAS), are needed to uncover additional genetic variants associated with lipedema. These efforts will not only expand our understanding of the genetic architecture of lipedema but also pave the way for future precision medicine strategies.

It is becoming apparent, however, that the genetic landscape of lipedema is complex and multifaceted, characterized by significant heritability, numerous potentially interacting candidate genes, and the overlaid influence of hormonal, immune, and epigenetic factors. Thus, the transcriptomic, metabolomic, and lipidomic approaches to studying lipedema hold great promise for enhancing our understanding of this complex disease, in conjunction with genetics. The interplay of disease processes involving inflammation, abnormal lipid metabolism, and genetic predispositions alludes to the multifaceted nature of lipedema and highlights the need for comprehensive and coordinated research approaches that integrate multiple lines of inquiry. Examining the epigenetic regulators that might have been key protagonists right under our noses during the early gene studies promises to unlock advances in our mechanistic understanding. As the field evolves, these insights will not only inform our understanding of lipedema but will also guide the development of innovative therapeutic strategies that can alleviate the burden faced by those affected by lipedema. Understanding lipedema through the lens of OMICs ultimately paves the way for a more holistic and informed approach to patient care in this often-overlooked disease.

References

1. Humenikova L, Gates GE. Body image perceptions in western and post-communist countries: a cross-cultural pilot study of children and parents. *Matern Child Nutr*. 2008 Jul;4(3):220–31. DOI: https://doi.org/10.1111/j.1740-8709.2007.00133.x
2. Ishaq M, Bandara N, Morgan S, Nowell C, Mehdi AM, Lyu R, et al. Key signaling networks are dysregulated in patients with the adipose tissue disease, lipedema. *Int J Obes*. 2022 Mar;46(3):502–14. DOI: https://doi.org/10.1038/s41366-021-01002-1
3. Morgan S, Reid I, Bendon C, Ishaq M, Shayan R, Pope B, et al. A family-based study of inherited genetic risk in lipedema. *Lymphat Res Biol*. 2024 Apr 1;22(2):106–11. DOI: https://doi.org/10.1089/lrb.2023.0065
4. Child AH, Gordon KD, Sharpe P, Brice G, Ostergaard P, Jeffery S, et al. Lipedema: An inherited condition. *Am J Med Genet A*. 2010;152A(4):970–6. DOI: https://doi.org/10.1002/ajmg.a.33313
5. Grigoriadis D, Sackey E, Riches K, van Zanten M, Brice G, England R, et al. Investigation of clinical characteristics and genome associations in the 'UK lipoedema' cohort. medRxiv. 2021 Jan 1;2021.06.15.21258988. DOI: https://doi.org/10.1371/journal.pone.0274867
6. Klimentidis YC, Chen Z, Gonzalez-Garay ML, Grigoriadis D, Sackey E, Pittman A, et al. Genome-wide association study of a lipedema phenotype among women in the UK Biobank identifies multiple genetic risk factors. *Eur J Hum Genet*. 2023 Mar;31(3):338–44. DOI: https://doi.org/10.1038/s41431-022-01231-6
7. Michelini S, Chiurazzi P, Marino V, Dell'Orco D, Manara E, Baglivo M, et al. Aldo-keto reductase 1C1 (AKR1C1) as the first mutated gene in a family with nonsyndromic primary lipedema. *Int J Mol Sci*. 2020 Jan;21(17):6264. DOI: https://doi.org/10.3390/ijms21176264
8. Michelini S, Herbst KL, Precone V, Manara E, Marceddu G, Dautaj A, et al. A multi-gene panel to identify lipedema-predisposing genetic variants by a next-generation sequencing strategy. *J Pers Med*. 2022 Feb 11;12(2):268. DOI: https://doi.org/10.3390/jpm12020268
9. van Gurp JE, Lechner RL, Micha D, Maugeri A, Dulfer E, van Dijk FS, et al. Tenascin-X deficiency causing classical-like Ehlers-Danlos syndrome type 1 in humans is a significant risk factor of gastrointestinal and tracheal ruptures. *Clin Transl Gastroenterol*. 2025 Mar;16(3):e00821. DOI: https://doi.org/10.14309/ctg.0000000000000821
10. Demirdas S, Dulfer E, Robert L, Kempers M, van Beek D, Micha D, et al. Recognizing the tenascin-X deficient type of Ehlers-Danlos syndrome: a cross-sectional study in 17 patients. *Clin Genet*. 2017;91(3):411–25. DOI: https://doi.org/10.1111/cge.12853
11. Brenner E, Forner-Cordero I, Faerber G, Rapprich S, Cornely M. Body mass index vs. waist-to-height-ratio in patients with lipohyperplasia dolorosa (vulgo lipedema). *J Dtsch Dermatol Ges*

J Ger Soc Dermatol JDDG. 2023 Oct;21(10):1179–85. DOI: https://doi.org/10.1111/ddg.15182

12. Farooqi IS, Drop S, Clements A, Keogh JM, Biernacka J, Lowenbein S, et al. Heterozygosity for a POMC-null mutation and increased obesity risk in humans. *Diabetes*. 2006 Sep;55(9):2549–53. DOI: https://doi.org/10.2337/db06-0214
13. Wolf S, Rannikko JH, Virtakoivu R, Cinelli P, Felmerer G, Burger A, et al. A distinct M2 macrophage infiltrate and transcriptomic profile decisively influence adipocyte differentiation in lipedema. *Front Immunol* . 2022 Dec 20;13. Available from: https://www.frontiersin.org/journals/immunology/articles/10.3389/fimmu.2022.1004609/full
14. Kruppa P, Gohlke S, Łapiński K, Garcia-Carrizo F, Soultoukis GA, Infanger M, et al. Lipedema stage affects adipocyte hypertrophy, subcutaneous adipose tissue inflammation and interstitial fibrosis. *Front Immunol* . 2023 Jul 28;14. Available from: https://www.frontiersin.org/journals/immunology/articles/10.3389/fimmu.2023.1223264/full
15. Di Renzo L, Gualtieri P, Alwardat N, De Santis G, Zomparelli S, Romano L, et al. The role of IL-6 gene polymorphisms in the risk of lipedema. *Eur Rev Med Pharmacol Sci*. 2020 Mar;24(6):3236–44. DOI: https://doi.org/10.26355/eurrev_202003_20690
16. Westcott GP, Rosen ED. Crosstalk Between adipose and lymphatics in health and disease. *Endocrinology*. 2022 Jan 1;163(1):bqab224. DOI: https://doi.org/10.1210/endocr/bqab224
17. Al-Ghadban S, Cromer W, Allen M, Ussery C, Badowski M, Harris D, et al. Dilated blood and lymphatic microvessels, angiogenesis, increased macrophages, and adipocyte hypertrophy in lipedema thigh skin and fat tissue. *J Obes*. 2019 Mar 3;2019:1–10. DOI: https://doi.org/10.1155/2019/8747461
18. Nankam PAN, Cornely M, Klöting N, Blüher M. Is subcutaneous adipose tissue expansion in people living with lipedema healthier and reflected by circulating parameters? *Front Endocrinol* . 2022 Oct 31;13. Available from: https://www.frontiersin.orghttps://www.frontiersin.org/journals/endocrinology/articles/10.3389/fendo.2022.1000094/full
19. Ünlü Z, Çavuşoğlu T, Kosova F, Aydin A. The relationship between adipokines and the thickness of subcutaneous adipose tissue in lipedema. *Celal Bayar Üniversitesi Sağlık Bilim Enstitüsü Derg.* 2022 Mar 2; 296-304. DOI: https://doi.org/10.34087/cbusbed.1062223
20. Kempa S, Buechler C, Föh B, Felthaus O, Prantl L, Günther UL, et al. Serum metabolomic profiling of patients with lipedema. *Int J Mol Sci*. 2023 Jan;24(24):17437. DOI: https://doi.org/10.3390/ijms242417437
21. Katzer K, Hill JL, McIver KB. Lipedema and the potential role of estrogen in excessive adipose tissue accumulation. *Int J Mol Sci*. 2021;22(21):11720. DOI: https://doi.org/10.3390/ijms222111720
22. Cione E, Michelini S, Abrego-Guandique DM, Vaia N, Michelini S, Puleo V, et al. Identification of specific microRNAs in adipose tissue affected by lipedema. *Curr Issues Mol Biol.* 2024 Nov;46(11):11957–74. DOI: https://doi.org/10.3390/cimb46110710

III
Lipedema differential diagnosis and co-morbidities

Chapter Six
Lymphedema

Kristiana Gordon

Introduction

Lymphedema is a neglected disease, not unlike lipedema. It is far more common than healthcare providers realize, with an estimated 250 million individuals affected worldwide, of which 10 million are in the United States.[1] Despite its prevalence, there is a lack of interest amongst many clinicians to diagnose, manage, and help patients with lymphedema, not a dissimilar situation to lipedema. Much of this perceived disinterest is likely due to a lack of education on lymphatic diseases, something the authors of this book are taking steps to change. This chapter aims to provide an overview of the biological importance of the lymphatic system, together with how and why lymphedema develops when it fails.

Lipedema is frequently misdiagnosed as lymphedema since both diseases can present with increased volume in the lower and sometimes upper limbs, leading healthcare providers to more often suspect lymphedema as the cause. Unlike lipedema, an adipose (fat) tissue disease, lymphedema occurs due to inadequate lymphatic drainage, resulting in a buildup of lymphatic fluid in the skin and subcutaneous tissues (Figure 6.1). It is a chronic debilitating disease that may lead to significant physical and psychological morbidity, as swelling results in discomfort, reduced mobility, and impaired function. Recurrent infections complicate many cases of lymphedema, regardless of the underlying cause, and add to the burden of disease. Lymphedema typically affects one or more limbs, but any body part can be affected, depending on the underlying cause. Primary lymphedema arises due to an intrinsic abnormality involving a genetically determined abnormal development of lymphatic vessels. Whereas secondary lymphedema results from lymphatic damage due to extrinsic factors such as surgical lymphadenectomy, radiotherapy, or chronic venous disease. There is currently no curative treatment, but compression therapy in combination with exercise and weight management is effective. Lymphedema surgery may be considered in select cases but is unlikely to be curative or allow the patient to discontinue wearing compression garments.

Anatomy and physiology of the lymphatic system

The lymphatic system plays a vital role in the regulation of the circulatory and immune systems. It has several functions, including 1) maintenance of fluid balance by returning interstitial fluid from the tissue spaces back to the blood circulation, 2) maintaining immune function with the help of

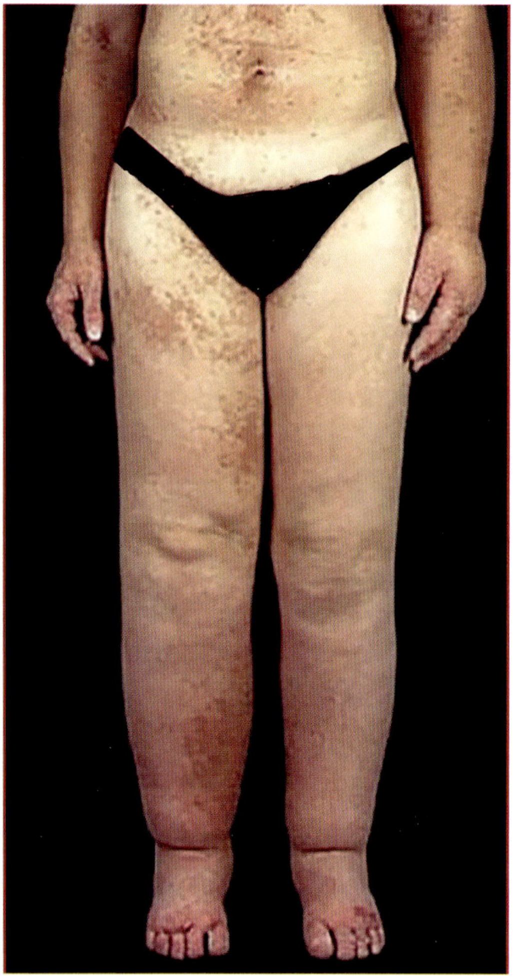

Figure 6.1: Lower limb lymphedema. (Note the left upper limb is also affected.) Adapted from Mansour et al., 2023.[2]

lymphoid organs, and 3) nutritional, as ingested fat is absorbed via intestinal lymphatics called lacteals.

The lymphatic system is not a circular system, unlike the blood vascular system. The lymphatic system is an extensive one-way network of lymphatic vessels and lymph nodes, whose primary function is to absorb and drain fluid and other materials from tissues (Figure 6.2).[3] These include capillary filtrate, plasma proteins, macrophages, lymphocytes, and malignant cells. The recently revised Starling model proves it is lymphatic drainage that prevents the accumulation of transcapillary plasma filtrate, and not via reabsorption in the venous system as originally thought.[4] The lymphatic system ensures that capillary filtrate is returned to the blood circulation system at the level of the subclavian vein via the thoracic duct.

Lymphatic vessels are present in almost all tissues in the body and are essentially of three types. Firstly, tiny initial lymphatic vessels absorb the capillary filtrate, leucocytes, and macrophages via gaps in their discontinuous basement membrane. This lymphatic fluid is then drained to the pre-collector lymphatic vessels, and then the larger collecting lymphatic vessels that actively pump lymphatic fluid towards the regional lymph nodes and beyond.[5] The lymphatic pre-collectors and collecting lymphatic vessels are covered by smooth muscle cells to permit vessel contraction and proximal propulsion of lymphatic fluid toward the thoracic duct.[6] Valves are present in the larger lymphatic vessels to ensure unidirectional flow of lymphatic fluid. Lymphedema develops when the volume of fluid filtered from the microvascular capillaries exceeds the capacity of the lymphatic system to drain it. This imbalance can result from:

1. Increased microvascular filtration, such as elevated venous pressure caused by varicose veins.
2. Reduced lymphatic drainage, often due to damage from cancer treatments; or
3. A combination of both factors.

The lymphatic system plays a vital role in our body's immune function. The lymphatic system includes primary and secondary lymphoid organs. In the primary lymphoid organs (bone marrow and thymus), immune cell production and maturation take place, whereas secondary lymphoid organs (lymph nodes, spleen, and mucosa-associated lymphoid organs such as the

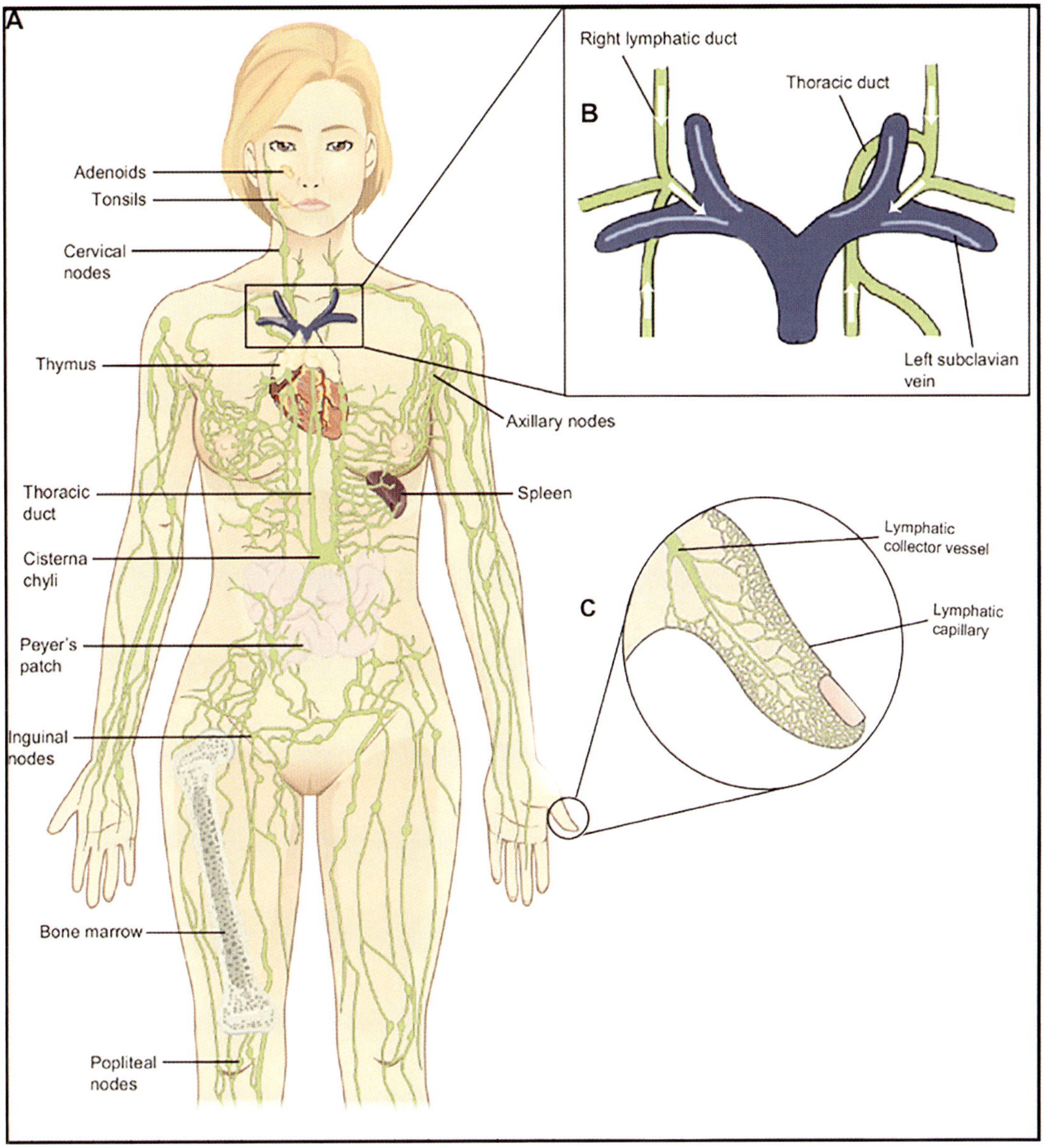

Figure 6.2: Anatomy of the lymphatic system: (A) the lymphatic system includes a series of lymphatic vessels, providing a one-way drainage route from all tissues back to the blood circulation via the great veins in the neck. The initial dermal lymphatic capillaries absorb interstitial material and fluid to make lymph, which drains into lymphatic collectors. Lymph is pumped from the gut and lower half of the body to the cisterna chyli, a sac-like structure situated below the diaphragm, and then on to the thoracic duct; (B) the thoracic duct is responsible for lymph drainage coming from most of the body, with the exception of the right side of the head and neck, the right side of the thorax, and the right upper limb, which drain primarily into the right lymphatic duct. Both ducts drain into the great veins of the neck; (C) the intricate dermal lymphatic capillary network drains downstream into the lymphatic collector vessels on route to the lymph nodes. Adapted from Martin-Almedina et al., 2021.[9]

tonsils and adenoids) are the sites for lymphocyte activation. The lymphatic system mediates the transport of antigens (i.e. a toxin or foreign substance), macrophages, lymphocytes, and dendritic cells to draining lymph nodes via afferent lymphatic vessels. It also assists with the trafficking of infection-fighting leucocytes to and from lymph nodes.[7] This lymphatic drainage and transport system allows for an adaptive immune response to be generated to pathogens constantly trying to invade us. Localized skin infections (e.g. warts, cellulitis, or athlete's foot) occur more often in people with lymphedema due to a disturbance in immune cell trafficking, which compromises local tissue immune surveillance. Lymphedema has been reported to convey a relative risk of 71 times the normal for the development of cellulitis.[8] Effective lymphedema treatment will significantly reduce this risk.

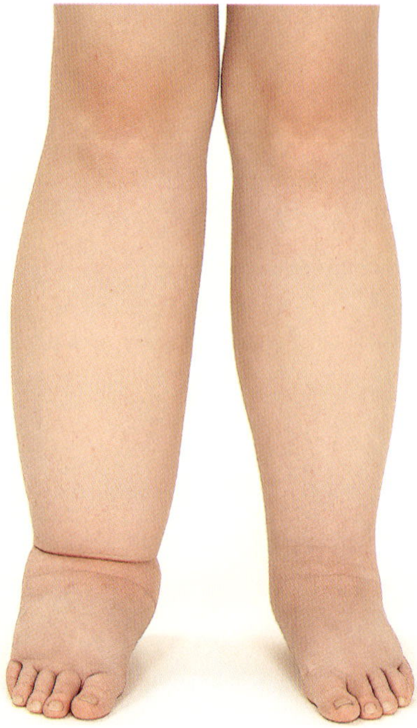

Figure 6.3: Lower limb lymphedema: note the asymmetrical swelling and involvement of the feet. Adapted from Gordon et al., 2020.[13]

Diagnosing lymphedema

The clinical signs of lymphedema range from mild swelling to that of a massive enlargement in chronic, untreated cases. Protein-rich materials, lipids, and debris accumulate in addition to the lymphatic fluid. This results in 'solid' and 'fluid' components to the swelling, giving rise to the brawny nature of chronic edema that resists pitting.[10] Lymphedema typically begins as mild, initially reversible swelling. In the early stages, the affected limb will exhibit 'pitting,' meaning that prolonged pressure from a clinician's thumb leaves a visible indentation due to fluid accumulation in the tissue.

Chronic accumulation of lymphatic fluid within the tissues eventually results in a more 'solid' swelling (Figure 6.3). Characteristic skin thickening and induration of the deeper tissues over time make pitting more difficult to elicit but may still be possible. The pathognomonic sign of lymphedema is a positive Stemmer sign, or the inability to pinch and lift a fold of skin at the base of the 2nd toe as a result of the thickened tissues.[11] Papillomatosis (small flesh-colored papules) develops in the untreated patient as a result of dilated lymphatic vessels and subsequent fibrosis within the dermal layer of the skin (Figure 6.4). Lymphangiectasia appears as small fluid-filled blisters on the skin surface. Lymphatic fluid may leak through the skin as a result of minimal trauma and is termed lymphorrhea.

The severity of lymphedema can be staged according to its clinical features, which may be useful in monitoring the response to treatment over a prolonged period (See Table 6.1 and Figures 6.5 and 6.6). These changes contrast with those seen in limb enlargement from lipedema, where the feet are spared, the tissues are invariably tender, soft, and non-pitting (See Table 6.2 and Figure 6.7).

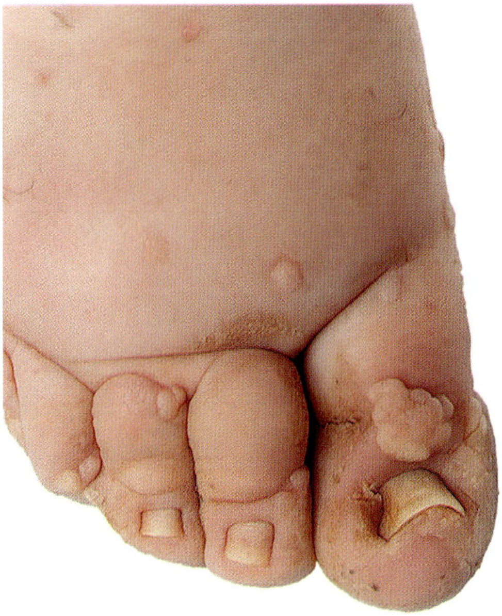

Figure 6.4: Skin changes associated with severe lymphedema. There is lymphedema of the dorsal foot and toes. Stemmer's sign will be positive. Papillomatosis and hyperkeratosis have occurred near the swollen toes. (Creative Commons license allows this image to be reproduced from: Gordon et al. 2020.[13])

Table 6.1: International staging of lymphedema (ISL). Adapted from the 2020 Consensus Document of the International Society of Lymphology.[14]

Lymphedema stage	Clinical features
0	Latent or subclinical where swelling is not yet evident despite impaired lymphatic drainage.
1	Mild pitting edema that resolves with limb elevation.
2	Pitting edema that does not resolve with elevation. Signs of tissue fibrosis and fat deposition may become apparent, resulting in less obvious pitting.
3	Development of elephantiasis skin changes, i.e. solid swelling (non-pitting) with associated skin changes, including hyperkeratosis and papillomatosis.

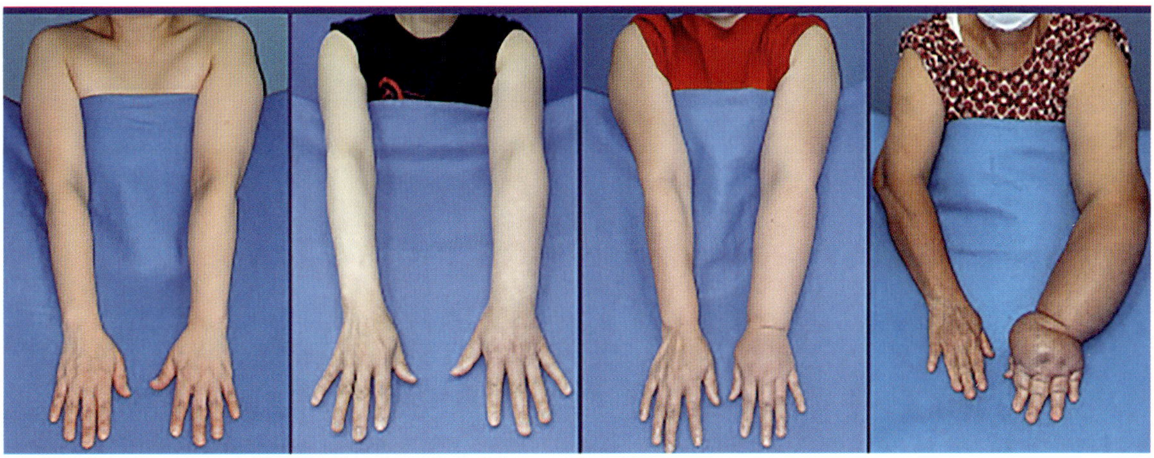

Figure 6.5: Stages 0–3 in upper extremity lymphedema. *Lymphedema staging for upper limbs* is licensed under CC BY 4.0.

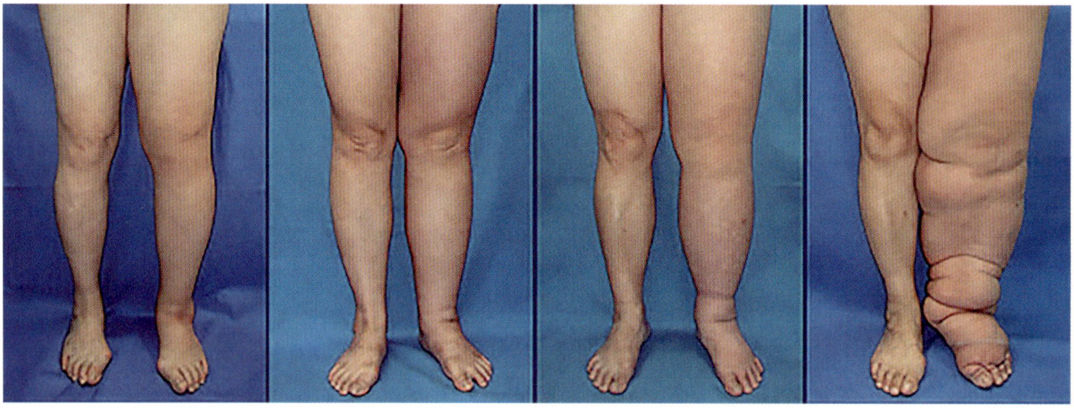

Figure 6.6: Stages 0–3 in lower extremity lymphedema stages. *Lymphedema staging for lower limbs* is licensed under CC BY 4.0.

Table 6.2: Clinical findings of lymphedema vs. lipedema.

Characteristics	**Lymphedema**	**Lipedema**
Gender	Any gender	Almost exclusively female
Age of onset of clinical signs	Any age (usually childhood/puberty for primary lymphedema, and adulthood for secondary lymphedema)	Usually between ages 10–30 yrs
Sparing of hands/feet	No	Yes
Areas affected	Any body site, but usually one or more limbs are affected (depending on the underlying cause), often asymmetrically	Symmetrical involvement of the lower limbs +/- upper limbs
Family history of similar issues	Rarely (unless for primary lymphedema)	Often
Effect of limb elevation	Initially results in limb volume reduction, but this effect reduces as the disease progresses, if left untreated	None
Presence of pitting	Present in the early stages of lymphedema	None
Tenderness/pain	Often absent, but can be present	Present
Skin changes	Solid/thicker skin +/- hyperkeratosis and papillomatosis in late-stage disease	Absent
Easy bruising	Absent	Present
Stemmer's sign (of 2nd toes)	Positive	Negative
History of cellulitis infections	Frequent	Absent
Effect of compression	Good compression results in significant limb volume reduction	Compression will not significantly reduce limb volumes, but may improve limb pain

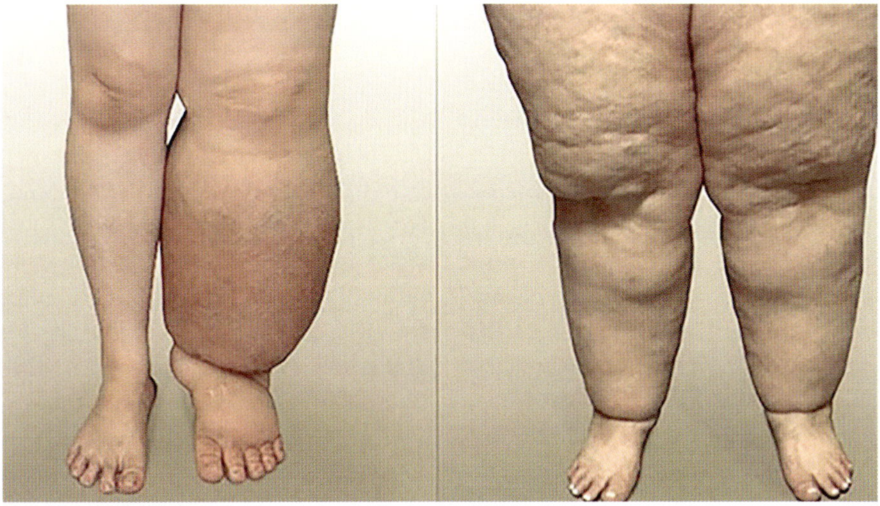

Figure 6.7: Left lower extremity lymphedema (left) is contrasted with bilateral lower extremity lipedema (right). Note the key differences of lymphedema i.e. involvement of the top of the foot, and asymmetrical limb involvement. ©2017, Lipedema Simplified LLC. Used with permission.

Most cases of lymphedema can be diagnosed from the history and clinical findings. The use of lymphatic imaging techniques is dependent on availability and expertise, but can be utilized to confirm lymphedema when necessary. Lymphoscintigraphy is the current gold standard diagnostic test for lymphedema. It involves injecting a radio-labeled protein or colloid, exclusively cleared by lymphatics, into the skin of the foot (for lower limb examination). Measurement of uptake in regional (inguinal) lymph nodes and transit through the lymphatics with a gamma camera allows for both crude imaging of lymphatic drainage pathways and functional measurement of lymphatic flow over 2 hours. Lymphoscintigraphy images can be helpful when investigating patients with suspected primary lymphedema, as it is possible to correlate abnormalities with a genetically diagnosed condition.[12]

Causes of lymphedema

Lymphedema occurs when the lymphatic system is unable to drain the interstitial fluid from the tissues adequately. This may be due to primary lymphedema (an intrinsic developmental abnormality of the lymphatic system present from birth) or due to secondary lymphedema, where an extrinsic issue has affected the lymphatic system. Secondary lymphedema is far more common than primary lymphedema; however, the latter should be considered as a differential diagnosis when a teenage girl is questioning whether lipedema is the cause of her pubertal-onset lower limb enlargement (Figure 6.3).

Primary lymphedema

Primary lymphedema occurs when there is an inborn weakness, usually genetically determined, in the lymphatic system. Onset early in life or the presence of a family history of similar swelling should make a clinician suspect primary lymphedema. However, primary lymphedema is not one disease but the presenting feature of several distinct clinical entities, and it can be challenging to make an accurate diagnosis. The subtypes of primary lymphedema vary in terms of age of onset of swelling, affected sites, possible associated diseases, and underlying genetic cause.

Primary lymphedema was historically classified according to the age of onset of swelling, i.e. lymphedema congenita (swelling present at birth); lymphedema praecox (swelling develops at puberty); and lymphedema tarda (swelling develops after 35 years of age).[15,16] However, it has become clear that this classification system, based purely on age of onset, is over-simplified and fails to consider associated health problems that may need to be excluded, such as the high risk of leukemia associated with Emberger syndrome, which is thankfully a rare cause of childhood-onset lower limb lymphedema. In addition, the discovery of causal genes has changed the way clinicians approach the diagnosis and management of primary lymphedema.

Connell et al.[17] created a new diagnostic classification pathway for primary lymphedema in 2010, founded on clinical phenotype (see Figure 6.8). It is based not simply on the age of onset of the lymphedema but also on the sites affected and the presence of associated features, such as dysmorphology, distichiasis (aberrant eyelashes), varicose veins, vascular malformations, and limb overgrowth. Systemic lymphatic involvement is also taken into consideration. Broadly speaking, there are five main subtypes of primary lymphedema presented within a color-coded algorithm to aid diagnosis and facilitate genetic testing. In recent times, the algorithm has proved invaluable in the interpretation of genetic results, as some clinicians readily request genetic panel testing without possessing the skills to interpret genetic variants of uncertain significance.

The five subtypes of primary lymphedema are listed in Table 6.3, and it is the 'late onset' group of primary lymphedemas that may need to be excluded when assessing a young woman with suspected lower limb lipedema. Within this group, lymphedema-distichiasis syndrome and Meige disease may both present with increased lower limb volumes around the time of puberty and are likely to have a strong family history of pubertal-onset swelling. However, clinical assessment should permit differentiation between the diseases without always needing to investigate with lymphoscintigraphy or genetic testing. Lymphedema-distichiasis syndrome occurs as a result of a mistake in the *FOXC2* gene. Clinical signs include the presence of distichiasis (additional eyelashes that are smaller and grow inwards, causing ocular irritation), varicose veins, and a history of congenital heart disease. It is inherited in an autosomal dominant pattern, so a family history will include affected males. Meige disease, however, is the most common form of primary lymphedema and affects females significantly more often than males.

It presents with pubertal, or later in life, onset of lower limb lymphedema. There are no other associated health problems, and an underlying genetic mistake is rarely identified (although mistakes in *GJC2, HGF*, and *CELSR1* genes have been identified in some individuals), making Meige disease harder to exclude as a differential diagnosis for lipedema based on the history alone.[13] However, a clinical examination should be able to differentiate Meige disease from lipedema, as Meige disease will involve the feet, and swelling is often asymmetrical, with pitting invariably present. These features should make the clinician strongly favor a diagnosis of primary lymphedema over lipedema. Table 6.2 compares the clinical signs of lymphedema and lipedema and can be used to aid in diagnosis. If doubt persists, then imaging with lymphoscintigraphy can confirm lymphedema if there are recognizable patterns of abnormal lymphatic drainage for the subtypes of primary lymphedema listed in Table 6.3.[12]

Knowing the genetic cause enables a better understanding of natural history, associated diseases, inheritance patterns, and how the different types of primary lymphedema develop. For example, a patient with primary lymphedema due to Milroy disease may only have problems with

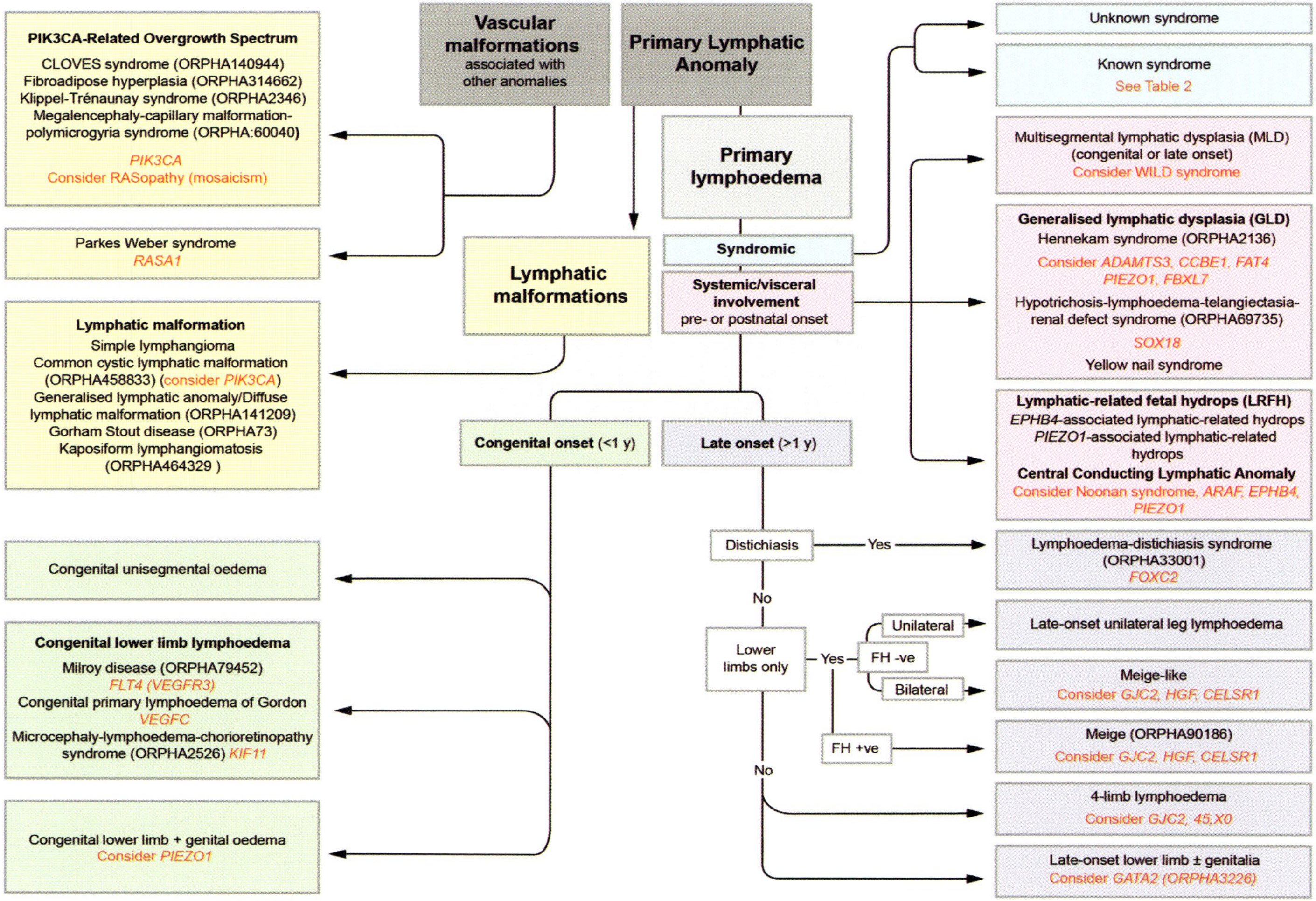

Figure 6.8: St George's classification algorithm for primary lymphatic anomalies. The five main groupings (colour coded) with their various clinical subtypes of disease. Primary lymphoedema is the major clinical feature in the green, pink and purple sections. Text in red indicates the suggested genetic test and/or differential diagnosis for the subgroup, however, the indicated genes do not explain the cause of disease in all patients in each grouping. For example, only 70% of patients with Milroy disease are explained by mutations in FLT4/ VEGFR3.33 FH, family history; +ve, positive; –ve, negative. (Image shared by St George's Lymphovascular Research Group under the CC BY-SA 4.0 International licence on Wikimedia Commons).

Table 6.3: Subtypes of primary lymphedema.

Subtype	Examples (gene mutations in italics)	Comment
Genetic syndromes associated with lymphedema	Turner syndrome Noonan syndrome	Swelling is not the predominant feature of the child's health problems, but simply part of their overall condition
Lymphedema with systemic (internal) lymphatic abnormalities	Hennekam syndrome (e.g. due to a mutation in the *CCBE1* gene)	A rare form of primary lymphedema. These children may be swollen at birth (usually affecting several limbs/body parts) and have internal lymphatic problems, e.g. fluid around the heart and/or lungs. They may also have abnormal lymphatic drainage of the small intestine, causing them to have diarrhea when they eat fatty foods
Lymphedema in association with overgrowth of tissues	*PIK3CA*-related overgrowth syndrome (PROS). There are several diseases within this group, including Klippel-Trenaunay syndrome	Lymphedema may develop in association with overgrowth of tissues within the swollen limb e.g. the muscle, bone, or fatty tissues are increased in size. These diseases are mosaic, with mutations confirmed on tissue biopsy of affected sites
Congenital lymphedema	Milroy disease (*VEGFR3*)	Lower limb lymphedema is present at birth (or develops within the first few months of life)
Late-onset primary lymphedema	Lymphedema distichiasis syndrome (*FOXC2*) Meige disease	Swelling of lower limbs (+/- upper limbs) develops after the first year of the patient's life. The majority are present after puberty

lower limb swelling from birth, but some forms of primary lymphedema occur in association with other health problems such as congenital heart disease, systemic/internal lymphatic abnormalities (pleural and/or pericardial effusions, ascites), or very rarely hematological malignancy.

Although mutations are identified in less than a quarter of patients, the development of genetic testing has made it easier to identify many of these patients and facilitate early treatment of associated health problems.[13] Unfortunately, there is no curative treatment for primary lymphedema. Hopefully, gene therapy will be available to treat some forms within the next decade. In the meantime, several repurposed medications have been successfully used in the management of complex cases of primary lymphedema with progressive, and often internal, lymphatic problems.[18, 19, 20]

Secondary lymphedema

Secondary lymphedema develops from an acquired disruption of lymphatic drainage pathways, such as damage to the lymphatic vessels and/or lymph nodes. While lymphatic filariasis is the most common cause of lymphedema, affecting an estimated 40 million people worldwide, cases are concentrated in the tropics and rarely present in the United States or Europe.[21] Filariasis occurs as a result of mosquitoes transmitting filarial larvae into the lymphatics, where they hatch into adult worms, causing damage to the lymphatic system.

More common causes of lymphedema presenting in the US and Europe include those secondary to necessary cancer treatment. Removal of lymph nodes, radiotherapy, and certain chemotherapy agents can damage and disrupt the lymphatic drainage pathways.[22] Perhaps the most recognized form of secondary lymphedema in the developed world is that of breast cancer-related lymphedema (BCRL). Despite recent advances in breast cancer treatment, including the introduction of minimal surgery guided by sentinel lymph node biopsy, the prevalence of BCRL remains stubbornly high at 15–20%.[23, 24] The reasons why some patients develop BCRL and others do not, despite similar treatment plans, remain a mystery, but an underlying genetically determined susceptibility has been proposed.[25]

Other causes of secondary lymphedema are listed in Table 6.4 and include surgery, inflammatory diseases, trauma, venous disease, and immobility.[26] Higher venous pressures from heart failure and/or venous disease, low plasma proteins (protein-losing states, liver disease), and chronic inflammation (infection, inflammatory skin disease) will increase lymphatic fluid production. Similarly, impaired lymphatic drainage from damage to the lymphatic system from surgery or infection, obesity, and poor mobility could be contributory factors. Certain medications can cause peripheral edema, such as calcium channel antagonists for hypertension, which cause lymphatic dysfunction by inhibiting the contractile function of the vessels.[27] Chronic lower limb edema in the elderly is not uncommon and is often a multi-factorial disease. Age and obesity independently impair lymphatic function. A patient who is older, immobile, and overweight with some chronic right-sided heart failure will have multiple physiological factors contributing to swollen legs.

Table 6.4: Causes of impaired lymphatic function.

Cause of impaired lymphatic function	Examples
Malignancy and cancer treatment	Lymph node biopsy/ clearance Radiotherapy Active/recurrent cancer
Infection	Filariasis Recurrent cellulitis
Elevated venous pressures	Varicose veins, deep vein thrombosis, Heart failure, Obstructive sleep apnea
Dependency	Immobility (e.g. post-CVA)
Obesity	
Medications	Calcium channel blockers Taxanes Corticosteroids Non-steroidal anti-inflammatory drugs
Trauma to lymphatic pathways	Accidental trauma to the lymphatic system, Surgical trauma
Chronic cutaneous inflammatory disease	Acne, rosacea, Hidradenitis suppurativa, Cutaneous Crohn's disease
Low protein states	Protein-losing enteropathy
Liver disease	
Nephrotic syndrome	

Management of lymphedema

Patients with lymphedema must be offered treatment and not be expected to 'live with' their disease. If possible, the underlying cause or exacerbating factor should be managed in the hope that it may reverse some lymphatic dysfunction, such as discontinuation of calcium channel blockers, or prescription of immunosuppressive therapy to reduce the inflammation from cutaneous Crohn's disease. However, the reality is that treatment of the underlying cause rarely leads to resolution of edema. Thereafter, cases of primary and secondary lymphedema share the same management pathway, utilizing noninvasive therapies to optimize lymphatic function. Lymphedema therapy can be very effective but requires a proactive and motivated patient to ensure the best results. To date, there is no drug therapy specific to lymphedema, and there is no surgical operation of proven benefit to all. Weight control is an essential component of long-term lymphedema management, as a high BMI has a negative impact on lymphatic function and mobility. While limb elevation and diuretics may partially reduce lymph production via capillary filtration, they cannot improve lymphatic drainage and function. Therefore, overnight elevation has little impact on chronic lymphedema, and there is no place for long-term diuretics in the management of lymphedema. The International Society of Lymphology has developed guidelines regarding the management of lymphedema.[14] The cornerstones of lymphedema treatment are summarized below.

Compression therapy

Compression is the most important component of lymphedema management. The physical treatment of lymphedema, often called complete decongestive therapy (CDT), should occur in two distinct stages. The goal of the intensive first stage, the reduction phase, is to 'disorganize' the fibrotic lymphedema and reduce the volume and discomfort. To do so, a combination of techniques should be used: multi-layered bandages, exercise, manual lymph drainage, and skin care. The intensive reduction phase of lymphedema treatment should be offered to patients with significant swelling of any body site to achieve considerable volume reduction. The duration of reduction phase therapy varies across the globe but typically involves daily manual lymphatic drainage massage (MLD), bandaging, and exercises once daily for an approximate duration of 2 to 4 weeks. Unlike the blood circulatory system, which has the power of the heart to pump fluid around, the lymphatic system relies on muscle movement to stimulate the flow of lymphatic fluid, especially in the lower limbs. Therefore, patients are encouraged to exercise while in compression, as external pressure forces from a bandage enhance the effect of movement on the flow of lymphatic fluid. Following this intensive treatment, the patient is then fitted with compression garments to maintain the reduced volumes.

The goal of the second stage of treatment, the maintenance phase, is to maintain the results achieved in the reduction phase. The techniques used in this phase are: compression with low-stretch elastic garments, specific exercises, and skin care. Patients with milder lymphedema may be able to skip the reduction phase bandaging and instead wear compression garments daily. Compression garments limit the amount of lymphatic fluid accumulation within the affected tissues. They have a graduated compression profile (more strength distally than at the proximal end of the garment), ensuring lymphatic fluid flows in the correct direction of drainage. As with compression bandages, the effects are enhanced when a patient exercises while wearing their compression garments. The patient's compliance with the daily use of their garments is crucial for a successful outcome.

Compression therapy can also be achieved with the use of Velcro strapping systems applied to swollen limbs.[28] These adjustable garments are often utilized in the maintenance phase of lymphedema treatment and are ideal for patients with significant co-morbidities who are unable to comply with donning standard compression garments.

Manual lymphatic drainage

Manual lymphatic drainage (MLD) is a massage technique performed by trained lymphedema therapists. The aim is to re-route the accumulation of lymphatic fluid from affected regions via collateral lymphatic vessels towards other lymphatic pathways that can drain normally. There is limited evidence in the literature to support its use.[29, 30, 31] However, MLD is widely practiced, and many patients, therapists, and physicians advocate the benefits.

Skincare and cellulitis management

Compromised lymphatic drainage results in localized tissue immunodeficiency as a result of disrupted immune cell trafficking. Disturbance to lymph drainage, therefore, increases the patient's risk of infection and also leads to difficulties in subsequent eradication of infection. Up to 50% of patients with lymphedema suffer one or more attacks of cellulitis. Acute cellulitis requires treatment with at least two weeks of antibiotics, or recurrence may develop due to inadequate treatment of the original infection. Education on skincare, including the use of emollients, is required to reduce portals of entry for infection, especially via interdigital tinea pedis (athlete's foot). Recurrent cellulitis may sometimes require lifelong prophylactic antibiotics and should be considered in patients with two or more attacks of cellulitis per year.[32]

Surgical management

Traditional excisional surgical procedures for the management of lymphedema, such as the Charles procedure, are now rarely employed as post-operative complications can cause more suffering than the pre-operative disease state (e.g. exacerbation of swelling and/or recurrent infections), and none have curative potential.[33] Less risky types of lymphedema surgery are available, but they are rarely curative or suitable for everyone with lymphedema. Careful patient selection must be undertaken by the treating physician to minimize harm and manage patient expectations of success. Three types of lymphedema surgery that are available in larger lymphedema treatment centers include lymphatic-venous anastomosis (LVA), lymph node transfer (LNT), and liposuction.

LVA surgery is a type of lymphovenous bypass, utilizing a supermicrosurgical technique to anastomose distal lymphatic vessels to nearby venules. The aim is to bypass the dysfunctional lymphatic system and improve regional lymph drainage via the redistribution of lymph within the venous system. It is popular amongst surgeons as it is performed via small incisions under local anesthesia. Post-operative complications are rare but include lymphatic vessel occlusion, possibly due to thrombus formation within the lumen.[34] A review of the literature suggests that the efficacy of LVA surgery is variable, with studies reporting mean post-operative volume reduction ranging from just 4% to 67%.[33, 35, 36] However, subjective symptom relief was found in the majority of patients, as well as a reduction in the number of cellulitis episodes.[37]

Lymph node transfer (LNT) surgery involves transplantation of normal lymphatic tissue within a flap from an unaffected site of the patient to the affected region. Fewer centers perform this type of surgery than LVA, but the reported results appear encouraging in patients with secondary lymphedema. For example, Becker et al.[38] reported a series of 24 patients receiving deep/superficial inferior epigastric perforator flap (DIEP/SIEP) transposition, with 10 patients reportedly cured of their lymphoedema (41.6%). An additional 6 patients experienced > 50% volume reduction, 6 patients achieved <50% reduction, and 2 patients had no improvement. Concerns still exist over its use in patients with primary lymphedema who may lack 'normal' lymph nodes or lymphatic vasculature, even at unaffected sites.

As previously mentioned, longstanding lymphedema may be associated with excess fatty tissue deposition within the swollen limb, with abnormal adipogenesis presumed secondary to inflammatory changes within lymphedematous tissue.[39] This abnormal fatty tissue cannot be reduced by decongestive lymphedema treatment, nor LVA or LNT surgeries. Liposuction can achieve significant volume reduction in these types of 'fatty lymphedema' when combined with lifelong compression therapy. However, liposuction must only be undertaken in compliant patients able to wear compression garments lifelong, as surgery will damage lymphatic vessels within the lymphedematous tissues that may have been functional.[40] Liposuction techniques, although not curative, offer an effective symptomatic treatment for patients with 'fatty lymphedema,' with Brorson reporting long-term limb volume reduction of more than 100% in compliant patients followed for up to 17 years.[41, 42]

Conclusion

In summary, our current understanding of lymphedema rests on several well-established principles. The lymphatic system plays a vital role in maintaining fluid balance and immune surveillance by returning interstitial fluid to the bloodstream. When this system fails – due either to congenital abnormalities (as in primary lymphedema) or external factors such as surgery, radiation, or trauma (as in secondary lymphedema) – fluid accumulates in the interstitial spaces, leading to swelling, inflammation, and increased risk of recurrent cellulitis. Despite its chronic nature, lymphedema can often be effectively managed with non-invasive physical therapies aimed at enhancing lymphatic flow through existing or collateral pathways. These treatments are applicable to both primary and secondary forms. In more advanced stages, where fibrotic or adipose tissue becomes dominant and unresponsive to compression, surgical options such as liposuction may be considered in carefully selected cases.

However, significant gaps in knowledge remain. One key question is why only some individuals develop lymphedema following lymphatic injury while others do not. The underlying genetic predispositions for primary lymphedema are also still being uncovered, and ongoing research is likely to reveal additional causal genes in the future.

Finally, several treatment approaches remain in the realm of conjecture. Surgical procedures, such as LVA and LNT, show promise in some cases but currently lack sufficient high-quality evidence to support their widespread use. Continued research and clinical trials will be necessary to clarify their role in long-term lymphedema management and determine which patients may benefit most from these emerging interventions.

References

1. Greene AK. Epidemiology and morbidity of lymphedema. In: Greene AK, Slavin SA, Brorson H, editors. *Lymphedema: Presentation, Diagnosis, and Treatment* . Cham: Springer International Publishing; 2015, p. 33–44. DOI: https://doi.org/10.1007/978-3-319-14493-1_4
2. Mansour S, Josephs KS, Ostergaard P, Gordon K, Zanten MV, Pearce J, et al. Redefining WILD syndrome: a primary lymphatic dysplasia with congenital multisegmental lymphoedema, cutaneous lymphovascular malformation, CD4

lymphopaenia and warts. *J Med Genet*. 2023 Jan 1;60(1):84–90. DOI: https://doi.org/10.1136/jmedgenet-2021-107820

3. Oliver G, Srinivasan RS. Lymphatic vasculature development: current concepts. *Ann N Y Acad Sci*. 2008; 1131:75–81. DOI: https://doi.org/10.1196/annals.1413.006
4. Levick JR, Michel CC. Microvascular fluid exchange and the revised Starling principle. *Cardiovasc Res*. 2010 Jul 15;87(2):198–210. DOI: https://doi.org/10.1093/cvr/cvq062
5. Pflicke H, Sixt M. Preformed portals facilitate dendritic cell entry into afferent lymphatic vessels. *J Exp Med*. 2009 Dec 21;206(13):2925–35. DOI: https://doi.org/10.1084/jem.20091739
6. Bridenbaugh EA, Gashev AA, Zawieja DC. Lymphatic muscle: a review of contractile function. *Lymphat Res Biol*. 2003 Apr;1(2):147–58. DOI: https://doi.org/10.1089/153968503321642633
7. Teijeira A, Russo E, Halin C. Taking the lymphatic route: dendritic cell migration to draining lymph nodes. *Semin Immunopathol*. 2014 Mar 1;36(2):261–74. DOI: https://doi.org/10.1007/s00281-013-0410-8
8. Dupuy A, Benchikhi H, Roujeau JC, Bernard P, Vaillant L, Chosidow O, et al. Risk factors for erysipelas of the leg (cellulitis): case-control study. *BMJ*. 1999 Jun 12;318(7198):1591–4. DOI: https://doi.org/10.1136/bmj.318.7198.1591
9. Martin-Almedina S, Mortimer PS, Ostergaard P. Development and physiological functions of the lymphatic system: insights from human genetic studies of primary lymphedema. *Physiol Rev*. 2021 Oct;101(4):1809–71. DOI: https://doi.org/10.1152/physrev.00006.2020
10. Mortimer PS. Managing lymphoedema. *Clin Exp Dermatol*. 1995 Mar;20(2):98–106. DOI: https://doi.org/10.1111/j.1365-2230.1995.tb02665.x
11. Stemmer R. [A clinical symptom for the early and differential diagnosis of lymphedema]. *VASA Z Gefasskrankheiten*. 1976 Jan 1;5(3):261–2. Available from: https://pubmed.ncbi.nlm.nih.gov/969857/
12. Connell F, Gordon K, Brice G, Keeley V, Jeffery S, Mortimer P, et al. The classification and diagnostic algorithm for primary lymphatic dysplasia: an update from 2010 to include molecular findings. *Clin Genet*. 2013;84(4):303–14. DOI: https://doi.org/10.1111/cge.12173
13. Gordon K, Varney R, Keeley V, Riches K, Jeffery S, Van Zanten M, et al. Update and audit of the St George's classification algorithm of primary lymphatic anomalies: a clinical and molecular approach to diagnosis. *J Med Genet*. 2020 Oct;57(10):653–9. DOI: https://doi.org/10.1136/jmedgenet-2019-106084
14. Executive Committee of the International Society of Lymphology. The diagnosis and treatment of peripheral lymphedema: 2020 consensus document of the International Society of Lymphology. *Lymphology*. 2020;53(1):3–19. DOI: https://doi.org/10.2458/lymph.4649
15. Allen EV. Lymphedema of the extremities: classification, etiology, and differential diagnosis: a study of 300 cases. *Arch Intern Med*. 1934 Oct 1;54(4):606–24. DOI: https://doi.org/10.1001/archinte.1934.00160160125008
16. Kinmonth JB, Taylor GW, Tracy GD, Marsh JD. Primary lymphœdema. Clinical and lymphangiographic studies of a series of 107 patients in which the lower limbs were affected. *Br J Surg*. 1957 Jul 1;45(189):1–10. DOI: https://doi.org/10.1002/bjs.18004518902
17. Connell F, Brice G, Jeffery S, Keeley V, Mortimer P, Mansour S. A new classification system for primary lymphatic dysplasias based on phenotype. *Clin Genet*. 2010;77(5):438–52. DOI: https://doi.org/10.1111/j.1399-0004.2010.01394.x
18. Ricci KW, Hammill AM, Mobberley-Schuman P, Nelson SC, Blatt J, Bender JLG, et al. Efficacy of systemic sirolimus in the treatment of generalized lymphatic anomaly and Gorham–Stout disease. *Pediatr Blood Cancer*. 2019;66(5):e27614. DOI: https://doi.org/10.1002/pbc.27614
19. Gordon K, Moore M, Van Zanten M, Pearce J, Itkin M, Madden B, et al. Case report: progressive central conducting lymphatic abnormalities in the RASopathies. Two case reports, including successful treatment by MEK inhibition. *Front Genet*. 2022 Sep 27;13. Available from: https://www.frontiersin.org/journals/genetics/articles/10.3389/fgene.2022.1001105/full
20. Torales LDG, Sempowski BA, Krikorian GL, Woodis KM, Paulissen SM, Smith CL, et al. Central conducting lymphatic anomaly: from

bench to bedside. *J Clin Invest*. 2024 Apr 15;134(8). Available from: https://www.jci.org/articles/view/172839

21. de Almeida AB, Freedman DO. Epidemiology and immunopathology of bancroftian filariasis. *Microbes Infect*. 1999 Oct 1;1(12):1015–22. DOI: https://doi.org/10.1016/S1286-4579(99)80519-X
22. Sakorafas GH, Peros G, Cataliotti L, Vlastos G. Lymphedema following axillary lymph node dissection for breast cancer. *Surg Oncol*. 2006 Nov 1;15(3):153–65. DOI: https://doi.org/10.1016/j.suronc.2006.11.003
23. DiSipio T, Rye S, Newman B, Hayes S. Incidence of unilateral arm lymphoedema after breast cancer: a systematic review and meta-analysis. *Lancet Oncol*. 2013 May;14(6):500–15. DOI: https://doi.org/10.1016/S1470-2045(13)70076-7
24. Lin Y, Xu Y, Wang C, Song Y, Huang X, Zhang X, et al. Loco-regional therapy and the risk of breast cancer-related lymphedema: a systematic review and meta-analysis. *Breast Cancer*. 2021 Nov 1;28(6):1261–72. DOI: https://doi.org/10.1007/s12282-021-01263-8
25. Finegold DN, Baty CJ, Knickelbein KZ, Perschke S, Noon SE, Campbell D, et al. Connexin 47 mutations increase risk for secondary lymphedema following breast cancer treatment. *Clin Cancer Res*. 2012 Apr 16;18(8):2382–90. DOI: https://doi.org/10.1158/1078-0432.CCR-11-2303
26. Nagai Y, Aoyama K, Endo Y, Ishikawa O. Lymphedema of the extremities developed as the initial manifestation of rheumatoid arthritis. *Eur J Dermatol EJD*. 2007;17(2):175–6. Available from: https://www.jle.com/en/revues/ejd/e-docs/lymphedema_of_the_extremities_developed_as_the_initial_manifestation_of_rheumatoid_arthritis_273513/article.phtml
27. Russell PS, Hong J, Trevaskis NL, Windsor JA, Martin ND, Phillips ARJ. Lymphatic contractile function: a comprehensive review of drug effects and potential clinical application. *Cardiovasc Res*. 2022 Jul 1;118(11):2437–57. DOI: https://doi.org/10.1093/cvr/cvab279
28. Damstra RJ, Partsch H. Prospective, randomized, controlled trial comparing the effectiveness of adjustable compression Velcro wraps versus inelastic multicomponent compression bandages in the initial treatment of leg lymphedema. *J Vasc Surg Venous Lymphat Disord*. 2013 Jan 1;1(1):13–9. DOI: https://doi.org/10.1016/j.jvsv.2012.05.001
29. Williams A f., Vadgama A, Franks P j., Mortimer P s. A randomized controlled crossover study of manual lymphatic drainage therapy in women with breast cancer-related lymphoedema. *Eur J Cancer Care (Engl)*. 2002;11(4):254–61. DOI: https://doi.org/10.1046/j.1365-2354.2002.00312.x
30. Woods M. The experience of manual lymph drainage as an aspect of treatment for lymphoedema. *Int J Palliat Nurs*. 2003 Aug;9(8):336–42; discussion 342. DOI: https://doi.org/10.12968/ijpn.2003.9.8.11524
31. McNeely ML, Magee DJ, Lees AW, Bagnall KM, Haykowsky M, Hanson J. The addition of manual lymph drainage to compression therapy for breast cancer related lymphedema: a randomized controlled trial. *Breast Cancer Res Treat*. 2004 Jul 1;86(2):95–106. DOI: https://doi.org/10.1023/B:BREA.0000032978.67677.9f
32. Thomas KS, Crook AM, Nunn AJ, Foster KA, Mason JM, Chalmers JR, et al. Penicillin to prevent recurrent leg cellulitis. N Engl J Med. 2013 May 2;368(18):1695–703. DOI: https://doi.org/10.1056/NEJMoa1206300
33. Dumanian GA, Futrell WJ. The Charles procedure: misquoted and misunderstood since 1950. *Plast Reconstr Surg*. 1996 Dec;98(7):1258. Available from: https://journals.lww.com/plasreconsurg/abstract/1996/12000/the_charles_procedure__misquoted_and_misunderstood.22.aspx
34. Nielubowicz J, Olszewski W. Surgical lymphaticovenous shunts in patients with secondary lymphoedema. *Br J Surg*. 1968 Jun 1;55(6):440–2. DOI: https://doi.org/10.1002/bjs.1800550609
35. Campisi C, Bellini C, Campisi C, Accogli S, Bonioli E, Boccardo F. Microsurgery for lymphedema: Clinical research and long-term results. *Microsurgery*. 2010;30(4):256–60. DOI: https://doi.org/10.1002/micr.20737
36. Damstra RJ, Voesten HGJ, van Schelven WD, van der Lei B. Lymphatic venous anastomosis (LVA) for treatment of secondary arm lymphedema. A prospective study of 11 LVA procedures in 10 patients with breast cancer related lymphedema and a critical review of the literature. *Breast Cancer Res Treat*. 2009 Jan 1;113(2):199–206.

DOI: https://doi.org/10.1007/s10549-008-9932-5
37. Forte AJ, Khan N, Huayllani MT, Boczar D, Saleem HY, Lu X, et al. Lymphaticovenous anastomosis for lower extremity lymphedema: a systematic review. *Indian J Plast Surg Off Publ Assoc Plast Surg India*. 2020 Mar;53(1):17–24. DOI: https://doi.org/10.1055/s-0040-1709372
38. Becker C, Assouad J, Riquet M, Hidden G. Postmastectomy lymphedema: long-term results following microsurgical lymph node transplantation. *Ann Surg*. 2006 Mar;243(3):313. DOI: https://doi.org/10.1097/01.sla.0000201258.10304.16
39. Zampell JC, Aschen S, Weitman ES, Yan A, Elhadad S, De Brot Andrade M, et al. Regulation of adipogenesis by lymphatic fluid stasis Part I: adipogenesis, fibrosis, and inflammation. *Plast Reconstr Surg*. 2012 Apr;129(4):825–34. DOI: https://doi.org/10.1097/PRS.0b013e3182450b2d
40. Warren AG, Brorson H, Borud LJ, Slavin SA. Lymphedema: a comprehensive review. *Ann Plast Surg*. 2007 Oct;59(4):464. DOI: https://doi.org/10.1097/01.sap.0000257149.42922.7e
41. Schaverien MV, Munnoch DA, Brorson H. Liposuction treatment of lymphedema. *Semin Plast Surg*. 2018 Feb;32(1):42–7. DOI: https://doi.org/10.1055/s-0038-1635116
42. Brorson H. From lymph to fat: complete reduction of lymphoedema. *Phlebology*. 2010 Oct 1;25(1_suppl):52–63. DOI: https://doi.org/10.1258/phleb.2010.010s08

Chapter Seven
Obesity

Rachel Huynh and Tracey McLaughlin

Introduction

Meg is a 52-year-old woman with a history of hypertension and prediabetes. She sits in your clinic, expressing frustration over her increasing belly size, persistent fatigue, low mood, and episodes of emotional eating. Her weight gain over the past several years has made it difficult for her to keep up with her kindergarten students, and she avoids plane travel due to shame about her large size. She shows you a photo of herself as a fit and active college cheerleader and says quietly, 'I would do anything to feel like that again'. Her story echoes that of countless patients who struggle not only with the physical health impacts of obesity but also with the emotional toll, societal judgment, and internalized stigma that accompany the disease.

This chapter focuses on the medical aspects of obesity. It addresses health risks and outlines current approaches to diagnosis and treatment. Meg's story reminds us that obesity is not a failure of willpower. It is a complex, chronic disease. Many factors contribute to it, including biology, psychology, environment, and social context. As clinicians, centering the lived experience of individuals with obesity helps challenge stigma, guide more compassionate care, and support more effective long-term management.

Epidemiology and prevalence of obesity

Obesity is present in one in eight adults worldwide.[1, 2] In the United States, 32.7% of adults are overweight and 40.4% have obesity, together affecting almost three-quarters of the adult population.[3] Childhood obesity is on the rise globally, with over 400 million children and adolescents affected by overweight or obesity (160 million with obesity).[4] The highest obesity prevalence is observed in the United States, Saudi Arabia, and several Pacific Island nations, while the most rapid increases are occurring in low- and middle-income countries, particularly in parts of southeast Asia, the Middle East, and sub-Saharan Africa.[5]

Obesity is a major driver of chronic disease and disability, contributing to over 4 million deaths per year worldwide, primarily from cardiovascular disease (CVD), type 2 diabetes mellitus (T2DM), and cancer.[6] In the US alone, the estimated annual medical cost of obesity exceeds $170 billion, and obesity is associated with over $1,800 in excess annual medical costs per person, placing a significant burden on the healthcare system and on individuals.[7] These realities underscore the urgency of advancing not only effective prevention and treatment strategies but also a deeper understanding of obesity's underlying biology, social determinants, and lived experience.

Classification and diagnosis of obesity

Obesity is defined by the World Health Organization (WHO)[1] as 'excess or abnormal fat accumulation that presents a risk to health,' and by the Centers for Disease Control and Prevention (CDC)[3] as 'weight that is higher than what is considered healthy for a given height.' Body mass index (BMI) remains the most widely used metric for classifying weight status and assessing obesity. It is imperfect because it does not measure body fat directly, nor does it provide information on body fat distribution, and it varies by age, sex, race, and ethnicity. Despite these limitations, BMI is a simple, inexpensive, and highly standardized tool, and thus is the recommended screening tool for overweight and obesity. It is calculated by dividing a person's weight in kilograms by the square of their height in meters (kg/m^2) and is categorized as shown in Table 7.1.

Table 7.1: Classification by BMI ranges by non-Asian and Asian race.

Classification by BMI	Non-Asian	Asian
Normal weight	18.5–24.9 kg/m^2	18.5–22.9 kg/m^2
Overweight	25.0–29.9 kg/m^2	23.0–24.9 kg/m^2
Obesity Class I	30.0–34.9 kg/m^2	25.0–29.9 kg/m^2
Obesity Class II	35.0–39.9 kg/m^2	≥30.0–34.9 kg/m^2
Obesity Class III	≥40.0 kg/m^2	≥35.0 kg/m^2

These cutoffs underestimate risks of metabolic disease, including diabetes, associated with excess body weight in the Asian population.[8, 9] Thus, the recommended BMI classifications adopted by the National Institutes of Health (NIH) and WHO for Asian individuals define overweight as a BMI of ≥23 to 24.9 kg/m^2 and obesity as a BMI of ≥25 kg/m^2.

Another measure of total adiposity is body fat percentage, which is typically measured by dual-energy X-ray absorptiometry (DXA) scan or bioelectrical impedance analysis (BIA). Of these two, DXA is more accurate but is costly and entails a low dose of radiation exposure, so it is not routinely used at this time to quantify adiposity. For patients with high muscle mass, such as athletes or bodybuilders, in whom BMI is likely to overestimate adiposity, DXA can be used. Similarly, metabolic risk related to excess adiposity could be underestimated in individuals with low muscle mass who might also benefit from DXA, but this is not routinely being done. Healthy body fat differs by sex and age, as shown in Table 7.2.

Table 7.2: Healthy per cent body fat ranges by sex and age.

Age	Women	Men
20–39 years	21–32%	8–19%
40–59 years	23–33%	11–21%
60–79 years	24–35%	13–24%

Central adiposity predicts T2DM, CVD, and mortality independent of BMI.[10, 11] Visceral adipose tissue (VAT), a type of central fat stored deep in the abdominal cavity around internal organs, particularly, may increase the risk of these adverse clinical outcomes.[12, 13] However, because it requires advanced imaging tools such as DXA, computed tomography, or magnetic resonance imaging, visceral fat mass is not readily measured. Clinicians often use waist circumference (WC) or waist-to-hip ratio (WtHR) as estimates that can, in part, capture visceral adiposity.

Independent of BMI, many studies have shown that WC or WtHR measurements predict diabetes, CVD, and total mortality. Thus, clinicians and researchers can incorporate WC or WtHR into routine assessments as shown in Table 7.3. These assessments are inexpensive and do not entail risk but are harder to perform in a standardized manner since measurement is influenced by the location of the tape measure and the patient's arm position. According to guidelines from The Obesity Society, the American Heart Association, and the American College of Cardiology, standard cutoff values for WC and WtHR are used to assess cardiometabolic risk. However, for Asian populations, the International Diabetes Federation (IDF) recommends lower thresholds (see Table 7.3) due to differences in body composition and a higher risk of metabolic complications at lower levels of adiposity.[14, 15]

Table 7.3: Healthy waist circumference and waist-to-hip ratio by sex and non-Asian or Asian race.

Sex/race	WC	WtHR
Men (non-Asian)	≥102 cm (40 in)	≥0.90
Women (non-Asian)	≥88 cm (35 in)	≥0.85
Men (Asian)	≥90 cm (35.5 in)	≥0.90
Women (Asian)	≥80 cm (31.5 in)	≥0.85

WC = waist circumference, WtHR = waist-to-hip ratio.

Etiology of obesity and determinants of fat distribution

Obesity is a multifactorial disease resulting from the complex interplay of behavioral, environmental, genetic, hormonal, and social influences. This section explores key contributors to the development of obesity, including genetic predisposition, racial and ethnic variations, and sex-based differences in fat distribution. Additional factors such as endocrine diseases, medication effects, lifestyle behaviors, environmental exposures, and broader social and structural determinants of health are also examined to provide a comprehensive understanding of obesity's etiology.

Genetic determinants

In a small subset of individuals, rare, highly penetrant genetic defects, such as pathogenic variants in the leptin–melanocortin pathway (e.g. *MC4R, LEP, LEPR, POMC*) or syndromic imprinting diseases like Prader-Willi syndrome, can cause severe, early-onset hyperphagic obesity.[16, 17, 18] These monogenic or syndromic forms are typically driven by high-impact loss-of-function mutations that severely disrupt appetite regulation and energy balance.

In contrast, most obesity cases involve polygenic influences, where common genetic variants, typically single-nucleotide polymorphisms (SNPs), in the same or related genes modestly increase obesity risk. Genome-wide association studies (GWAS) have identified hundreds of loci associated with BMI, many of which affect appetite regulation, energy homeostasis, and adipocyte biology.[19, 20, 21]

While genetics accounts for up to 50% of obesity risk, it plays an even more important role in governing fat distribution, as shown in multiple GWAS studies.[13, 22, 23, 24, 25] Routine genetic testing is not recommended for adults with obesity and is generally reserved for children and adolescents with hyperphagia and features suggesting an obesity syndrome, such as intellectual disability, delayed growth or puberty, and specific physical stigmata.

Race and ethnicity

In considering race, while there may be biological differences in adipose tissue and the propensity for metabolic diseases, we must also remember that race may also serve as a proxy for lived experiences of racism, healthcare access, and socioeconomic disadvantage – factors that can significantly influence the risk of obesity.

Notably, obesity prevalence in the US shows marked racial and ethnic disparities. Non-Hispanic Black (NHB) adults have the highest rates,[26, 27] followed by Hispanic adults,[26, 28] American Indian/Alaska Native (AI/AN) adults,[28, 29] non-Hispanic White (NHW) adults.[26, 28] Non-Hispanic Asian (NHA) adults have the lowest rates using the standard BMI ≥30 kg/m^2, though prevalence rises when using the lower BMI cutoff of ≥27.5 kg/m^2.[30] These data underscore persistent disparities, particularly among women and communities of color.

Such disparities may be simplistically attributed to race/ethnicity, but complex social and structural determinants must be considered as well. Access to affordable, healthy food and safe environments for physical activity is often limited in low-income or inner-city neighborhoods, where high crime rates, lack of green space, and financial barriers to gym memberships pose significant challenges.[31, 32, 33] In addition, cultural norms, including dietary traditions and attitudes toward exercise and body size, affect behaviors around food and physical activity.[34, 35, 36, 37, 38] Access to safe places to exercise, healthy food, and dependence on technology significantly influence obesity rates. Neighborhoods with limited access to recreational facilities and healthy food options are associated with higher obesity rates.[39, 40]

Race and ethnicity intersect with global geography. Obesity rates exceed 40% in countries such as the United States, Saudi Arabia, and several Pacific Island nations, whereas rates remain relatively lower in Japan and South Korea despite increasing westernization. These differences reflect that while genetic predisposition plays a role, the built environment, food availability, and cultural practices are critical determinants of obesity prevalence across different regions.[5, 41]

Hispanic individuals demonstrate higher VAT accumulation and significantly greater prevalence[42] of metabolic dysfunction-associated steatotic liver disease (MASLD), compared to NHB individuals, even at equivalent BMI levels.[43, 44] Body fat distribution patterns differ substantially by ancestry. Individuals of East Asian, South Asian, and Latino descent tend to have greater central and VAT accumulation relative to total body fat, as compared to White individuals at the same BMI, thus placing them at elevated risk for insulin resistance, MASLD, and CVD.[28, 44] Asian populations exhibit higher levels of VAT and increased cardiometabolic risk starting at lower BMI, prompting the adoption of lower BMI cutoffs for assessing health risk in these groups.[28, 45]

Metabolic syndrome affects approximately 50–55% of AI/AN adults, well above the 34.7% seen in the general US population.[46] This elevated burden is accompanied by disproportionately high rates of obesity (affecting nearly half of AI/AN adults), diabetes (about three times higher than in NHW populations), and CVD, which is the leading cause of death.[28, 47] In AI/AN populations, CVD develops earlier and leads to higher death rates, especially in younger adults.[46, 48, 49]

Sex determinants

Sex influences nearly every aspect of body fat. Total amount, regional distribution, adipose cell function, and the relationship to metabolic outcomes differ by sex. The prevalence of obesity is higher in women than in men globally (18.5% vs. 14%).[5] In the US, 40.3% of adults have obesity (BMI ≥30), with no significant difference between men and women; however, among those with severe obesity (BMI ≥40), which affects 9.4% of US adults, prevalence is notably higher in women

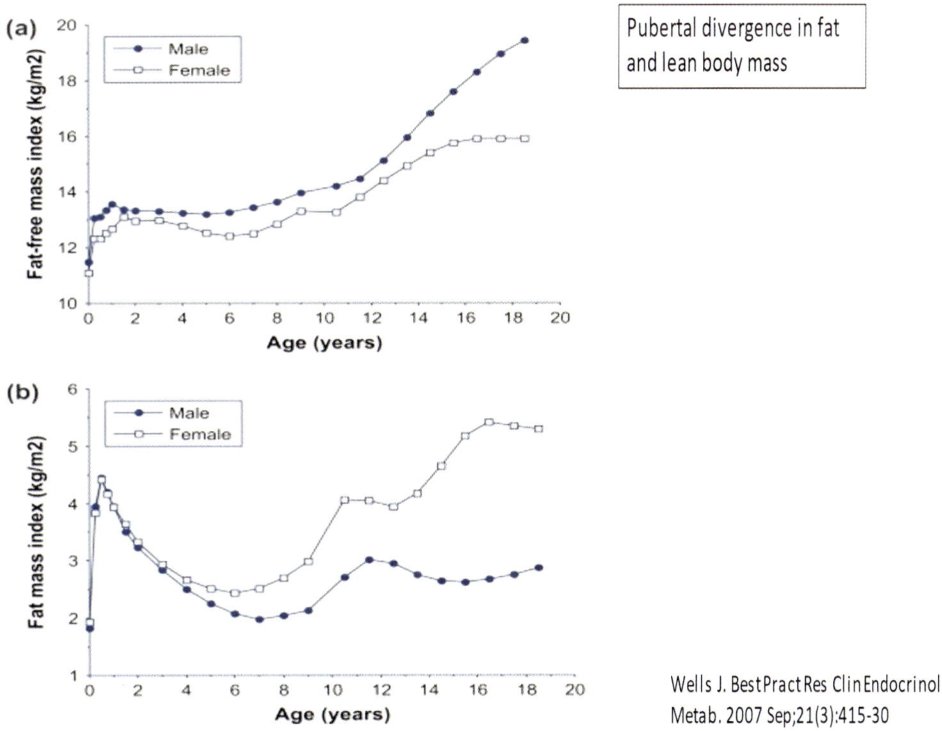

Figure 7.1: Pubertal divergence of lean and fat body mass by sex showing (a) males have higher lean mass (fat-free mass index) after puberty, with relatively lower fat mass; (b) females have higher fat mass after puberty, with relatively lower fat-free mass. Taken together, these graphs represent pubertal sexual dimorphism in body composition, with boys showing greater gains in lean mass and girls showing greater gains in fat mass. Courtesy of Dr. McLaughlin's Lab.

(11.1%) than in men (6.5%) during the 2021–2023 period.[50, 51]

Compared to males, females have a higher percentage of body fat, which begins at puberty (Figure 7.1) and persists through the lifespan, whereas males have a higher percentage of lean mass.[52] Women accumulate relatively more subcutaneous fat, whereas men accumulate more visceral fat, starting in puberty (Figure 7.2).[53, 54] Furthermore, women are more likely to exhibit a gynoid (lower body, or gluteofemoral) fat distribution, whereas males are more likely to exhibit an android (upper body, or central) fat distribution.[55, 56]

After menopause, this sex difference in fat distribution diminishes or reverses. Women experience a shift toward central adiposity, characterized by increased visceral and trunk fat, reduced leg fat, and a higher trunk-to-leg fat ratio compared to premenopausal women.[57, 58] These sex-based differences are also reflected at the cellular and molecular level. Although the mechanisms that govern the size and function of adipose depots and adipocytes remain incompletely understood and are sometimes conflicting, several consistent findings have emerged:

1. Women have larger fat cells in the gluteofemoral region.[57] This may be due to

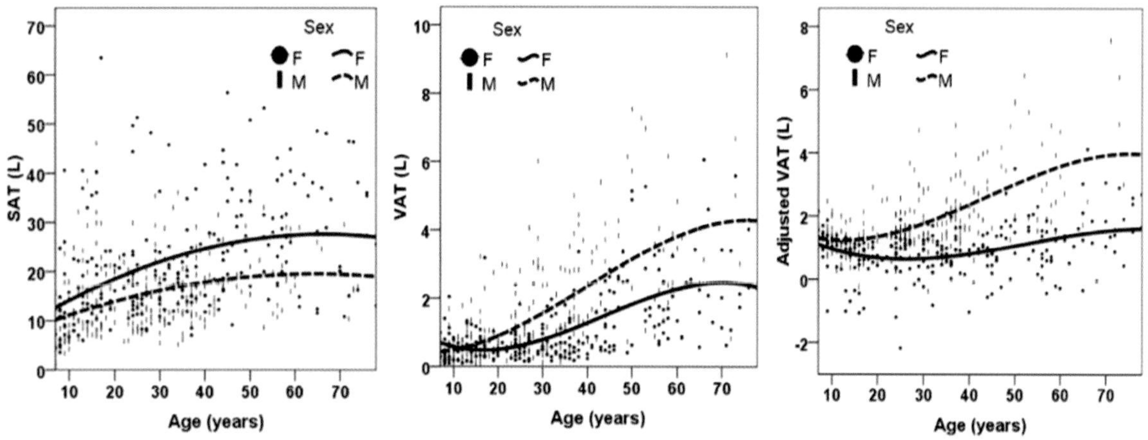

Figure 7.2: Sexual dimorphism of adipose tissue distribution across the lifespan: on the left, total body subcutaneous (SAT); on the right visceral (VAT). Volume in liters (L). Courtesy of Dr. McLaughlin's Lab.

differences in lipoprotein lipase, which allows circulating fat to enter fat cells in adipose tissue, and/or to enzymes such as diglyceride acyltransferase that promote fat storage in the fat cells by allowing free fatty acids to bind glycerol and form a lipid droplet.[58]

2. Women demonstrate greater insulin-mediated glucose uptake in adipose tissue.[59]
3. Insulin suppresses lipolysis more effectively in women, meaning fat breakdown is more inhibited.[60]

Traditionally, larger fat cells have been associated with inflammation, insulin resistance, and T2DM. However, this association may not hold true in females. In mouse models, females fed a high-fat diet show less inflammation than males.[61] In humans, for any given degree of adiposity, women tend to have lower plasma glucose, triglycerides, and blood pressure, further supporting the notion that female adipose tissue may confer protection against metabolic dysregulation.[57] Together, these findings support the idea of sexual dimorphism in the capacity for adipose cell expansion. Specifically, findings demonstrate that women may be able to accommodate adipose cell enlargement to a greater extent before triggering pathological processes such as inflammation, ectopic and visceral fat accumulation, and metabolic disease. This may help explain observed associations between female sex and a more protective fat distribution pattern, characterized by greater gluteofemoral fat and a higher proportion of subcutaneous fat relative to visceral fat.

These sex-specific differences, while not fully understood, are shaped by both chromosomal (XX vs. XY) and hormonal influences.[62, 63, 64] Sex steroids play a key role in fat distribution, with evidence indicating that estrogen promotes fat storage in the lower body (glutofemoral region) primarily in premenopausal women.[53, 54] Women experience hormonal transitions during pregnancy, perimenopause, and menopause, which contribute to changes in body fat distribution.[65] Indeed, pregnancy is associated with subcutaneous fat gain due to elevated estrogen and progesterone.[66] In contrast, the decline in estrogen during perimenopause and menopause promotes visceral fat accumulation. This shift may help explain why the risk of CVD increases ten years later in women than in men, rising primarily in the postmenopausal period.[65, 67]

Men, on the other hand, tend to have more visceral fat throughout life due to their android pattern of fat distribution, which may partly explain why they develop T2DM and CVD at an earlier age than women.[68, 69, 70] Further evidence for the role of sex steroids in regulating fat distribution and function comes from studies in transgender individuals: male-to-female patients (trans women) treated with estrogen exhibit an increased fat-to-lean mass ratio and decreased visceral-to-subcutaneous fat ratio, while female-to-male patients (trans men) on testosterone may experience greater VAT accumulation.[71]

Environmental and behavioral contributors

Lifestyle factors contribute significantly to overweight and obesity. Food quantity and quality, physical inactivity, sleep disturbances, and chronic stress interact with genetic predisposition to influence adiposity and metabolic risk.[72, 73, 74] Diet is a primary driver in obesity and is discussed in detail in Chapter 14 of this text. Regular physical activity supports weight management by increasing energy expenditure, preserving lean body mass, and improving insulin sensitivity and cardiovascular health. Aerobic and resistance training are both beneficial: aerobic exercise enhances glucose uptake and lipid metabolism, while resistance training maintains muscle mass and improves insulin sensitivity. [75, 76, 77, 78] The American College of Sports Medicine recommends at least 150 minutes of moderate aerobic activity per week, with greater benefits seen at 200–300 minutes, especially for reducing visceral fat and improving cardiometabolic health.[78]

Other contributors to obesity include eating disorders. Binge eating disorder and night eating syndrome are recognized psycho-behavioral contributors that exacerbate weight gain and complicate management.[79] One study found that over one-third of individuals with overweight and obesity are affected by binge eating disorder, carbohydrate addiction, or both, underscoring the need for routine screening and integrated treatment approaches in patients with obesity.[80] Weight cycling, or repeated episodes of weight loss and regain, is often driven by restrictive dieting and unrealistic goals, and is particularly common among individuals with binge eating disorder and night eating syndrome. Studies have shown that weight cycling is associated with binge eating behaviors, psychological distress, and worsened weight outcomes in individuals with obesity. [81, 82, 83]

Endocrine and iatrogenic contributors

When evaluating patients with obesity or atypical fat distribution, it's essential to consider secondary causes such as endocrine diseases (e.g. hypothyroidism, Cushing's syndrome) and iatrogenic factors (e.g. corticosteroids, hormone therapies, beta-blockers).[84] These diseases can promote weight gain and/or altered fat distribution. Clinical stigmata such as rounded or 'moon' face, purple/pink striae on the skin, and muscle weakness can point to underlying Cushing's syndrome, while dry skin, low energy, and constipation might indicate underlying hypothyroidism, and darkening of the skin around the back and sides of the neck often indicate insulin resistance and polycystic ovary syndrome. Evaluation should be pursued with a physician. Additionally, exposure to endocrine-disrupting chemicals such as bisphenol A (BPA) and phthalates may exacerbate obesity by altering hormonal signaling, inducing chronic inflammation in adipose tissue, and promoting adipogenesis.[85, 86]

Social and structural determinants of health

Social determinants of health, including socioeconomic status, access to healthcare, education, and neighborhood environment, play a crucial role in obesity risk and management. Limited access to healthy foods, safe spaces for physical activity, and healthcare resources can contribute to weight gain and hinder effective treatment. In the context of lipedema, although the disease itself is primarily genetic and hormonal, coexisting overweight/obesity, which exists in 3 out of 4 patients with lipedema,[87] and limited healthcare access can delay diagnosis, reduce quality of life, and complicate management. These barriers can lead to worsened symptoms and reduced quality of life, highlighting the importance of addressing social and structural factors alongside medical care.

Obesity and metabolic disease

Not all overweight/obese individuals are at equal risk for metabolic complications of obesity. Indeed, metabolically healthy and unhealthy subgroups have been well described.[88, 89, 90, 91] At the center of this distinction is insulin resistance.[92] Insulin resistance generally refers to resistance to insulin-mediated glucose uptake (IMGU) into cells in the body, where glucose is stored or metabolized to fuel cellular metabolism. Despite the fact that 80–90% of total-body IMGU occurs in skeletal muscle,[93, 94, 95] it has long been noted that IMGU correlates more highly with fat mass than with muscle mass.[96] Clearly, it is related to excess body weight: the higher the body weight, the higher the risk of having insulin resistance.

However, there is quite a bit of heterogeneity, and thus not all obese people are insulin resistant, and not all normal body weight individuals are insulin sensitive.[12, 97, 98, 99] IMGU varies sixfold among normoglycemic individuals of the same body weight.[100] Furthermore, when followed prospectively for up to 14 years, the most insulin-resistant subgroup of weight-matched individuals demonstrates an eightfold increased incidence of diabetes/impaired glucose tolerance, a fourfold increased incidence of CVD, and a twofold increased risk of hypertension.[98, 101, 102] When otherwise healthy obese individuals are stratified according to the degree of insulin resistance, marked differences in metabolic and cardiovascular risk factors are apparent, with the insulin-resistant subgroup exhibiting significantly higher blood pressure, higher fasting plasma triglyceride and lower HDL cholesterol concentrations, elevations in fasting and 2-hour plasma glucose, as well as circulating markers of inflammation and vascular dysfunction.[97, 103]

Despite the heterogeneity in metabolic risk factors described above, it is clear that in susceptible individuals, insulin resistance is responsive to weight loss, whether dietary, medical, or surgical. The clearest example of this is the observation that when insulin-resistant and insulin-sensitive individuals lose an equal amount of body weight via dietary intervention, it is the insulin-resistant, but not the insulin-sensitive, subgroup that experiences statistically significant improvements in insulin sensitivity, as well as in biomarkers of CVD risk such as plasma triglycerides, hsCRP, and ADMA.[103, 104, 105] Thus, those individuals who develop insulin resistance as a result of weight gain can also reverse it with weight loss,[104, 106, 107] whereas insulin-sensitive people appear largely impervious to developing these metabolic changes in response to increased body fat.[97, 99, 108] This important observation implies that (1) factors other than fat mass *per se* are important in determining insulin resistance and associated metabolic consequences of obesity, and that (2) the insulin-resistant subgroup of overweight/obese individuals should be targeted for intensive weight-loss interventions given their higher risk profile and documented metabolic improvements in response to weight loss.

Regional fat distribution and metabolic disease

The relationship between body fat distribution and metabolic disease was first published in the 1950s. It was noted that an android versus a gynoid distribution of fat was associated with diabetes, atherosclerotic CVD, and gout, all of which are related to insulin resistance.[109, 110] Since that time, numerous studies have confirmed that upper-body or truncal fat distribution is associated with a greater risk for these diseases than lower-body fat or peripheral fat distribution.[111, 112, 113]

Perhaps more important is VAT: this fat, which represents only 5–15% of total body fat, surrounds organs like the intestine, heart, pancreas, kidney, and others. It has different cellular and molecular characteristics and is speculated to have different biological functions than subcutaneous fat, the primary function of which is to store and mobilize energy. Even after adjusting for BMI and waist circumference, VAT is independently associated with insulin resistance[114, 115] and adverse cardiometabolic outcomes, including diabetes, hypertension, and metabolic syndrome.[13, 115, 116]

How does VAT contribute to these metabolic consequences? One theory is called the portal hypothesis. This theory contends that free fatty acids released from fat cells in VAT drain directly into the portal vein, where they are delivered to the liver, where they cause hepatic steatosis and liver insulin resistance, which leads to elevated fasting glucose. These changes contribute to the development of MASLD,[117] T2DM, and elevated hepatic production of VLDL-triglycerides.[118] Finally, VAT releases pro-inflammatory cytokines such as IL-6, which drain directly to the liver, where they augment hepatic secretion of hsCRP and impair liver metabolic function. Adiponectin, an anti-inflammatory and insulin-sensitizing adipokine primarily secreted by subcutaneous fat, is typically reduced in individuals with high visceral fat, further exacerbating metabolic disturbances.[119] Visceral fat drives hormonal and inflammatory disruptions that promote insulin resistance and dysregulated lipid metabolism. This metabolic dysfunction exacerbates adipose tissue health, fueling a vicious cycle of fat accumulation and chronic inflammation.[120]

Dysfunctional adipose tissue ('sick fat'): cellular and molecular mechanisms

When body fat mass expands, adipose cells must either increase in size (hypertrophy) or number (hyperplasia) (see Figure 7.3). Although it was once thought that adipocyte number did not increase after adolescence, there is now data showing that the adipose number in adult humans is not fixed.[121, 122, 123] The ability to make new fat cells, likely from a reservoir of dormant preadipocytes, is critically important in the setting of weight gain, because already-large adipocytes cannot enlarge indefinitely. As adipocytes enlarge beyond this capacity, they can outgrow their blood supply, leading to local hypoxia. This hypoxic environment triggers the release of hypoxia-inducible factors (e.g. HIF-1α), which stimulate the release of chemokines such

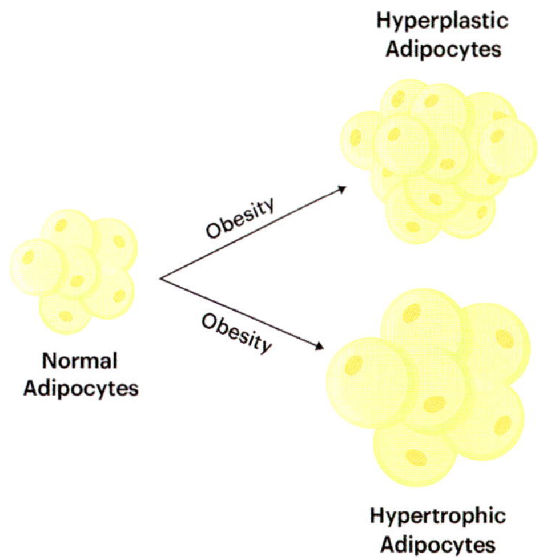

Figure 7.3: Adipocyte hyperplasia versus hypertrophy. Courtesy of Dr. McLaughlin's Lab.

as MCP-1, which attract macrophages into the adipose tissue.[124, 125] The infiltrating macrophages, along with dying adipocytes undergoing necrosis or apoptosis, create a state of chronic low-grade inflammation characterized by increased secretion of pro-inflammatory cytokines like TNF-α and IL-6.[126, 127] This process is similar to acute injury and wound healing, but in the case of obesity, it is chronic. Additionally, the continued inflammation leads to fibrosis, which makes the adipose tissue stiffer and less flexible. This stiffness restricts healthy expansion of adipose tissue, so fat cells cannot expand properly to store lipids effectively, and/or new fat cells cannot form properly. The increased mechanical stress and rigidity from extracellular matrix remodeling and fibrosis can thus impair their capacity to store fat and promote inflammation, further contributing to adipose tissue dysfunction[128, 129, 130] and systemic metabolic disturbances.[131]

Free fatty acids can spill over into surrounding tissue in a process termed 'lipotoxicity,' with deposition in non-adipose organs such as liver, muscle, and other organs, impairment of insulin action (insulin resistance), and stimulation of inflammatory pathways. Clinical consequences include visceral obesity, MASLD, and fatty heart (leading to heart failure), and fatty pancreas (contributing to beta-cell dysfunction and diabetes).[131,132] Other adverse effects of adipocyte hypertrophy include mitochondrial dysfunction and endoplasmic reticulum stress, both of which impair insulin signaling pathways and cause insulin resistance.[133, 134] These dysfunctions result from reduced fatty acid oxidation, decreased ATP production, increased reactive oxygen species (ROS), ROS-mediated signaling interference of insulin receptors, and a 'pseudohypoxic' state that promotes fibrosis and inflammation.[135, 136]

Clinical consequences and co-morbidities of obesity and dysfunctional adipose tissue

Obesity is a complex disease that touches nearly every part of the body, quietly shaping health in ways that often go unnoticed until complications arise. The excess fat that accumulates around the organs is not just stored energy; it is an active, disruptive organ, contributing to metabolic and organ dysfunction through ectopic lipid deposition in tissues such as the liver, muscle, and pancreas.

Metabolic consequences

Obesity is associated with a number of metabolic co-morbidities, most notably insulin resistance, prediabetes, and T2DM. These conditions emerge from complex interactions between excess nutrient intake, dysfunctional adipose tissue, and systemic inflammation.

Metabolic disease occurs via lipotoxicity as described above, with fat deposition in non-adipose tissues such as skeletal muscle, liver, heart, and pancreas, as well as expansion of visceral fat depots. Adipocyte hypertrophy with consequent adipocyte necrosis induces a state of chronic low-grade inflammation within adipose tissue, leading to adipocyte dysfunction and systemic insulin resistance. Fat deposition in non-adipose tissues also induces inflammation and cellular dysfunction.

Insulin resistance initially manifests as impaired glucose uptake in skeletal muscle, increased hepatic gluconeogenesis, and reduced suppression of lipolysis in adipose tissue. The pancreas compensates with increased insulin secretion (hyperinsulinemia), which can maintain normoglycemia for a time. However, as β-cell function declines under the stress of ongoing lipotoxicity, glucotoxicity, and inflammation, blood glucose levels begin to rise.

This transition from normoglycemia to hyperglycemia defines the spectrum from insulin resistance to prediabetes (characterized by impaired fasting glucose or impaired glucose tolerance), and ultimately to T2DM. T2DM is a chronic metabolic disease characterized by insulin resistance and progressive β-cell insufficiency, resulting in hyperglycemia. It is a progressive disease with wide-ranging microvascular and macrovascular complications, including retinopathy, nephropathy, neuropathy, CVD, and increased risk of infection. Importantly, insulin resistance is characterized by a cluster of abnormalities including atherogenic dyslipidemia (low HDL cholesterol, high triglycerides, and high small-dense LDL cholesterol), hypertension, impaired glucose tolerance, and a prothrombotic state that collectively define metabolic syndrome.[137, 138]

Consequences to the liver

These systemic metabolic disturbances extend their impact to the liver, where insulin resistance and ectopic fat deposition give rise to MASLD, the hepatic manifestation of metabolic syndrome. MASLD may be clinically silent in its early stages and is often incidentally discovered or remains undetected until advanced fibrosis or cirrhosis develops, underscoring the importance of early recognition and vigilant screening in at-risk individuals, particularly those with obesity, metabolic syndrome, or T2DM.[139]

Cardiovascular consequences

Obesity is strongly associated with hypertension, atherosclerotic CVD, heart failure, and stroke.[11, 140, 141, 142] Excess adiposity, particularly the pro-inflammatory VAT, contributes to heightened sympathetic nervous system activity, vascular endothelial dysfunction and atherogenesis, and systemic inflammation, which collectively elevate cardiovascular risk.[143] The progression from endothelial dysfunction to atherosclerotic CVD is a hallmark of obesity-related cardiometabolic risk. Chronic inflammation, dyslipidemia, and insulin resistance promote plaque formation and instability, increasing the risk of myocardial infarction, stroke, and peripheral artery disease.[11, 144] Obesity is also closely linked to heart failure, particularly heart failure with preserved ejection fraction. This is believed to result in part from fat infiltration into cardiomyocytes, promoting myocardial stiffness and diastolic dysfunction even in the setting of preserved systolic function.[11, 145] Insulin resistance and chronic low-grade inflammation further exacerbate cardiomyocyte changes in obesity-related heart failure by impairing endothelial function and promoting microvascular disease and cardiac remodeling.[145, 146, 147]

Consequences to fertility

Obesity significantly contributes to reproductive dysfunction, particularly in individuals assigned female at birth. It is strongly associated with polycystic ovary syndrome (PCOS), a disease marked by ovulatory dysfunction and hyperandrogenism.[148, 149, 150, 151] Excess adiposity contributes to hormonal imbalances by enhancing peripheral conversion of androgens to estrogen and disrupting hypothalamic-pituitary-ovarian axis signaling, leading to impaired ovulation, irregular menstruation, and reduced fertility.[152] Even outside of PCOS, obesity independently lowers fertility by affecting oocyte quality, endometrial receptivity, and pregnancy maintenance.[153, 154] Clinical evidence shows that a preconception weight loss of just 5–10% can improve ovulatory function and enhance fertility outcomes.[152, 155]

Respiratory system consequences

Obstructive sleep apnea is highly prevalent in patients with obesity and is linked to intermittent hypoxia, oxidative stress, and increased cardiovascular morbidity.[156, 157] Additionally, obesity-related mechanical restriction and inflammation can exacerbate asthma and other respiratory diseases, impairing pulmonary function and quality of life, and decreasing responsiveness to corticosteroid treatment.[158]

Musculoskeletal consequences

The increased mechanical load imposed by excess body weight accelerates degenerative joint disease, particularly osteoarthritis of weight-bearing joints such as the knees and hips, with obesity-related systemic inflammation further contributing to cartilage degradation. Additionally, the prevalence of gout is significantly associated with obesity and metabolic disturbances, which may contribute to hyperuricemia.[159, 160]

Management strategies targeting dysfunctional fat and metabolic risk

Effective management of dysfunctional adipose tissue and its metabolic consequences requires a multifaceted approach. This section outlines key intervention strategies, including lifestyle modifications, pharmacological therapies, and surgical options. Emphasis is also placed on the importance of compassionate, comprehensive counseling and appropriate referrals to support long-term weight management and overall health.

Lifestyle and weight loss

Lifestyle interventions remain foundational, with diet and exercise playing critical roles in reducing visceral fat. Evidence shows that lifestyle changes can significantly improve metabolic health even without large amounts of weight loss. A randomized controlled trial found that a 12-month lifestyle intervention reduced the prevalence of metabolic syndrome by 31%, lowered waist circumference, and decreased inflammatory markers such as hsCRP, despite weight loss of less than 5% of initial body weight.[161] Similarly, a meta-analysis of randomized controlled trials showed that lifestyle modification doubled the likelihood of metabolic syndrome resolution and significantly improved blood pressure, triglycerides, fasting glucose, and waist circumference over one year.[162] Additionally, getting enough sleep and engaging in regular physical activity have been linked to better metabolic profiles and healthier fat tissue function, even in people with higher BMI.[89, 163]

While lifestyle change without weight loss can improve metabolic health, achieving clinically meaningful weight loss (a sustained reduction of 5% or more of initial body weight) yields even stronger improvements in metabolic health and reduction of obesity-related complications. Losing 5–10% of initial body weight has been shown to improve glycemic control, blood pressure, lipid profiles, and inflammatory markers, thereby reducing the risk of T2DM, CVD, and other co-morbidities.[164] One study found that a 5% weight loss significantly improves insulin sensitivity in adipose tissue, liver, and muscle, as well as pancreatic beta cell function.[165] The same study found that greater weight loss (10–16%) leads to additional, dose-dependent metabolic benefits, including further improvements in muscle insulin sensitivity and beta cell function, reductions in intrahepatic fat, and favorable changes in adipose tissue biology, such as reduction of systemic inflammation and fibrosis, restoring healthier fat cell function, and favorable adipokine profiles. Larger weight loss of more than 10% is associated with remission of T2DM, improvement in sleep apnea, and reduction in MASLD severity.[166, 167, 168, 169] Overall, these findings underscore that while lifestyle changes alone are beneficial, achieving and maintaining clinically meaningful weight loss will produce powerful and lasting impacts on metabolic health and quality of life.

Medications for weight loss

Pharmacologic therapies such as glucagon-like peptide-1 (GLP-1) receptor agonists, dual agonists targeting GLP-1 and glucose-dependent insulinotropic polypeptide (GIP) receptors have become integral to managing obesity and metabolic dysfunction by reducing body weight, targeting visceral fat reduction, and improving insulin sensitivity.[170] GLP-1 receptor agonists, including liraglutide, dulaglutide, and semaglutide, have demonstrated not only significant weight loss but also the ability to modulate adipose tissue inflammation and promote healthier adipocyte function.[171, 172] They work by mimicking the incretin hormone GLP-1, enhancing glucose-dependent insulin secretion, delaying gastric emptying, and reducing appetite via central nervous system pathways.

Dual agonists like tirzepatide, which activate both GLP-1 and GIP receptors, have shown greater efficacy than GLP-1 receptor agonists alone in achieving weight loss and improving glycemic control[173, 174] They may also enhance adipose tissue remodeling and restore adipocyte function, promoting more effective lipid storage and reducing ectopic fat accumulation and inflammation in organs, such as the liver and skeletal muscle.[175, 176]

Semaglutide can lead to an average weight loss of approximately 15%, while tirzepatide can result in 20% or more body weight reduction.[174, 177] Common side effects include nausea, vomiting, diarrhea, and constipation, which are typically dose-dependent and may improve with time.[178, 179] Acute pancreatitis and gallbladder disease, including cholelithiasis and cholecystitis, are rare risks, but clinicians should counsel patients on these before prescribing.[180, 181, 182] Additionally, these agents carry a boxed warning and are contraindicated in patients with a personal or family history of medullary thyroid carcinoma or multiple endocrine neoplasia type 2, due to a theoretical risk of C-cell tumors seen in rodents, though not confirmed in humans.[183]

Several FDA-approved medications are available as adjuncts to lifestyle modification in patients with overweight or obesity. Orlistat, a gastrointestinal lipase inhibitor, works by reducing dietary fat absorption by approximately 30%, leading to an average weight loss of about 5–7%. Common side effects include oily stools, flatulence, and fecal urgency.[184, 185, 186] Phentermine/topiramate, a combination of a sympathomimetic and an anticonvulsant, enhances appetite suppression and satiety and is associated with 8–10% weight loss. Side effects may include paresthesia, insomnia, dry mouth, and constipation, and it is contraindicated in pregnancy due to teratogenicity.[185, 187, 188] Bupropion/naltrexone, which combines a dopamine-norepinephrine reuptake inhibitor and an opioid antagonist, targets appetite and food cravings, producing around 5–9% weight loss. However, it may cause nausea, headache, and insomnia, and is contraindicated in individuals with seizure diseases or uncontrolled hypertension.[185, 189, 190, 191]

Surgery for weight loss

For patients with severe obesity or refractory metabolic disease, bariatric surgery may be an effective intervention for achieving substantial and durable weight loss and metabolic improvement. Sleeve gastrectomy and Roux-en-Y gastric bypass (RYGB) are the most commonly performed procedures, with average total body weight loss of approximately 25% for sleeve gastrectomy and 30–35% for RYGB, though most studies report 20–30% for both procedures, with RYGB generally achieving slightly greater and more durable weight loss.[192, 193] These procedures lead to substantial and sustained weight loss, improvements in adipose tissue inflammation, and reversal of adipocyte fibrosis, which are critical for restoring adipose tissue function and improving insulin sensitivity.[194]

Long-term data from the Swedish Obese Subjects study demonstrate durable reductions in cardiovascular risk and mortality, as well as remission of T2DM, in bariatric surgery patients.[195, 196] However, there are limitations to surgery and the different surgical approaches. Post-operative weight gain is still possible and is more common with sleeve gastrectomy. Current clinical guidelines, including those from the American Gastroenterological Association, recommend the use of anti-obesity medications like GLP-1 receptor agonists as adjunctive therapy in patients who experience weight regain or an incomplete metabolic response after bariatric surgery.

Bariatric surgery is generally safe, but it does carry procedure-specific risks: anastomotic leak, bleeding, and bowel obstruction. Roux-en-Y gastric bypass in particular is associated with higher rates of nutritional deficiencies (notably vitamin B12, iron) and perioperative complications, as compared to sleeve gastrectomy.[185, 197, 198] Thus, lifelong micronutrient supplementation and careful monitoring for individuals with RYGB is essential.[199, 200, 201, 202]

Patient counseling and engagement in obesity care

Managing obesity effectively goes beyond selecting medications or recommending surgery. To truly engage a patient requires skilled, empathetic counseling that respects the chronic, biologically complex nature of obesity while balancing the societal and financial barriers to care. Many patients experience shame, low motivation, or prior healthcare stigma that impedes adherence. Clinicians play a critical role in building (and rebuilding) trust in a pervasively anti-fat healthcare system, supporting gradual behavior change, and framing obesity care as a long-term but worthwhile journey. Please see Chapter 8 for further discussion of weight stigma.

Below, we include some techniques and phrases that clinicians may use when discussing the importance of obesity care with their patients. Use non-judgmental, weight-neutral language and focus on health improvements, rather than just the scale. Connecting lab values to tangible impacts on health can be helpful for patients. You may say something like, 'Even a 5–10% weight loss can make a big difference in how your body functions. Before the mirror shows it, your organs feel it,' and explain any of the following:

- Lower HbA1c (~0.6–1.0%) → 'This reduces your risk of diabetes complications like vision loss, nerve damage, and kidney issues – and might mean fewer or lower doses of medications.'
- Lower systolic blood pressure (5–10 mmHg) → 'That's enough to cut your risk of stroke or heart attack significantly.'
- Better cholesterol (↓ triglycerides, ↑HDL) → 'This helps prevent plaque buildup in your arteries and protects your heart.'
- Decrease insulin resistance (by up to 25%) → 'Your body uses food more efficiently, so you have more energy and are less fatigued after meals.'
- Decrease inflammation (↓CRP) → 'Chronic inflammation contributes to joint pain, fatigue, and disease risk. Reducing inflammation helps you feel better and live longer.'

Clinicians should emphasize that improvements in these lab values are evidence of physiologic improvement and a decrease in disease, even when weight loss appears modest. Set realistic, patient-driven goals tied to specific health priorities, such as mobility, energy, fertility, or reducing medication burden. Provide support by collaborating to brainstorm sustainable and culturally appropriate lifestyle changes. Help patients identify small, consistent actions that fit their routines. Leverage multidisciplinary teams, including dietitians, therapists, counselors, and community resources like local food banks or community nutrition programs, to reinforce changes and support patients longitudinally, especially when on anti-obesity medications or pursuing surgery.

At each encounter, assess for psychosocial contributors, including depression, binge eating, food insecurity, and trauma. These are not peripheral. Rather, they are often central to obesity pathophysiology and treatment adherence. Incorporating behavioral health and/or social support referrals early can improve outcomes and reduce patient dropout. Table 7.4 provides several sample screening questions.

During weight management conversations, use frameworks like motivational interviewing or the

Table 7.4: Sample questions to screen for psychosocial contributors to weight loss interference.

Screening for…	Why screen?	Questions to ask
Depression	Depression can drive overeating, fatigue, low motivation, and disengagement from self-care	PHQ-2 'Over the past two weeks, have you been feeling down, depressed, or hopeless?' 'Have you lost interest or pleasure in doing things you used to enjoy?' If positive, proceed to PHQ-9 questions.
Binge eating	Uncontrolled eating episodes are common in obesity and may affect treatment planning, especially if patients regularly 'override' their hunger and fullness cues	'Do you ever eat a large amount of food in a short time and feel out of control while eating?' 'Do you feel guilt, shame, or distress afterward?' 'Do you sometimes eat in secret or when you're not physically hungry?' (Consider follow-up with binge eating scale or SCOFF questionnaire if appropriate.)
Food insecurity	Food insecurity can drive consumption of calorie-dense, low-nutrient foods and erratic eating patterns	USDA 2-item screener; a 'yes' to either is positive for food insecurity: 'In the past 12 months, have you worried that your food would run out before you had money to buy more?' 'Did the food you bought ever just not last, and you didn't have money to get more?'
Trauma, especially adverse childhood events (ACEs) and/or weight-related	Trauma can shape eating behavior, body image, and emotional regulation	'Have you experienced any stressful or traumatic events that you think still affect how you feel about your body, eating, or health?' 'Has anyone or any event ever made you feel unsafe [especially around food, your body, or weight]?'

PHQ = Patient Health Questionnare; USDA = United States Department of Agriculture; SCOFF = Eating Disorders Questionnaire

5 As (Ask, Assess, Advise, Agree, Assist/Arrange) to structure brief counseling sessions, and aim to revisit patient goals regularly.[203, 204, 205] Table 7.5 below provides examples of each step in the 5 As approach for weight management counseling.

Table 7.5: The 5 As approach for weight management counseling.

Step	Description	Example sentence for clinicians
Ask	Obtain permission to discuss weight; explore the patient's readiness and concerns	'Would it be okay if we talked about your weight and how it might be affecting your health?'
Assess	Evaluate obesity severity, related complications, barriers, and patient motivation	'Can you describe a typical day of eating and physical activity for you?' 'Are there any particular challenges you've noticed in making changes?'
Advise	Provide clear, personalized advice on health risks and benefits of weight management	'Losing even 5% of your body weight can improve your blood sugar and blood pressure'
Agree	Collaborate to set realistic, achievable goals focusing on behavior change and health outcomes	'What do you think about setting a goal to walk 20 minutes three times a week? Does that feel doable?'
Assist/ Arrange	Offer resources, education, referrals, and support to overcome barriers Schedule a follow-up to monitor progress and adjust the plan	'I can refer you to a dietitian who can help create a meal plan that fits your lifestyle' 'Let's schedule a follow-up in a month to see how things are going and make any needed changes'

Special populations and considerations

Comprehensive obesity and weight management must account for the unique needs of diverse populations. This includes tailored approaches across the lifespan – from childhood to older adulthood – as well as considerations during pregnancy and among different racial and ethnic groups. Addressing these factors is essential for providing equitable and effective care.

Children and adolescents

Early patterns of fat distribution established in childhood and adolescence can influence lifelong metabolic risk.[206, 207, 208] Excess adiposity during these formative years often tracks into adulthood, increasing the risk of T2DM, dyslipidemia, and CVD later in life. Importantly, even those who were overweight or obese during childhood but achieved a normal BMI by adulthood had risks similar to those who maintained a normal BMI throughout their lives.[208] Prevention of inappropriately high childhood weight gain, early identification, and prompt intervention focusing on healthy lifestyle habits are critical to altering the metabolic trajectory of our youth.

Elderly: sarcopenic obesity and metabolic risk

In older adults, the coexistence of sarcopenia (age-related loss of muscle mass and strength) and obesity, termed sarcopenic obesity, poses unique clinical challenges. Sarcopenic obesity is associated with greater insulin resistance, systemic inflammation, and a higher prevalence of metabolic syndrome compared to obesity or sarcopenia alone.[209] Mechanistically, ectopic fat accumulation within skeletal muscle impairs mitochondrial function and promotes inflammatory cytokine production, exacerbating muscle loss and metabolic dysfunction.[106] This phenotype increases the risk of frailty, CVD, and mortality, underscoring the importance of combined nutritional intervention (adequate protein intake) and physical activity interventions (especially resistance training) to preserve muscle mass and improve metabolic health in this population.[210]

Pregnancy: gestational adiposity and metabolic complications

Pregnancy is a critical window where excessive gestational weight gain and adiposity increase risks for gestational diabetes, hypertensive diseases, and adverse perinatal outcomes. These complications not only affect maternal health but also predispose offspring to obesity and metabolic diseases, highlighting the need for careful monitoring and management of weight and metabolic parameters during pregnancy.[211, 212, 213, 214]

Ethnic differences in fat distribution and metabolic thresholds

Ethnic variations in body fat distribution and metabolic risk are well-recognized. As discussed previously, individuals of South Asian descent tend to accumulate more central adiposity and associated VAT at lower BMI levels; this phenotype was associated with a higher risk of insulin resistance, metabolic syndrome, T2DM, and CVD, at comparatively lower body weights than Caucasian populations.[215] One study found that 43.6% of normal-weight South Asians had two or more cardiometabolic abnormalities, compared to 21.0% of Caucasian populations.[216] Based on this evidence, in 2004, the WHO recommended lowering BMI cut-off points for defining overweight (BMI $\geq$23 kg/m^2) and obesity (BMI $\geq$27.5 kg/m^2) in Asian populations to better identify those at risk for cardiometabolic diseases.[217]

Prevention and public health perspectives

Critical to long-term obesity management is prevention through community health and primary care initiatives. Community and policy interventions that address obesogenic environments, such as improving access to healthy foods, creating safe spaces for physical activity, and regulating marketing of unhealthy products, are essential to reducing population-level risk factors.[218, 219]

A strong childhood obesity prevention program example is the Communities Creating Healthy Environments (CCHE) initiative (2009–2012), led by the Robert Wood Johnson Foundation. The CCHE supported 21 grassroots groups and tribal nations to address childhood obesity in communities of color. It secured 72 policy wins, with 37.5% of grants aimed at improving access to healthy food and 33.3% supporting safe recreation.[220] Clinicians can support such efforts by referring patients to local programs, partnering with community organizations, and being political advocates for policies that promote healthier environments.

Another exemplary program is Eat Better South Africa (EBSA), a transformative community health initiative dedicated to combating diet-related diseases in under-resourced South African communities. As the outreach arm of The Noakes Foundation, EBSA empowers individuals, particularly women, with practical, culturally relevant nutrition education focused on reducing sugar and processed food intake while promoting affordable, nutrient-dense whole foods. Through its 6-week programs, EBSA has achieved significant health improvements among participants.

A mixed-methods study reported average weight loss of 5.6 kg, reductions in BMI and waist circumference, and improved blood pressure and blood glucose levels six months post-intervention.[221] These outcomes underscore the program's effectiveness in addressing metabolic health issues.

Reducing obesity's burden, particularly in underserved populations, requires more than clinical treatment; it demands culturally relevant, community-driven prevention efforts and societal understanding that obesity is a disease with contributions from environmental, genetic, and behavioral factors. By fostering supportive environments, engaging local voices, and integrating prevention into primary care, we can build a more equitable and effective foundation for long-term obesity management.

Conclusion

Obesity is a heterogeneous disease characterized by excess body weight, alterations in regional fat distribution, and dysfunctional adipose tissue. The pathological expansion of adipose tissue – marked by adipocyte hypertrophy, hypoxia, chronic low-grade inflammation, fibrosis limiting proper lipid storage, and impaired vascularization – disrupts metabolic homeostasis and contributes to insulin resistance, dyslipidemia, and cardiovascular risk. Critically, fat distribution (central/visceral vs. subcutaneous) and adipocyte metabolic health significantly shape disease risk. This underscores the need for nuanced clinical assessment beyond BMI, with the most low-hanging fruit being WC and WtHR.

The case of 'Meg,' a 52-year-old woman experiencing progressive weight gain, fatigue, and metabolic co-morbidities who longs for a healthier past self, exemplifies the multifactorial challenges faced by patients with obesity. Her story highlights the importance of comprehensive evaluation and multidisciplinary care that integrates lifestyle modification, behavioral support, and when appropriate, pharmacologic therapies and surgical interventions.

Beyond biology, an integrated, patient-centered framework is essential – one that addresses not only the pathophysiological underpinnings of obesity but also the emotional, social, and systemic factors that shape a patient's lived experience. Recognizing obesity as a disease rather than a character flaw enables clinicians to offer more equitable, effective, and compassionate care. This approach not only improves metabolic health but also restores dignity, function, and long-term quality of life for patients navigating the burden of this complex disease.

References

1. WHO. *Obesity and overweight.* Available from: https://www.who.int/news-room/fact-sheets/detail/obesity-and-overweight
2. Boutari C, Mantzoros CS. A 2022 update on the epidemiology of obesity and a call to action: as its twin COVID-19 pandemic appears to be receding, the obesity and dysmetabolism pandemic continues to rage on. *Metabolism.* 2022 Aug 1;133:155217. DOI: https://doi.org/10.1016/j.metabol.2022.155217
3. CDC. Obesity. 2025. *Adult Obesity Facts.* Available from: https://www.cdc.gov/obesity/adult-obesity-facts/index.html
4. Kerr JA, Patton GC, Cini KI, Abate YH, Abbas N, Magied AHAAA, et al. Global, regional, and national prevalence of child and adolescent overweight and obesity, 1990–2021, with forecasts to 2050: a forecasting study for the Global Burden of Disease Study 2021. *The Lancet.* 2025 Mar 8;405(10481):785–812. DOI: https://doi.org/10.1016/S0140-6736(25)00397-6
5. Ng M, Gakidou E, Lo J, Abate YH, Abbafati C, Abbas N, et al. Global, regional, and national prevalence of adult overweight and obesity, 1990–2021, with forecasts to 2050: a forecasting study for the Global Burden of Disease Study 2021. *The Lancet.* 2025 Mar 8;405(10481):813–38. DOI: https://doi.org/10.1016/S0140-6736(25)00355-1

6. The GBD 2015 Obesity Collaborators. Health effects of overweight and obesity in 195 countries over 25 years. *N Engl J Med*. 2017 Jul 6;377(1):13–27.
DOI: https://doi.org/10.1056/NEJMoa1614362
7. Ward ZJ, Bleich SN, Long MW, Gortmaker SL. Association of body mass index with health care expenditures in the United States by age and sex. *PloS One*. 2021;16(3):e0247307. DOI: https://doi.org/10.1371/journal.pone.0247307
8. Razak F, Anand SS, Shannon H, Vuksan V, Davis B, Jacobs R, et al. Defining obesity cut points in a multiethnic population. *Circulation*. 2007 Apr 24;115(16):2111–8. DOI: https://doi.org/10.1161/CIRCULATIONAHA.106.635011
9. Caleyachetty R, Barber TM, Mohammed NI, Cappuccio FP, Hardy R, Mathur R, et al. Ethnicity-specific BMI cutoffs for obesity based on type 2 diabetes risk in England: a population-based cohort study. *Lancet Diabetes Endocrinol*. 2021 Jul 1;9(7):419–26. DOI: https://doi.org/10.1016/S2213-8587(21)00088-7
10. Jayedi A, Soltani S, Motlagh SZT, Emadi A, Shahinfar H, Moosavi H, et al. Anthropometric and adiposity indicators and risk of type 2 diabetes: systematic review and dose-response meta-analysis of cohort studies. *BMJ*. 2022 Jan 18;376:e067516.
DOI: https://doi.org/10.1136/bmj-2021-067516
11. Powell-Wiley TM, Poirier P, Burke LE, Després JP, Gordon-Larsen P, Lavie CJ, et al. Obesity and cardiovascular disease: a scientific statement from the American Heart Association. *Circulation*. 2021 May 25;143(21):e984–1010. DOI: https://doi.org/10.1161/CIR.0000000000000973
12. Neeland IJ, Ross R, Després JP, Matsuzawa Y, Yamashita S, Shai I, et al. Visceral and ectopic fat, atherosclerosis, and cardiometabolic disease: a position statement. *Lancet Diabetes Endocrinol*. 2019 Sep;7(9):715–25. DOI: https://doi.org/10.1016/S2213-8587(19)30084-1
13. Agrawal S, Klarqvist MDR, Diamant N, Stanley TL, Ellinor PT, Mehta NN, et al. BMI-adjusted adipose tissue volumes exhibit depot-specific and divergent associations with cardiometabolic diseases. *Nat Commun*. 2023 Jan 17;14(1):266.
DOI: https://doi.org/10.1038/s41467-022-35704-5
14. Rosenzweig JL, Bakris GL, Berglund LF, Hivert MF, Horton ES, Kalyani RR, et al. Primary prevention of ASCVD and T2DM in patients at metabolic risk: an Endocrine Society clinical practice guideline. *J Clin Endocrinol Metab*. 2019 Sep 1;104(9):3939–85.
DOI: https://doi.org/10.1210/jc.2019-01338
15. Zhu L, Spence C, Yang JW, Ma GX. The IDF definition is better suited for screening metabolic syndrome and estimating risks of diabetes in Asian American adults: evidence from NHANES 2011–2016. *J Clin Med*. 2020 Nov 28;9(12):3871.
DOI: https://doi.org/10.3390/jcm9123871
16. Hampl SE, Hassink SG, Skinner AC, Armstrong SC, Barlow SE, Bolling CF, et al. Clinical practice guideline for the evaluation and treatment of children and adolescents with obesity. *Pediatrics*. 2023 Feb 1;151(2):e2022060640.
DOI: https://doi.org/10.1542/peds.2022-060640
17. Bouchard C. Genetics of Obesity: What we have learned over decades of research. *Obes Silver Spring Md*. 2021 May;29(5):802–20.
DOI: https://doi.org/10.1002/oby.23116
18. Mahmoud R, Kimonis V, Butler MG. Genetics of obesity in humans: a clinical review. *Int J Mol Sci*. 2022 Sep 20;23(19):11005.
DOI: https://doi.org/10.3390/ijms231911005
19. Huang J, Huffman JE, Huang Y, Do Valle Í, Assimes TL, Raghavan S, et al. Genomics and phenomics of body mass index reveals a complex disease network. *Nat Commun*. 2022 Dec 29;13(1):7973.
DOI: https://doi.org/10.1038/s41467-022-35553-2
20. Locke AE, Kahali B, Berndt SI, Justice AE, Pers TH, Day FR, et al. Genetic studies of body mass index yield new insights for obesity biology. *Nature*. 2015 Feb;518(7538):197–206.
DOI: https://doi.org/10.1038/nature14177
21. Hoffmann TJ, Choquet H, Yin J, Banda Y, Kvale MN, Glymour M, et al. A large multiethnic genome-wide association study of adult body mass index identifies novel loci. *Genetics*. 2018 Oct;210(2):499–515.
DOI: https://doi.org/10.1534/genetics.118.301479
22. Schleinitz D, Böttcher Y, Blüher M, Kovacs P. The genetics of fat distribution. *Diabetologia*. 2014 Jul 1;57(7):1276–86.
DOI: https://doi.org/10.1007/s00125-014-3214-z
23. Rask-Andersen M, Karlsson T, Ek WE, Johansson

Å. Genome-wide association study of body fat distribution identifies adiposity loci and sex-specific genetic effects. *Nat Commun.* 2019 Jan 21;10(1):339.
DOI: https://doi.org/10.1038/s41467-018-08000-4

24. Shungin D, Winkler TW, Croteau-Chonka DC, Ferreira T, Locke AE, Mägi R, et al. New genetic loci link adipose and insulin biology to body fat distribution. *Nature.* 2015 Feb;518(7538):187–96. DOI: https://doi.org/10.1038/nature14132
25. Pulit SL, Stoneman C, Morris AP, Wood AR, Glastonbury CA, Tyrrell J, et al. Meta-analysis of genome-wide association studies for body fat distribution in 694 649 individuals of European ancestry. *Hum Mol Genet.* 2019 Jan 1;28(1):166–74. DOI: https://doi.org/10.1093/hmg/ddy327
26. US Preventive Services Task Force, Curry SJ, Krist AH, Owens DK, Barry MJ, Caughey AB, et al. Behavioral weight loss interventions to prevent obesity-related morbidity and mortality in adults: US Preventive Services Task Force recommendation statement. *JAMA.* 2018 Sep 18;320(11):1163–71.
DOI: https://doi.org/10.1001/jama.2018.13022
27. Cornier MA, Després JP, Davis N, Grossniklaus DA, Klein S, Lamarche B, et al. Assessing adiposity: a scientific statement from the American Heart Association. *Circulation.* 2011 Nov 1;124(18):1996–2019. DOI: https://doi.org/10.1161/CIR.0b013e318233bc6a
28. Mehta LS, Velarde GP, Lewey J, Sharma G, Bond RM, Navas-Acien A, et al. Cardiovascular disease risk factors in women: the impact of race and ethnicity: a scientific statement from the American Heart Association. *Circulation.* 2023 May 9;147(19):1471–87. DOI: https://doi.org/10.1161/CIR.0000000000001139
29. Office of Minority Health. *Obesity and American Indians/Alaska Natives.* Available from: https://minorityhealth.hhs.gov/obesity-and-american-indiansalaska-natives
30. Shah NS, Luncheon C, Kandula NR, Khan SS, Pan L, Gillespie C, et al. Heterogeneity in obesity prevalence among Asian American adults. *Ann Intern Med.* 2022 Nov;175(11):1493–500.
DOI: https://doi.org/10.7326/M22-0609
31. Mozaffarian D, Afshin A, Benowitz NL, Bittner V, Daniels SR, Franch HA, et al. Population approaches to improve diet, physical activity, and smoking habits: a scientific statement from the American Heart Association. *Circulation.* 2012 Sep 18;126(12):1514–63. DOI: https://doi.org/10.1161/CIR.0b013e318260a20b
32. Rock CL, Thomson C, Gansler T, Gapstur SM, McCullough ML, Patel AV, et al. American Cancer Society guideline for diet and physical activity for cancer prevention. *CA Cancer J Clin.* 2020 Jul;70(4):245–71.
DOI: https://doi.org/10.3322/caac.21591
33. Mui Y, Ballard E, Lopatin E, Thornton RLJ, Pollack Porter KM, Gittelsohn J. A community-based system dynamics approach suggests solutions for improving healthy food access in a low-income urban environment. *PloS One.* 2019;14(5):e0216985. DOI: https://doi.org/10.1371/journal.pone.0216985
34. Carnethon MR, Pu J, Howard G, Albert MA, Anderson CAM, Bertoni AG, et al. Cardiovascular health in African Americans: a scientific statement from the American Heart Association. *Circulation.* 2017 Nov 21;136(21):e393–423. DOI: https://doi.org/10.1161/CIR.0000000000000534
35. Min J, Goodale H, Xue H, Brey R, Wang Y. Racial-Ethnic Disparities in obesity and biological, behavioral, and sociocultural influences in the United States: a systematic review. *Adv Nutr Bethesda Md.* 2021 Jul 30;12(4):1137–48.
DOI: https://doi.org/10.1093/advances/nmaa162
36. Caprio S, Daniels SR, Drewnowski A, Kaufman FR, Palinkas LA, Rosenbloom AL, et al. Influence of race, ethnicity, and culture on childhood obesity: implications for prevention and treatment: a consensus statement of Shaping America's Health and the Obesity Society. *Diabetes Care.* 2008 Nov;31(11):2211–21.
DOI: https://doi.org/10.2337/dc08-9024
37. Stovall T, Mitchell NA, Smith F, Jones R. An exploratory study on the sociocultural consequences of food consumption patterns among African American girls. *Appetite.* 2021 Nov 1;166:105429.
DOI: https://doi.org/10.1016/j.appet.2021.105429
38. James DCS, Pobee JW, Oxidine D, Brown L, Joshi G. Using the health belief model to develop culturally appropriate weight-management materials

for African-American women. *J Acad Nutr Diet.* 2012 May;112(5):664–70. DOI: https://doi.org/10.1016/j.jand.2012.02.003

39. Mylona EK, Shehadeh F, Fleury E, Kalligeros M, Mylonakis E. Neighborhood-level analysis on the impact of accessibility to fast food and open green spaces on the prevalence of obesity. *Am J Med.* 2020 Mar;133(3):340–346.e1. DOI: https://doi.org/10.1016/j.amjmed.2019.08.024
40. Oh JI, Lee KJ, Hipp A. Food deserts exposure, density of fast-food restaurants, and park access: exploring the association of food and recreation environments with obesity and diabetes using global and local regression models. *PloS One.* 2024;19(4):e0301121. DOI: https://doi.org/10.1371/journal.pone.0301121
41. Oudat Q, Messiah SE, Ghoneum AD. A Multi-level approach to childhood obesity prevention and management: lessons from Japan and the United States. *Nutrients.* 2025 Feb 28;17(5):838. DOI: https://doi.org/10.3390/nu17050838
42. Tesfai K, Pace J, El-Newihi N, Martinez ME, Tincopa MA, Loomba R. Disparities for Hispanic adults with metabolic dysfunction-associated steatotic liver disease in the United States: a systematic review and meta-analysis. *Clin Gastroenterol Hepatol.* 2025 Feb 1;23(2):236–49. DOI: https://doi.org/10.1016/j.cgh.2024.06.038
43. Fu CE, Teng M, Tung D, Ramadoss V, Ong C, Koh B, et al. Sex and race-ethnic disparities in metabolic dysfunction-associated steatotic liver disease: an analysis of 40,166 individuals. *Dig Dis Sci.* 2024 Sep 1;69(9):3195–205. DOI: https://doi.org/10.1007/s10620-024-08540-4
44. Lim U, Monroe KR, Buchthal S, Fan B, Cheng I, Kristal BS, et al. Propensity for intra-abdominal and hepatic adiposity varies among ethnic groups. *Gastroenterology.* 2019 Mar 1;156(4):966–975.e10. DOI: https://doi.org/10.1053/j.gastro.2018.11.021
45. Li Z, Daniel S, Fujioka K, Umashanker D. Obesity among Asian American people in the United States: a review. *Obes Silver Spring Md.* 2023 Feb;31(2):316–28. DOI: https://doi.org/10.1002/oby.23639
46. Godfrey TM, Cordova-Marks FM, Jones D, Melton F, Breathett K. Metabolic syndrome among American Indian and Alaska Native populations: implications for cardiovascular health. *Curr Hypertens Rep.* 2022 May;24(5):107–14. DOI: https://doi.org/10.1007/s11906-022-01178-5
47. Sharma G, Kelliher A, Deen J, Parker T, Hagerty T, Choi EE, et al. Status of maternal cardiovascular health in American Indian and Alaska Native individuals: a scientific statement from the American Heart Association. *Circ Cardiovasc Qual Outcomes.* 2023 Jun;16(6):e000117. DOI: https://doi.org/10.1161/HCQ.0000000000000117
48. Breathett K, Sims M, Gross M, Jackson EA, Jones EJ, Navas-Acien A, et al. Cardiovascular health in American Indians and Alaska Natives: a scientific statement from the American Heart Association. *Circulation.* 2020 Jun 23;141(25):e948–59. DOI: https://doi.org/10.1161/CIR.0000000000000773
49. Sinclair KA, Bogart A, Buchwald D, Henderson JA. The prevalence of metabolic syndrome and associated risk factors in Northern Plains and Southwest American Indians. *Diabetes Care.* 2011 Jan;34(1):118–20. DOI: https://doi.org/10.2337/dc10-0221
50. Emmerich SD, Fryar CD, Stierman B, Ogden CL. Obesity and severe obesity prevalence in adults: United States, August 2021–August 2023. *NCHS Data Brief.* 2024 Sep;(508). DOI: https://doi.org/10.15620/cdc/159281
51. Zhao L, Park S, Ward ZJ, Cradock AL, Gortmaker SL, Blanck HM. State-specific prevalence of severe obesity among adults in the US using bias correction of self-reported body mass index. *Prev Chronic Dis.* 2023 Jul 13;20:E61. DOI: https://doi.org/10.5888/pcd20.230005
52. Wells JCK. Sexual dimorphism of body composition. *Best Pract Res Clin Endocrinol Metab.* 2007 Sep;21(3):415–30. DOI: https://doi.org/10.1016/j.beem.2007.04.007
53. Shen W, Punyanitya M, Silva AM, et al. Sexual dimorphism of adipose tissue distribution across the lifespan: a cross-sectional whole-body magnetic resonance imaging study. *Nutrition & Metabolism* 2009 Apr 16;6:17. DOI:10.1186/1743-7075-6-17
54. Koceva A, Herman R, Janez A, Rakusa M, Jensterle M. Sex- and gender-related differences in obesity: from pathophysiological mechanisms to clinical implications. *Int J Mol Sci.* 2024 Jul 4;25(13):7342. DOI: https://doi.org/10.3390/ijms25137342

55. Bredella MA. Sex differences in body composition. In: Mauvais-Jarvis F, editor. *Sex and Gender Factors Affecting Metabolic Homeostasis, Diabetes and Obesity* . Cham: Springer International Publishing; 2017, p. 9–27. DOI: https://doi.org/10.1007/978-3-319-70178-3_2
56. Blouin K, Boivin A, Tchernof A. Androgens and body fat distribution. *J Steroid Biochem Mol Biol.* 2008 Feb;108(3–5):272–80. DOI: https://doi.org/10.1016/j.jsbmb.2007.09.001
57. Krotkiewski M, Björntorp P, Sjöström L, Smith U. Impact of obesity on metabolism in men and women. Importance of regional adipose tissue distribution. *J Clin Invest.* 1983 Sep 1;72(3):1150–62. DOI: https://doi.org/10.1172/JCI111040
58. Tchernof A, Bélanger C, Morisset AS, Richard C, Mailloux J, Laberge P, et al. Regional differences in adipose tissue metabolism in women: minor effect of obesity and body fat distribution. *Diabetes.* 2006 May 1;55(5):1353–60. DOI: https://doi.org/10.2337/db05-1439
59. Foley JE, Kashiwagi A, Chang H, Huecksteadt TP, Lillioja S, Verso MA, et al. Sex difference in insulin-stimulated glucose transport in rat and human adipocytes. *Am J Physiol-Endocrinol Metab.* 1984 Mar;246(3):E211–5. DOI: https://doi.org/10.1152/ajpendo.1984.246.3.E211
60. Arner P, Viguerie N, Massier L, Rydén M, Astrup A, Blaak E, et al. Sex differences in adipose insulin resistance are linked to obesity, lipolysis and insulin receptor substrate 1. *Int J Obes.* 2024 Jul;48(7):934–40. DOI: https://doi.org/10.1038/s41366-024-01501-x
61. Grove KL, Fried SK, Greenberg AS, Xiao XQ, Clegg DJ. A microarray analysis of sexual dimorphism of adipose tissues in high-fat-diet-induced obese mice. *Int J Obes.* 2010 Jun;34(6):989–1000. DOI: https://doi.org/10.1038/ijo.2010.12
62. Link JC, Wiese CB, Chen X, Avetisyan R, Ronquillo E, Ma F, et al. X chromosome dosage of histone demethylase KDM5C determines sex differences in adiposity. *J Clin Invest.* 2020 Nov 2;130(11):5688–702. DOI: https://doi.org/10.1172/JCI140223
63. Zore T, Palafox M, Reue K. Sex differences in obesity, lipid metabolism, and inflammation – a role for the sex chromosomes? *Mol Metab.* 2018 Sep 1;15:35–44. DOI: https://doi.org/10.1016/j.molmet.2018.04.003
64. Palmer BF, Clegg DJ. The sexual dimorphism of obesity. *Mol Cell Endocrinol.* 2015 Feb 15;402:113–9. DOI: https://doi.org/10.1016/j.mce.2014.11.029
65. El Khoudary SR, Aggarwal B, Beckie TM, Hodis HN, Johnson AE, Langer RD, et al. Menopause transition and cardiovascular disease risk: implications for timing of early prevention: a scientific statement from the American Heart Association. *Circulation.* 2020 Dec 22;142(25):e506–32. DOI: https://doi.org/10.1161/CIR.0000000000000912
66. O'Sullivan AJ, Crampton LJ, Freund J, Ho KK. The route of estrogen replacement therapy confers divergent effects on substrate oxidation and body composition in postmenopausal women. *J Clin Invest.* 1998 Sep 1;102(5):1035–40. DOI: https://doi.org/10.1172/JCI2773
67. Ko SH, Jung Y. Energy metabolism changes and dysregulated lipid metabolism in postmenopausal women. *Nutrients.* 2021 Dec;13(12):4556. DOI: https://doi.org/10.3390/nu13124556
68. Kammerlander AA, Lyass A, Mahoney TF, Massaro JM, Long MT, Vasan RS, et al. Sex differences in the associations of visceral adipose tissue and cardiometabolic and cardiovascular disease risk: the Framingham Heart Study. *J Am Heart Assoc.* 2021 Jun;10(11):e019968. DOI: https://doi.org/10.1161/JAHA.120.019968
69. Baarts RB, Jensen MR, Hansen OM, Haddock B, Prescott E, Hovind P, et al. Age- and sex-specific changes in visceral fat mass throughout the life-span. *Obesity.* 2023;31(7):1953–61. DOI: https://doi.org/10.1002/oby.23779
70. Nordström A, Hadrévi J, Olsson T, Franks PW, Nordström P. Higher prevalence of type 2 diabetes in men than in women is associated with differences in visceral fat mass. *J Clin Endocrinol Metab.* 2016 Oct 1;101(10):3740–6. DOI: https://doi.org/10.1210/jc.2016-1915
71. Elbers JMH, Asscheman H, Seidell JC, Megens JAJ, Gooren LJG. Long-term testosterone administration increases visceral fat in female to male transsexuals. *J Clin Endocrinol Metab.* 1997 Jul 1;82(7):2044–7. DOI: https://doi.org/10.1210/jcem.82.7.4078
72. Kim MS, Shim I, Fahed AC, Do R, Park WY, Natarajan P, et al. Association of genetic risk,

lifestyle, and their interaction with obesity and obesity-related morbidities. *Cell Metab.* 2024 Jul 2;36(7):1494–1503.e3. DOI: https://doi.org/10.1016/j.cmet.2024.06.004

73. Zhang M, Ward J, Strawbridge RJ, Anderson JJ, Celis-Morales C, Pell JP, et al. Genetic predisposition to adiposity, and type 2 diabetes: the role of lifestyle and phenotypic adiposity. *Eur J Endocrinol.* 2025 Apr 30;192(5):549–57. DOI: https://doi.org/10.1093/ejendo/lvaf084
74. Isasi CR, Moon JY, Gallo LC, Qi Q, Wang T, Sotres-Alvarez D, et al. Chronic stress, genetic risk, and obesity in US Hispanic/Latinos: results from the Hispanic Community Health Study/Study of Latinos. *Psychosom Med.* 2022 Sep 1;84(7):822–7. DOI: https://doi.org/10.1097/PSY.0000000000001107
75. Colberg SR, Sigal RJ, Yardley JE, Riddell MC, Dunstan DW, Dempsey PC, et al. Physical activity/exercise and diabetes: a position statement of the American Diabetes Association. *Diabetes Care.* 2016 Nov;39(11):2065–79. DOI: https://doi.org/10.2337/dc16-1728
76. Fletcher GF, Ades PA, Kligfield P, Arena R, Balady GJ, Bittner VA, et al. Exercise standards for testing and training: a scientific statement from the American Heart Association. *Circulation.* 2013 Aug 20;128(8):873–934. DOI: https://doi.org/10.1161/cir.0b013e31829b5b44
77. Oppert JM, Ciangura C, Bellicha A. Physical activity and exercise for weight loss and maintenance in people living with obesity. *Rev Endocr Metab Disord.* 2023 Oct;24(5):937–49. DOI: https://doi.org/10.1007/s11154-023-09805-5
78. Jakicic JM, Powell KE, Campbell WW, Dipietro L, Pate RR, Pescatello LS, et al. Physical activity and the prevention of weight gain in adults: a systematic review. *Med Sci Sports Exerc.* 2019 Jun;51(6):1262–9. DOI: https://doi.org/10.1249/MSS.0000000000001938
79. McCuen-Wurst C, Ruggieri M, Allison KC. Conditioned eating and obesity: associations between binge-eating disease, night-eating syndrome, and weight-related comorbidities. *Ann N Y Acad Sci.* 2018 Jan;1411(1):96–105. DOI: https://doi.org/10.1111/nyas.13467
80. Ivezaj V, White MA, Grilo CM. Examining binge-eating disease and food addiction in adults with overweight and obesity. *Obes Silver Spring Md.* 2016 Oct;24(10):2064–9. DOI: https://doi.org/10.1002/oby.21607
81. Venditti EM, Wing RR, Jakicic JM, Butler BA, Marcus MD. Weight cycling, psychological health, and binge eating in obese women. *J Consult Clin Psychol.* 1996;64(2):400–5. DOI: https://doi.org/10.1037/0022-006X.64.2.400
82. Madigan CD, Pavey T, Daley AJ, Jolly K, Brown WJ. Is weight cycling associated with adverse health outcomes? A cohort study. *Prev Med.* 2018 Mar;108:47–52. DOI: https://doi.org/10.1016/j.ypmed.2017.12.010
83. Zwaan M, Engeli S, Müller A. Temperamental factors in severe weight cycling. A cross-sectional study. *Appetite.* 2015;91:336–42. DOI: https://doi.org/10.1016/j.appet.2015.04.064
84. van der Valk ES, van den Akker ELT, Savas M, Kleinendorst L, Visser JA, Van Haelst MM, et al. A comprehensive diagnostic approach to detect underlying causes of obesity in adults. *Obes Rev Off J Int Assoc Study Obes.* 2019 Jun;20(6):795–804. DOI: https://doi.org/10.1111/obr.12836
85. Dalamaga M, Kounatidis D, Tsilingiris D, Vallianou NG, Karampela I, Psallida S, et al. The role of endocrine disruptors bisphenols and phthalates in obesity: current evidence, perspectives and controversies. *Int J Mol Sci.* 2024 Jan 4;25(1):675. DOI: https://doi.org/10.3390/ijms25010675
86. Veiga-Lopez A, Pu Y, Gingrich J, Padmanabhan V. Obesogenic endocrine disrupting chemicals: identifying knowledge gaps. trends *Endocrinol Metab TEM.* 2018 Sep;29(9):607–25. DOI: https://doi.org/10.1016/j.tem.2018.06.003
87. Czerwińska M, Ostrowska P, Hansdorfer-Korzon R. Lipoedema as a social problem. a scoping review. *Int J Environ Res Public Health.* 2021 Jan;18(19):10223. DOI: https://doi.org/10.3390/ijerph181910223
88. Smith GI, Mittendorfer B, Klein S. Metabolically healthy obesity: facts and fantasies. *J Clin Invest.* 2019 Oct 1;129(10):3978–89. DOI: https://doi.org/10.1172/JCI129186
89. Farabi SS, Smith GI, Schweitzer GG, Stein RI, Klein S. Do lifestyle factors and quality of life differ in people with metabolically healthy and unhealthy obesity? *Int J Obes* 2005. 2022

Oct;46(10):1778–85.
DOI: https://doi.org/10.1038/s41366-022-01180-6
90. Iacobini C, Pugliese G, Blasetti Fantauzzi C, Federici M, Menini S. Metabolically healthy versus metabolically unhealthy obesity. *Metabolism*. 2019 Mar;92:51–60. DOI: https://doi.org/10.1016/j.metabol.2018.11.009
91. Petersen MC, Smith GI, Palacios HH, Farabi SS, Yoshino M, Yoshino J, et al. Cardiometabolic characteristics of people with metabolically healthy and unhealthy obesity. *Cell Metab*. 2024 Apr 2;36(4):745–761.e5.
DOI: https://doi.org/10.1016/j.cmet.2024.03.002
92. McLaughlin T, Abbasi F, Lamendola C, Reaven G. Heterogeneity in the prevalence of risk factors for cardiovascular disease and type 2 diabetes mellitus in obese individuals: effect of differences in insulin sensitivity. *Arch Intern Med*. 2007 Apr 9;167(7):642–8.
DOI: https://doi.org/10.1001/archinte.167.7.642
93. Fujimoto BA, Young M, Carter L, Pang APS, Corley MJ, Fogelgren B, et al. The exocyst complex regulates insulin-stimulated glucose uptake of skeletal muscle cells. *Am J Physiol Endocrinol Metab*. 2019 Dec 1;317(6):E957–72.
DOI: https://doi.org/10.1152/ajpendo.00109.2019
94. Keske MA, Dwyer RM, Russell RD, Blackwood SJ, Brown AA, Hu D, et al. Regulation of microvascular flow and metabolism: an overview. *Clin Exp Pharmacol Physiol*. 2017 Jan;44(1):143–9.
DOI: https://doi.org/10.1111/1440-1681.12688
95. Merz KE, Thurmond DC. Role of skeletal muscle in insulin resistance and glucose uptake. *Compr Physiol*. 2020 Jul 8;10(3):785–809.
DOI: https://doi.org/10.1002/cphy.c190029
96. Koh HCE, van Vliet S, Meyer GA, Laforest R, Gropler RJ, Klein S, et al. Heterogeneity in insulin-stimulated glucose uptake among different muscle groups in healthy lean people and people with obesity. *Diabetologia*. 2021 May;64(5):1158–68. DOI: https://doi.org/10.1007/s00125-021-05383-w
97. Chen DL, Liess C, Poljak A, Xu A, Zhang J, Thoma C, et al. Phenotypic characterization of insulin-resistant and insulin-sensitive obesity. *J Clin Endocrinol Metab*. 2015 Nov;100(11):4082–91. DOI: https://doi.org/10.1210/jc.2015-2712
98. Bo S, Musso G, Gambino R, Villois P, Gentile L, Durazzo M, et al. Prognostic implications for insulin-sensitive and insulin-resistant normal-weight and obese individuals from a population-based cohort. *Am J Clin Nutr*. 2012 Nov;96(5):962–9.
DOI: https://doi.org/10.3945/ajcn.112.040006
99. McLaughlin T, Craig C, Liu LF, Perelman D, Allister C, Spielman D, et al. Adipose cell size and regional fat deposition as predictors of metabolic response to overfeeding in insulin-resistant and insulin-sensitive humans. *Diabetes*. 2016 May;65(5):1245–54.
DOI: https://doi.org/10.2337/db15-1213
100. Yeni-Komshian H, Carantoni M, Abbasi F, Reaven GM. Relationship between several surrogate estimates of insulin resistance and quantification of insulin-mediated glucose disposal in 490 healthy nondiabetic volunteers. *Diabetes Care*. 2000 Feb;23(2):171–5.
DOI: https://doi.org/10.2337/diacare.23.2.171
101. Wang T, Li M, Zeng T, Hu R, Xu Y, Xu M, et al. Association between insulin resistance and cardiovascular disease risk varies according to glucose tolerance status: a nationwide prospective cohort study. *Diabetes Care*. 2022 Aug 1;45(8):1863–72.
DOI: https://doi.org/10.2337/dc22-0202
102. Meigs JB, Rutter MK, Sullivan LM, Fox CS, D'Agostino RB, Wilson PWF. Impact of insulin resistance on risk of type 2 diabetes and cardiovascular disease in people with metabolic syndrome. *Diabetes Care*. 2007 May;30(5):1219–25. DOI: https://doi.org/10.2337/dc06-2484
103. Ferrannini E, Balkau B, Coppack SW, Dekker JM, Mari A, Nolan J, et al. Insulin resistance, insulin response, and obesity as indicators of metabolic risk. *J Clin Endocrinol Metab*. 2007 Aug;92(8):2885–92.
DOI: https://doi.org/10.1210/jc.2007-0334
104. McLaughlin T, Abbasi F, Lamendola C, Yee G, Carter S, Cushman SW. Dietary weight loss in insulin-resistant non-obese humans: metabolic benefits and relationship to adipose cell size. *Nutr Metab Cardiovasc Dis NMCD*. 2019 Jan;29(1):62–8. DOI: https://doi.org/10.1016/j.numecd.2018.09.014
105. McLaughlin T, Stühlinger M, Lamendola C, Abbasi F, Bialek J, Reaven GM, et al. Plasma asymmetric dimethylarginine concentrations are

elevated in obese insulin-resistant women and fall with weight loss. *J Clin Endocrinol Metab.* 2006 May;91(5):1896–900.
DOI: https://doi.org/10.1210/jc.2005-1441

106. Shulman GI. Ectopic fat in insulin resistance, dyslipidemia, and cardiometabolic disease. *N Engl J Med.* 2014 Sep 18;371(12):1131–41.
DOI: https://doi.org/10.1056/NEJMra1011035
107. Samuel VT, Shulman GI. The pathogenesis of insulin resistance: integrating signaling pathways and substrate flux. *J Clin Invest.* 126(1):12–22.
DOI: https://doi.org/10.1172/JCI77812
108. Klöting N, Fasshauer M, Dietrich A, Kovacs P, Schön MR, Kern M, et al. Insulin-sensitive obesity. *J Physiol Endocrinol Metab.* 2010 Sep;299(3):E506–515.
DOI: https://doi.org/10.1152/ajpendo.00586.2009
109. Vague J. The degree of masculine differentiation of obesities. *Obes Res.* 1996;4(2):204–12.
DOI: https://doi.org/10.1002/j.1550-8528.1996.tb00536.x
110. Vague J. The degree of masculine differentiation of obesities: a factor determining predisposition to diabetes, atherosclerosis, gout, and uric calculous disease. *Am J Clin Nutr.* 1956;4(1):20–34.
DOI: https://doi.org/10.1093/ajcn/4.1.20
111. Karpe F, Pinnick KE. Biology of upper-body and lower-body adipose tissue – link to whole-body phenotypes. *Nat Rev Endocrinol.* 2015 Feb;11(2):90–100.
DOI: https://doi.org/10.1038/nrendo.2014.185
112. Lotta LA, Wittemans LBL, Zuber V, Stewart ID, Sharp SJ, Luan J, et al. Association of genetic variants related to gluteofemoral vs. abdominal fat distribution with type 2 diabetes, coronary disease, and cardiovascular risk factors. *JAMA.* 2018 Dec 25;320(24):2553–63.
DOI: https://doi.org/10.1001/jama.2018.19329
113. Yang Y, Xie M, Yuan S, Zeng Y, Dong Y, Wang Z, et al. Sex differences in the associations between adiposity distribution and cardiometabolic risk factors in overweight or obese individuals: a cross-sectional study. *BMC Public Health.* 2021 Jun 26;21(1):1232.
DOI: https://doi.org/10.1186/s12889-021-11316-4
114. Preis SR, Massaro JM, Robins SJ, Hoffmann U, Vasan RS, Irlbeck T, et al. Abdominal subcutaneous and visceral adipose tissue and insulin resistance in the Framingham Heart Study. *Obes Silver Spring Md.* 2010 Nov;18(11):2191–8.
DOI: https://doi.org/10.1038/oby.2010.59
115. Fox CS, Massaro JM, Hoffmann U, Pou KM, Maurovich-Horvat P, Liu CY, et al. Abdominal visceral and subcutaneous adipose tissue compartments: association with metabolic risk factors in the Framingham Heart Study. *Circulation.* 2007 Jul 3;116(1):39–48. DOI: https://doi.org/10.1161/CIRCULATIONAHA.106.675355
116. Mongraw-Chaffin M, Hairston KG, Hanley AJG, Tooze JA, Norris JM, Palmer ND, et al. Association of visceral adipose tissue and insulin resistance with incident metabolic syndrome independent of obesity status: the IRAS Family Study. *Obes Silver Spring Md.* 2021 Jul;29(7):1195–202.
DOI: https://doi.org/10.1002/oby.23177
117. Bansal SK, Bansal MB. Pathogenesis of MASLD and MASH – role of insulin resistance and lipotoxicity. *Aliment Pharmacol Ther.* 2024 Jun;59 Suppl 1:S10–22.
DOI: https://doi.org/10.1111/apt.17930
118. Yanai H, Adachi H, Hakoshima M, Iida S, Katsuyama H. Metabolic–dysfunction-associated steatotic liver disease-its pathophysiology, association with atherosclerosis and cardiovascular disease, and treatments. *Int J Mol Sci.* 2023 Oct 23;24(20):15473.
DOI: https://doi.org/10.3390/ijms242015473
119. Jung UJ, Choi MS. Obesity and its metabolic complications: the role of adipokines and the relationship between obesity, inflammation, insulin resistance, dyslipidemia and nonalcoholic fatty liver disease. *Int J Mol Sci.* 2014 Apr 11;15(4):6184–223.
DOI: https://doi.org/10.3390/ijms15046184
120. Lee MJ, Kim J. The pathophysiology of visceral adipose tissues in cardiometabolic diseases. *Biochem Pharmacol.* 2024 Apr;222:116116.
DOI: https://doi.org/10.1016/j.bcp.2024.116116
121. Cypess AM. Reassessing human adipose tissue. *N Engl J Med.* 2022 Feb 23;386(8):768–79.
DOI: https://doi.org/10.1056/NEJMra2032804
122. Arner P, Rydén M. Human white adipose tissue: a highly dynamic metabolic organ. *J Intern Med.* 2022 May;291(5):611–21.
DOI: https://doi.org/10.1111/joim.13435

123. Spalding KL, Arner E, Westermark PO, Bernard S, Buchholz BA, Bergmann O, et al. Dynamics of fat cell turnover in humans. *Nature*. 2008 Jun 5;453(7196):783–7. DOI: https://doi.org/10.1038/nature06902
124. Lee YS, Kim JW, Osborne O, Oh DY, Sasik R, Schenk S, et al. Increased adipocyte O2 consumption triggers HIF-1α, causing inflammation and insulin resistance in obesity. *Cell*. 2014 Jun 5;157(6):1339–52. DOI: https://doi.org/10.1016/j.cell.2014.05.012
125. Trayhurn P, Wang B, Wood IS. Hypoxia in adipose tissue: a basis for the dysregulation of tissue function in obesity? *Br J Nutr*. 2008 Aug;100(2):227–35. DOI: https://doi.org/10.1017/S0007114508971282
126. Lindhorst A, Raulien N, Wieghofer P, Eilers J, Rossi FMV, Bechmann I, et al. Adipocyte death triggers a pro-inflammatory response and induces metabolic activation of resident macrophages. *Cell Death Dis*. 2021 Jun 5;12(6):579. DOI: https://doi.org/10.1038/s41419-021-03872-9
127. Suganami T, Nishida J, Ogawa Y. A paracrine loop between adipocytes and macrophages aggravates inflammatory changes: role of free fatty acids and tumor necrosis factor alpha. *Arterioscler Thromb Vasc Biol*. 2005 Oct;25(10):2062–8. DOI: https://doi.org/10.1161/01.ATV.0000183883.72263.13
128. Sun K, Li X, Scherer PE. Extracellular matrix (ECM) and fibrosis in adipose tissue: overview and perspectives. *Compr Physiol*. 2023 Jan 30;13(1):4387–407. DOI: https://doi.org/10.1002/cphy.c220020
129. Crewe C, An YA, Scherer PE. The ominous triad of adipose tissue dysfunction: inflammation, fibrosis, and impaired angiogenesis. *J Clin Invest*. 2017 Jan 3;127(1):74–82. DOI: https://doi.org/10.1172/JCI88883
130. Gliniak CM, Pedersen L, Scherer PE. Adipose tissue fibrosis: the unwanted houseguest invited by obesity. *J Endocrinol*. 2023 Dec 1;259(3):e230180. DOI: https://doi.org/10.1530/JOE-23-0180
131. Fuster JJ, Ouchi N, Gokce N, Walsh K. Obesity-induced changes in adipose tissue microenvironment and their impact on cardiovascular disease. *Circ Res*. 2016 May 27;118(11):1786–807. DOI: https://doi.org/10.1161/CIRCRESAHA.115.306885
132. Xu S, Lu F, Gao J, Yuan Y. Inflammation-mediated metabolic regulation in adipose tissue. *Obes Rev Off J Int Assoc Study Obes*. 2024 Jun;25(6):e13724. DOI: https://doi.org/10.1111/obr.13724
133. Wang CH, Wang CH, Hung PJ, Wei YH. Disruption of mitochondria-associated ER membranes impairs insulin sensitivity and thermogenic function of adipocytes. *Front Cell Dev Biol* . 2022 Sep 9;10. Available from: https://www.frontiersin.org/journals/cell-and-developmental-biology/articles/10.3389/fcell.2022.965523/full
134. Guilherme A, Virbasius JV, Puri V, Czech MP. Adipocyte dysfunctions linking obesity to insulin resistance and type 2 diabetes. *Nat Rev Mol Cell Biol*. 2008 May;9(5):367–77. DOI: https://doi.org/10.1038/nrm2391
135. Kim JA, Wei Y, Sowers JR. Role of mitochondrial dysfunction in insulin resistance. *Circ Res*. 2008 Feb 29;102(4):401–14. DOI: https://doi.org/10.1161/CIRCRESAHA.107.165472
136. Jackisch L, Murphy AM, Kumar S, Randeva H, Tripathi G, McTernan PG. Tunicamycin-induced endoplasmic reticulum stress mediates mitochondrial dysfunction in human adipocytes. *J Clin Endocrinol Metab*. 2020 Sep 1;105(9):dgaa258. DOI: https://doi.org/10.1210/clinem/dgaa258
137. Kahn SE, Hull RL, Utzschneider KM. Mechanisms linking obesity to insulin resistance and type 2 diabetes. *Nature*. 2006 Dec 14;444(7121):840–6. DOI: https://doi.org/10.1038/nature05482
138. Ellulu MS, Patimah I, Khaza'ai H, Rahmat A, Abed Y. Obesity and inflammation: the linking mechanism and the complications. *Arch Med Sci AMS*. 2017 Jun;13(4):851–63. DOI: https://doi.org/10.5114/aoms.2016.58928
139. Younossi ZM, Golabi P, Paik JM, Henry A, Van Dongen C, Henry L. The global epidemiology of nonalcoholic fatty liver disease (NAFLD) and nonalcoholic steatohepatitis (NASH): a systematic review. *Hepatol Baltim Md*. 2023 Apr;77(4):1335–47. DOI: https://doi.org/10.1097/HEP.0000000000000004
140. Whelton PK, Carey RM, Aronow WS, Casey DE, Collins KJ, Dennison Himmelfarb C, et al. 2017

ACC/AHA/AAPA/ABC/ACPM/AGS/APhA/ASH/ASPC/NMA/PCNA Guideline for the prevention, detection, evaluation, and management of high blood pressure in adults: executive summary: a report of the American College of Cardiology/American Heart Association Task Force on Clinical Practice Guidelines. *Hypertens Dallas Tex 1979*. 2018 Jun;71(6):1269–324. DOI: https://doi.org/10.1161/HYP.0000000000000066

141. Kim MS, Kim WJ, Khera AV, Kim JY, Yon DK, Lee SW, et al. Association between adiposity and cardiovascular outcomes: an umbrella review and meta-analysis of observational and Mendelian randomization studies. *Eur Heart J*. 2021 Sep 7;42(34):3388–403. DOI: https://doi.org/10.1093/eurheartj/ehab454
142. Hall ME, Cohen JB, Ard JD, Egan BM, Hall JE, Lavie CJ, et al. Weight-loss strategies for prevention and treatment of hypertension: a scientific statement from the American Heart Association. *Hypertens Dallas Tex 1979*. 2021 Nov;78(5):e38–50. DOI: https://doi.org/10.1161/HYP.0000000000000202
143. Koenen M, Hill MA, Cohen P, Sowers JR. Obesity, adipose tissue and vascular dysfunction. *Circ Res*. 2021 Apr 2;128(7):951–68. DOI: https://doi.org/10.1161/CIRCRESAHA.121.318093
144. Henein MY, Vancheri S, Longo G, Vancheri F. The role of inflammation in cardiovascular disease. *Int J Mol Sci*. 2022 Oct 26;23(21):12906. DOI: https://doi.org/10.3390/ijms232112906
145. Ren J, Wu NN, Wang S, Sowers JR, Zhang Y. Obesity cardiomyopathy: evidence, mechanisms, and therapeutic implications. *Physiol Rev*. 2021 Oct 1;101(4):1745–807. DOI: https://doi.org/10.1152/physrev.00030.2020
146. Li C, Qin D, Hu J, Yang Y, Hu D, Yu B. Inflamed adipose tissue: A culprit underlying obesity and heart failure with preserved ejection fraction. *Front Immunol*. 2022 Nov 22;13:947147. DOI: https://doi.org/10.3389/fimmu.2022.947147
147. Nakamura M, Sadoshima J. Cardiomyopathy in obesity, insulin resistance and diabetes. *J Physiol*. 2020 Jul;598(14):2977–93. DOI: https://doi.org/10.1113/JP276747
148. Barber TM, Dimitriadis GK, Andreou A, Franks S. Polycystic ovary syndrome: insight into pathogenesis and a common association with insulin resistance. *Clin Med Lond Engl*. 2015 Dec;15 Suppl 6:s72–76. DOI: https://doi.org/10.7861/clinmedicine.15-6-s72
149. Ollila MME, Piltonen T, Puukka K, Ruokonen A, Järvelin MR, Tapanainen JS, et al. Weight gain and dyslipidemia in early adulthood associate with polycystic ovary syndrome: prospective cohort study. *J Clin Endocrinol Metab*. 2016 Feb;101(2):739–47. DOI: https://doi.org/10.1210/jc.2015-3543
150. Diamanti-Kandarakis E. Role of obesity and adiposity in polycystic ovary syndrome. *Int J Obes 2005*. 2007 Nov;31 Suppl 2:S8–13; discussion S31–32. DOI: https://doi.org/10.1038/sj.ijo.0803730
151. Messinis IE, Messini CI, Anifandis G, Dafopoulos K. Polycystic ovaries and obesity. *Best Pract Res Clin Obstet Gynaecol*. 2015 May;29(4):479–88. DOI: https://doi.org/10.1016/j.bpobgyn.2014.11.001
152. Practice Committee of the American Society for Reproductive Medicine. Obesity and reproduction: a committee opinion. *Fertil Steril*. 2015 Nov;104(5):1116–26. DOI: https://doi.org/10.1016/j.fertnstert.2015.08.018
153. Broughton DE, Moley KH. Obesity and female infertility: potential mediators of obesity's impact. *Fertil Steril*. 2017 Apr;107(4):840–7. DOI: https://doi.org/10.1016/j.fertnstert.2017.01.017
154. Medenica S, Spoltore ME, Ormazabal P, Marina LV, Sojat AS, Faggiano A, et al. Female infertility in the era of obesity: the clash of two pandemics or inevitable consequence? *Clin Endocrinol (Oxf)*. 2023 Feb;98(2):141–52. DOI: https://doi.org/10.1111/cen.14785
155. Haase CL, Varbo A, Laursen PN, Schnecke V, Balen AH. Association between body mass index, weight loss and the chance of pregnancy in women with polycystic ovary syndrome and overweight or obesity: a retrospective cohort study in the UK. *Hum Reprod Oxf Engl*. 2023 Mar 1;38(3):471–81. DOI: https://doi.org/10.1093/humrep/deac267
156. Drager LF, Togeiro SM, Polotsky VY, Lorenzi-Filho G. Obstructive sleep apnea: a cardiometabolic risk in obesity and the metabolic syndrome. *J Am Coll Cardiol*. 2013 Aug 13;62(7):569–76.

DOI: https://doi.org/10.1016/j.jacc.2013.05.045
157. Alterki A, Abu-Farha M, Al Shawaf E, Al-Mulla F, Abubaker J. Investigating the relationship between obstructive sleep apnoea, inflammation and cardio-metabolic diseases. *Int J Mol Sci*. 2023 Apr 6;24(7):6807. DOI: https://doi.org/10.3390/ijms24076807
158. Reyes Noriega N, Del-Río-Navarro BE, Berber A, de Jesús Romero Tapia S, Molina Díaz DJM. Effect of obesity on lung function in the pediatric and adult populations with asthma: a review. *J Clin Med*. 2023 Aug 19;12(16):5385. DOI: https://doi.org/10.3390/jcm12165385
159. Eun Y, Han K, Lee SW, Kim K, Kang S, Lee S, et al. Altered risk of incident gout according to changes in metabolic syndrome status: a nationwide, population-based cohort study of 1.29 million young men. *Arthritis Rheumatol Hoboken NJ*. 2023 May;75(5):806–15. DOI: https://doi.org/10.1002/art.42381
160. Yang Y, Xian W, Wu D, Huo Z, Hong S, Li Y, et al. The role of obesity, type 2 diabetes, and metabolic factors in gout: a Mendelian randomization study. *Front Endocrinol*. 2022;13:917056. DOI: https://doi.org/10.3389/fendo.2022.917056
161. Bo S, Ciccone G, Baldi C, Benini L, Dusio F, Forastiere G, et al. Effectiveness of a lifestyle intervention on metabolic syndrome. A randomized controlled trial. *J Gen Intern Med*. 2007 Dec;22(12):1695–703. DOI: https://doi.org/10.1007/s11606-007-0399-6
162. Yamaoka K, Tango T. Effects of lifestyle modification on metabolic syndrome: a systematic review and meta-analysis. *BMC Med*. 2012 Nov 14;10:138. DOI: https://doi.org/10.1186/1741-7015-10-138
163. Potter GDM, Cade JE, Hardie LJ. Longer sleep is associated with lower BMI and favorable metabolic profiles in UK adults: findings from the National Diet and Nutrition Survey. *PloS One*. 2017;12(7):e0182195. DOI: https://doi.org/10.1371/journal.pone.0182195
164. Wing RR, Lang W, Wadden TA, Safford M, Knowler WC, Bertoni AG, et al. Benefits of modest weight loss in improving cardiovascular risk factors in overweight and obese individuals with type 2 diabetes. *Diabetes Care*. 2011 Jul;34(7):1481–6. DOI: https://doi.org/10.2337/dc10-2415
165. Magkos F, Fraterrigo G, Yoshino J, Luecking C, Kirbach K, Kelly SC, et al. Effects of moderate and subsequent progressive weight loss on metabolic function and adipose tissue biology in humans with obesity. *Cell Metab*. 2016 Apr 12;23(4):591–601. DOI: https://doi.org/10.1016/j.cmet.2016.02.005
166. Kuna ST, Reboussin DM, Strotmeyer ES, Millman RP, Zammit G, Walkup MP, et al. Effects of weight loss on obstructive sleep apnea severity. ten-year results of the Sleep AHEAD study. *Am J Respir Crit Care Med*. 2021 Jan 15;203(2):221–9. DOI: https://doi.org/10.1164/rccm.201912-2511OC
167. Tahrani AA, Morton J. Benefits of weight loss of 10% or more in patients with overweight or obesity: a review. *Obes Silver Spring Md*. 2022 Apr;30(4):802–40. DOI: https://doi.org/10.1002/oby.23371
168. Koutoukidis DA, Astbury NM, Tudor KE, Morris E, Henry JA, Noreik M, et al. Association of weight loss interventions with changes in biomarkers of nonalcoholic fatty liver disease: a systematic review and meta-analysis. *JAMA Intern Med*. 2019 Sep 1;179(9):1262–71. DOI: https://doi.org/10.1001/jamainternmed.2019.2248
169. Takawy MW, Abdelmalek MF. Impact of weight loss on metabolic dysfunction associated steatohepatitis and hepatic fibrosis. *Curr Diab Rep*. 2025 Feb 18;25(1):23. DOI: https://doi.org/10.1007/s11892-025-01579-1
170. Tschöp M, Nogueiras R, Ahrén B. Gut hormone-based pharmacology: novel formulations and future possibilities for metabolic disease therapy. *Diabetologia*. 2023 Oct;66(10):1796–808. DOI: https://doi.org/10.1007/s00125-023-05929-0
171. Szekeres Z, Nagy A, Jahner K, Szabados E. Impact of selected glucagon-like peptide-1 receptor agonists on serum lipids, adipose tissue, and muscle metabolism – a narrative review. *Int J Mol Sci*. 2024 Jul 27;25(15):8214. DOI: https://doi.org/10.3390/ijms25158214
172. Stafeev I, Sorkina E, Koksharova E, Tumanyan T, Sklyanik I, Menshikov M, et al. The effects of glucagon-like peptide type 1 (GLP-1) and its analogues in adipose tissue: is there a way to thermogenesis? *Curr Mol Med*. 2021;21(7):527–38.

DOI: https://doi.org/10.2174/1566524020666201201095029
173. Campbell DB, Sobol CG, Stacy MR, Atway S, Teng X, Haurani MJ, et al. Revascularization outcomes stratified by glycemic control in patients with diabetes mellitus and chronic limb-threatening ischemia. *Ann Vasc Surg*. 2024 Mar;100:91–100.
DOI: https://doi.org/10.1016/j.avsg.2023.10.018
174. Aronne LJ, Horn DB, le Roux CW, Ho W, Falcon BL, Gomez Valderas E, et al. Tirzepatide as compared with semaglutide for the treatment of obesity. *N Engl J Med*. 2025 May 11;
DOI: https://doi.org/10.1056/NEJMoa2416394
175. Regmi A, Aihara E, Christe ME, Varga G, Beyer TP, Ruan X, et al. Tirzepatide modulates the regulation of adipocyte nutrient metabolism through long-acting activation of the GIP receptor. *Cell Metab*. 2024 Jul 2;36(7):1534–1549.e7.
DOI: https://doi.org/10.1016/j.cmet.2024.05.010
176. Nauck MA, Müller TD. Incretin hormones and type 2 diabetes. *Diabetologia*. 2023 Oct;66(10):1780–95.
DOI: https://doi.org/10.1007/s00125-023-05956-x
177. Wilding JPH, Batterham RL, Calanna S, Davies M, Van Gaal LF, Lingvay I, et al. Once-weekly semaglutide in adults with overweight or obesity. *N Engl J Med*. 2021 Mar 18;384(11):989–1002.
DOI: https://doi.org/10.1056/NEJMoa2032183
178. De Block CEM, Dirinck E, Verhaegen A, Van Gaal LF. Efficacy and safety of high-dose glucagon-like peptide-1, glucagon-like peptide-1/glucose-dependent insulinotropic peptide, and glucagon-like peptide-1/glucagon receptor agonists in type 2 diabetes. *Diabetes Obes Metab*. 2022 May;24(5):788–805.
DOI: https://doi.org/10.1111/dom.14640
179. Bettge K, Kahle M, Abd El Aziz MS, Meier JJ, Nauck MA. Occurrence of nausea, vomiting and diarrhoea reported as adverse events in clinical trials studying glucagon-like peptide-1 receptor agonists: a systematic analysis of published clinical trials. *Diabetes Obes Metab*. 2017 Mar;19(3):336–47.
DOI: https://doi.org/10.1111/dom.12824
180. He L, Wang J, Ping F, Yang N, Huang J, Li Y, et al. Association of glucagon-like peptide-1 receptor agonist use with risk of gallbladder and biliary diseases: a systematic review and meta-analysis of randomized clinical trials. *JAMA Intern Med*. 2022 May 1;182(5):513–9. DOI: https://doi.org/10.1001/jamainternmed.2022.0338
181. Kelly CA, Sipos JA. Approach to the patient with nodules: considering thyroid GLP-1 receptor agonists. *J Clin Endocrinol Metab*. 2025 May 19;110(6):e2080–7.
DOI: https://doi.org/10.1210/clinem/dgae722
182. Faillie JL, Yu OH, Yin H, Hillaire-Buys D, Barkun A, Azoulay L. Association of bile duct and gallbladder diseases with the use of incretin-based drugs in patients with type 2 diabetes mellitus. *JAMA Intern Med*. 2016 Oct 1;176(10):1474–81. DOI: https://doi.org/10.1001/jamainternmed.2016.1531
183. Blonde L, Umpierrez GE, Reddy SS, McGill JB, Berga SL, Bush M, et al. American Association of Clinical endocrinology clinical practice guideline: developing a diabetes mellitus comprehensive care plan – 2022 update. *Endocr Pract Off J Am Coll Endocrinol Am Assoc Clin Endocrinol*. 2022 Oct;28(10):923–1049.
DOI: https://doi.org/10.1016/j.eprac.2022.08.002
184. Torgerson JS, Hauptman J, Boldrin MN, Sjöström L. XENical in the prevention of diabetes in obese subjects (XENDOS) study: a randomized study of orlistat as an adjunct to lifestyle changes for the prevention of type 2 diabetes in obese patients. *Diabetes Care*. 2004 Jan;27(1):155–61.
DOI: https://doi.org/10.2337/diacare.27.1.155
185. Grunvald E, Shah R, Hernaez R, Chandar AK, Pickett-Blakely O, Teigen LM, et al. AGA clinical practice guideline on pharmacological interventions for adults with obesity. *Gastroenterology*. 2022 Nov;163(5):1198–225.
DOI: https://doi.org/10.1053/j.gastro.2022.08.045
186. DailyMed. *XENICAL – orlistat capsule*. Available from: https://dailymed.nlm.nih.gov/dailymed/drugInfo.cfm?setid=6240792b-9224-2d10-e053-2a91aa0a2c3e
187. American Diabetes Association Professional Practice Committee. 8. Obesity and weight management for the prevention and treatment of type 2 diabetes: standards of care in diabetes –2025. *Diabetes Care*. 2025 Jan 1;48(1 Suppl 1):S167–80.
DOI: https://doi.org/10.2337/dc25-S008
188. Lei XG, Ruan JQ, Lai C, Sun Z, Yang X. Efficacy

and safety of phentermine/topiramate in adults with overweight or obesity: a systematic review and meta-analysis. *Obes Silver Spring Md.* 2021 Jun;29(6):985–94. DOI: https://doi.org/10.1002/oby.23152

189. Onakpoya IJ, Lee JJ, Mahtani KR, Aronson JK, Heneghan CJ. Naltrexone-bupropion (Mysimba) in management of obesity: a systematic review and meta-analysis of unpublished clinical study reports. *Br J Clin Pharmacol.* 2020 Apr;86(4):646–67. DOI: https://doi.org/10.1111/bcp.14210
190. Greenway FL, Fujioka K, Plodkowski RA, Mudaliar S, Guttadauria M, Erickson J, et al. Effect of naltrexone plus bupropion on weight loss in overweight and obese adults (COR-I): a multicentre, randomised, double-blind, placebo-controlled, phase 3 trial. *Lancet Lond Engl.* 2010 Aug 21;376(9741):595–605. DOI: https://doi.org/10.1016/S0140-6736(10)60888-4
191. DailyMed. *CONTRAVE EXTENDED – RELEASE– naltrexone hydrochloride and bupropion hydrochloride tablet, extended release.* Available from: https://dailymed.nlm.nih.gov/dailymed/drugInfo.cfm?setid=9889a75d-4197-496c-aae1-15c9058c1d1b
192. Arterburn DE, Telem DA, Kushner RF, Courcoulas AP. Benefits and risks of bariatric surgery in adults: a review. *JAMA.* 2020 Sep 1;324(9):879–87. DOI: https://doi.org/10.1001/jama.2020.12567
193. Courcoulas AP, Daigle CR, Arterburn DE. Long term outcomes of metabolic/bariatric surgery in adults. *BMJ.* 2023 Dec 18; DOI: https://doi.org/10.1136/bmj-2022-071027
194. Thorell A. The 2020 ESPEN Arvid Wretlind lecture: metabolic response in bariatric surgery – mechanisms and clinical implications. *Clin Nutr.* 2021 May 1;40(5):2602–8. DOI: https://doi.org/10.1016/j.clnu.2021.03.044
195. Sjöström L. Review of the key results from the Swedish Obese Subjects (SOS) trial – a prospective controlled intervention study of bariatric surgery. *J Intern Med.* 2013;273(3):219–34. DOI: https://doi.org/10.1111/joim.12012
196. Carlsson LMS, Sjöholm K, Jacobson P, Andersson-Assarsson JC, Svensson PA, Taube M, et al. Life expectancy after bariatric surgery in the Swedish Obese Subjects study. *N Engl J Med.* 2020 Oct 15;383(16):1535–43. DOI: https://doi.org/10.1056/NEJMoa2002449
197. Nie Y, Zhang Y, Liu B, Meng H. Glucagon-like peptide-1 receptor agonists for the treatment of suboptimal initial clinical response and weight gain recurrence after bariatric surgery: a systematic review and meta-analysis. *Obes Surg.* 2025 Mar;35(3):808–22. DOI: https://doi.org/10.1007/s11695-025-07733-8
198. Esparham A, Mehri A, Dalili A, Richards J, Khorgami Z. Safety and efficacy of glucagon-like peptide-1 (GLP-1) receptor agonists in patients with weight regain or insufficient weight loss after metabolic bariatric surgery: a systematic review and meta-analysis. *Obes Rev Off J Int Assoc Study Obes.* 2024 Nov;25(11):e13811. DOI: https://doi.org/10.1111/obr.13811
199. Chang SH, Freeman NLB, Lee JA, Stoll CRT, Calhoun AJ, Eagon JC, et al. Early major complications after bariatric surgery in the USA, 2003–2014: a systematic review and meta-analysis. *Obes Rev Off J Int Assoc Study Obes.* 2018 Apr;19(4):529–37. DOI: https://doi.org/10.1111/obr.12647
200. Wunker C, Kumar S, Hallowell P, Collings A, Loss L, Bansal V, et al. Bariatric surgery and relevant comorbidities: a systematic review and meta-analysis. *Surg Endosc.* 2025 Mar 1;39(3):1419–48. DOI: https://doi.org/10.1007/s00464-025-11528-4
201. Kwon Y, Ha J, Lee YH, Kim D, Lee CM, Kim JH, et al. Comparative risk of anemia and related micronutrient deficiencies after Roux-en-Y gastric bypass and sleeve gastrectomy in patients with obesity: an updated meta-analysis of randomized controlled trials. *Obes Rev Off J Int Assoc Study Obes.* 2022 Apr;23(4):e13419. DOI: https://doi.org/10.1111/obr.13419
202. Liang L, Liang L, Huang Y, Liang H, Su J, Zhou Y. Incidence and risk factors of in-hospital gastrointestinal-related complications following bariatric surgery: a retrospective nationwide inpatient sample database study. *Obes Surg.* 2025 May;35(5):1790–9. DOI: https://doi.org/10.1007/s11695-025-07840-6
203. Acosta A, Streett S, Kroh MD, Cheskin LJ, Saunders KH, Kurian M, et al. White Paper AGA: POWER – Practice guide on obesity and

weight management, education, and resources. *Clin Gastroenterol Hepatol Off Clin Pract J Am Gastroenterol Assoc*. 2017 May;15(5):631–649.e10. DOI: https://doi.org/10.1016/j.cgh.2016.10.023

204. Gallagher C, Corl A, Dietz WH. Weight can't wait: a guide to discussing obesity and organizing treatment in the primary care setting. *Obes Silver Spring Md*. 2021 May;29(5):821–4. DOI: https://doi.org/10.1002/oby.23154
205. Vallis M, Piccinini-Vallis H, Sharma AM, Freedhoff Y. Clinical review: modified 5 As: minimal intervention for obesity counseling in primary care. *Can Fam Physician Med Fam Can*. 2013 Jan;59(1):27–31. Available from: https://pubmed.ncbi.nlm.nih.gov/23341653/
206. Marketou ME, Buechler NS, Fragkiadakis K, Plevritaki A, Zervakis S, Maragkoudakis S, et al. Visceral fat and cardiometabolic future in children and adolescents: a critical update. *Pediatr Res*. 2023 Nov;94(5):1639–47. DOI: https://doi.org/10.1038/s41390-023-02709-9
207. Aris IM, Rifas-Shiman SL, Li LJ, Kleinman KP, Coull BA, Gold DR, et al. Patterns of body mass index milestones in early life and cardiometabolic risk in early adolescence. *Int J Epidemiol*. 2019 Feb 1;48(1):157–67. DOI: https://doi.org/10.1093/ije/dyy286
208. Juonala M, Magnussen CG, Berenson GS, Venn A, Burns TL, Sabin MA, et al. Childhood adiposity, adult adiposity, and cardiovascular risk factors. *N Engl J Med*. 2011 Nov 17;365(20):1876–85. DOI: https://doi.org/10.1056/NEJMoa1010112
209. Batsis JA, Mackenzie TA, Jones JD, Lopez-Jimenez F, Bartels SJ. Sarcopenia, sarcopenic obesity and inflammation: results from the 1999–2004 National Health and Nutrition Examination Survey. *Clin Nutr Edinb Scotl*. 2016 Dec;35(6):1472–83. DOI: https://doi.org/10.1016/j.clnu.2016.03.028
210. Agostini D, Gervasi M, Ferrini F, Bartolacci A, Stranieri A, Piccoli G, et al. An integrated approach to skeletal muscle health in aging. *Nutrients*. 2023 Apr 7;15(8):1802. DOI: https://doi.org/10.3390/nu15081802
211. Catalano PM, Shankar K. Obesity and pregnancy: mechanisms of short term and long term adverse consequences for mother and child. *BMJ*. 2017 Feb 8;356:j1. DOI: https://doi.org/10.1136/bmj.j1
212. Grieger JA, Bianco-Miotto T, Grzeskowiak LE, Leemaqz SY, Poston L, McCowan LM, et al. Metabolic syndrome in pregnancy and risk for adverse pregnancy outcomes: a prospective cohort of nulliparous women. *PLoS Med*. 2018 Dec;15(12):e1002710. DOI: https://doi.org/10.1371/journal.pmed.1002710
213. Creanga AA, Catalano PM, Bateman BT. Obesity in Pregnancy. *N Engl J Med*. 2022 Jul 21;387(3):248–59. DOI: https://doi.org/10.1056/NEJMra1801040
214. Heslehurst N, Ngongalah L, Bigirumurame T, Nguyen G, Odeniyi A, Flynn A, et al. Association between maternal adiposity measures and adverse maternal outcomes of pregnancy: systematic review and meta-analysis. *Obes Rev Off J Int Assoc Study Obes*. 2022 Jul;23(7):e13449. DOI: https://doi.org/10.1111/obr.13449
215. Misra A, Khurana L. Obesity-related noncommunicable diseases: South Asians vs. White Caucasians. *Int J Obes*. 2005. 2011 Feb;35(2):167–87. DOI: https://doi.org/10.1038/ijo.2010.135
216. Gujral UP, Vittinghoff E, Mongraw-Chaffin M, Vaidya D, Kandula NR, Allison M, et al. Cardiometabolic abnormalities among normal-weight persons from five racial/ethnic groups in the United States. *Ann Intern Med*. 2017 May 2;166(9):628–36. DOI: https://doi.org/10.7326/M16-1895
217. WHO Expert Consultation. Appropriate body-mass index for Asian populations and its implications for policy and intervention strategies. *Lancet Lond Engl*. 2004 Jan 10;363(9403):157–63. DOI: https://doi.org/10.1016/S0140-6736(03)15268-3
218. Temple NJ. A proposed strategy against obesity: how government policy can counter the obesogenic environment. *Nutrients*. 2023 Jun 27;15(13):2910. DOI: https://doi.org/10.3390/nu15132910
219. Souza LMS, Chaves SCL, Santana JM, Pereira M. Public policy interventions for preventing and treating obesity: scoping review. *Nutr Rev*. 2023 Nov 10;81(12):1653–64. DOI: https://doi.org/10.1093/nutrit/nuad028
220. Subica AM, Grills CT, Villanueva S, Douglas JA. Community organizing for healthier

communities: environmental and policy outcomes of a national initiative. *Am J Prev Med.* 2016 Dec;51(6):916–25. DOI: https://doi.org/10.1016/j.amepre.2016.06.020

221. Pujol-Busquets G, Smith J, Fàbregues S, Bach-Faig A, Larmuth K. Mixed methods evaluation of a low-carbohydrate high-fat nutrition education program for women from underserved communities in South Africa. *Appetite.* 2025 Jan 1;204:107725.
DOI: https://doi.org/10.1016/j.appet.2024.107725

Chapter Eight
The challenge of weight stigma in recognizing lipedema

Joanna Dudek

Introduction

Weight stigma is a particular type of stigmatization – a process of being marked negatively, devalued, and ostracized due to a specific characteristic – in this case, increased body weight or size.[1] People labeled as 'fat' are stereotypically judged as lazier, inferior, less intelligent, weak-willed, unhealthy, food-focused, and less active, and they are often treated according to these stereotypes.[2]

Stigmatization and associated discrimination, where individuals with excess body fat are treated less favorably or persecuted due to their body weight or size, are prevalent in almost every domain,[3] including policy and law-making,[4] media,[5, 6] education,[7] the workplace,[8, 9] sports and fitness,[10, 11, 12] social and family life,[13, 14] and healthcare.[13, 15, 16] One of the most common sources of weight stigma is from healthcare professionals, second only to family members.[17] Evidence shows that weight bias is prevalent among health professionals, including physicians, nurses, nutritionists, psychologists, physiotherapists, exercise physiologists, and health profession students.[13] Negative attitudes toward individuals with excess fat tissue in healthcare settings can be both explicit – consciously expressed, and directly influencing decisions – and implicit, operating automatically and outside of conscious awareness. The latter can affect non-verbal communication and decisions made under cognitive burden.[13, 18]

Researchers estimate that 40 to 60 per cent of adults around the world, across a range of body sizes, have experienced weight stigma at some point in their lives,[16, 19] with higher rates among women and those with higher body mass index (BMI).[14] Weight stigma is also highly prevalent among youth, with parents, peers, and teachers being its main sources.[20]

Facing societal weight stigma, either directly or indirectly (when one suspects or anticipates stigma), can affect an individual's psychological, behavioral, and physiological functioning, leading to negative health consequences. Moreover, it can lead to weight bias internalization, also called self-directed weight stigma, when an individual starts blaming or devaluing oneself. Weight bias internalization is common, especially among those with higher BMI, females, and those who experienced weight stigma in their childhood.[19]

Consequences of weight stigma

Numerous studies show that misconceptions and stereotypes associated with higher body weight/excessive fat tissue and associated mistreatment lead to multiple negative psychological and physical consequences to the extent that weight stigma has been called a psychosocial contributor to obesity,[20] a social determinant of health, and a human rights issue.[21]

Contrary to popular belief that weight stigma may be a beneficial incentive for weight loss, studies indicate that experiencing stigmatization doubles the risk of developing obesity and triples the likelihood of maintaining obesity.[2] Stigmatized individuals are more likely to binge eat, choose unhealthy foods, engage less in physical activity, have a more negative attitude towards sports, and resort to unhealthy weight control methods. Facing weight stigma increases the risk of depression, eating disorders, and other psychological difficulties, such as lower self-esteem, worsened mood, higher dissatisfaction with one's appearance, and avoidance of public places and social interactions, leading to social isolation.[3, 20] Moreover, it produces specific physiological stress responses, e.g. increased levels of cortisol or pro-inflammatory factors that can exacerbate diseases associated with chronic stress and worsen the general health of an individual.[3, 22, 23, 24] Not surprisingly, there are also several research studies providing evidence for the negative consequences of weight bias internalization for mental and physical health.[19, 25]

Weight stigma and lipedema

Despite the lack of direct research on the prevalence of weight stigma among individuals with lipedema, existing data on weight stigma and the characteristics of lipedema suggest that these individuals likely experience weight stigma and are susceptible to internalizing weight bias. Excessive fat tissue, often distributed disproportionately and therefore difficult to conceal, might make individuals with lipedema even more vulnerable to stigmatization. Moreover, within the context of little knowledge about lipedema among healthcare professionals,[26] and misdiagnosing it as obesity[27] as well as obesity that coexists with lipedema[28] we may expect that individuals with lipedema will or have been exposed to weight stigma throughout their lives.

Recent studies provide preliminary results confirming these assumptions. In the qualitative study by Christoffersen and Tennfjord,[29] individuals with lipedema have reported stigma in healthcare settings – being asked about BMI, labeled as lazy, and told that their problems will be resolved once they lose weight. They reported feeling pressured to seek treatment for increased weight despite meeting criteria for obesity, and some of them felt disrespected. In another qualitative study, several women reported that they were fat-shamed during healthcare encounters, were given unsupportive advice, judged as weak-willed, and mistreated. Some of them had to see many healthcare professionals before obtaining the diagnosis. Others mentioned blaming themselves and feeling guilty for having lipedema.[30] In a quantitative study conducted in Sweden, participants with lipedema reported lower satisfaction with healthcare than the general Swedish female population. Furthermore, higher levels of stigma among participants were related to lower physical and social functioning and emotional well-being.[31] Common sources of weight stigma and examples are shown in Table 8.1.

Table 8.1: Common sources of weight stigma.

Source	Examples
Healthcare providers	Judgmental comments, misdiagnosis, bias during exams
Family members	Shaming, pressure to lose weight, negative comparisons
Media	Stereotypical portrayals, unrealistic body images
Peers and teachers	Bullying, exclusion, labeling
Workplace	Discrimination in hiring, pay inequity

Lipedema diagnosis

Individuals with lipedema report that the prolonged time to obtain the right diagnosis, typically taking decades from when the first symptoms occur, is connected with the effort of visiting numerous specialists.[27, 32, 33] Without the diagnosis, they may be offered or may try ineffective treatment options. This can have multiple negative consequences for physical health (such as the risk of progression, loss of mobility, secondary lymphedema, and other problems), as well as mental health (depression, eating disorders, lowered self-esteem). Therefore, researchers emphasize the need for early diagnosis.[32]

One of the challenges on an already difficult path to obtaining the right diagnosis might be weight stigma. Although there is no research looking precisely into the role of weight stigma in recognizing lipedema, we believe that it may pose a challenge in three ways: one connected to the over-attribution of symptoms to obesity, another to the mistreatment caused by the pervasiveness of weight stigma in general and especially in healthcare settings, and finally, one related to weight bias internalization.

Over-attribution of symptoms to excessive weight/fat tissue

Due to explicit or implicit negative attitudes toward people with excessive fat tissue, healthcare professionals are overly focused on BMI. They tend to over-attribute symptoms and problems to obesity and fail to consider treatment options beyond advising the patient to lose weight.[34] They may miss important symptoms reported by the patient, which further prolongs the time to obtain the right diagnosis. If healthcare professionals are not familiar with lipedema and unaware of the impact of weight stigma on their behavior, they may overlook the need for further diagnosis, and dismiss the patient's concerns, attributing them solely to high body weight (e.g. concerns such as chronic pain, heaviness, and swelling associated with lipedema). Furthermore, this can be exacerbated by gender bias related to how we perceive pain.[35, 36, 37, 38] Pain reported by women is often invalidated, seen as less severe than reported, unimportant, or treated as a symptom attributed to psychological factors. Due to this bias common in healthcare, pain, as one of the important symptoms of lipedema,[39,40] may be overlooked or disregarded.

Some of the biases discussed in this chapter may contribute to the fact that women are, on average, diagnosed later than men with various chronic conditions,[41,42] or have to wait longer for the correct diagnosis.[43] Cleghorn[44] has thoroughly investigated this topic, examining the historical roots of the prolonged misdiagnosis and mistreatment of women's bodies. Lipedema, which could be included as an example of a misdiagnosed disease, is discussed in her book.

Mistreatment caused by the pervasiveness of weight stigma

Another potential pathway to explain the negative role of weight stigma in recognizing lipedema is the mistreatment related to the pervasiveness of weight stigma in general, and especially in healthcare settings. If healthcare workers have negative attitudes towards individuals with excess body fat and perceive them as less disciplined, non-compliant, and more irritating, they also tend to treat them differently.[45] The higher the patient's BMI, the less patience and respect they received, the less willingness to help them, and the more the meeting with the patient was seen as a waste of time.[2, 18, 46] It was shown that the higher the BMI, the lower the 'patient-doctor' alliance.[47] The patient, feeling that they are perceived in terms of their stigmatized identity (excessive weight), can change the way they perceive their health provider, and in turn, it can affect their compliance.[18] Individuals experiencing such stigmatization often start avoiding medical visits and check-ups, which leads to a deterioration of their overall health and makes it harder to obtain help.[18, 45, 48] It is then possible that some individuals with lipedema, having experienced stigmatization (directly or indirectly), decide to stop looking for medical help for their symptoms as they want to avoid another unpleasant experience or mistreatment.

Weight bias internalization

Finally, there is also a possibility that self-directed weight stigma can affect the process of obtaining a diagnosis. When an individual starts to blame themselves for their weight, to think negatively about themselves and their body, and to believe they are lazy or just need to work harder to lose weight, they can experience a decrease in mood, lower self-esteem, depression, and other mental health problems.[25] Eventually, they may give up on any actions to improve their well-being and health whatsoever. Once stigma is internalized, a person may invalidate their own experiences and miss important signals from their body by attributing symptoms to poor self-control or laziness and thereby minimizing pain or other physical sensations by treating them as a punishment for 'bad' behavior. They might avoid the healthcare system not solely because of fear of being mistreated but rather because they do not believe they can be offered anything useful. Therefore, they do not actively seek help, can underreport their symptoms or report them inaccurately, and avoid opportunities to learn about the diagnosis (see Table 8.2).

Table 8.2: Effects of internalized weight stigma.

Effect	Description
Low self-esteem	Chronic self-criticism and negative self-image
Avoidance of healthcare	Skipping medical appointments due to fear of judgment
Social isolation	Avoidance of public spaces or activities
Disordered eating	Binge eating, starvation, or emotional eating
Reduced treatment-seeking	Belief that symptoms are deserved or self-inflicted

Strategies for bias reduction

Raising awareness about lipedema among healthcare professionals and the general public is essential to ensure timely and accurate diagnoses, which can expedite patients' access to proper treatment and improve their quality of life. Yet, we cannot forget about the role of weight stigma, weight bias internalization, and gender bias related to pain. Without addressing them, lipedema symptoms may still be overlooked or dismissed. The first crucial step to change is raising awareness of weight stigma and other biases among healthcare professionals, students, and the general public. Being aware of one's attitudes, their consequences, and their impact on decisions and behaviors is necessary to change one's behavior.[21]

Researchers have proposed numerous interventions for weight stigma in healthcare, such as education early in the students' training and continuously afterwards, about empathy-evoking or weight-inclusive approaches (see review in Talumaa et al, 2022[16]), and internalized weight stigma.[49, 50, 51] Public health policy changes have also been suggested; for example, those related to language usage, changing laws to address weight discrimination, and using media to correct misinformation and change narratives about body weight.[3, 14] Nutter and colleagues[21] proposed a number of recommendations for a global effort to reduce stigma: raising awareness of weight stigma, focusing on weight-neutral health promotion, using non-stigmatizing, inclusive language, distinguishing between body size and obesity (BMI being an insufficient tool for diagnosis), and finally, conducting further research.

Conclusion

In conclusion, increasing knowledge about lipedema and targeting weight stigma and gender bias related to pain might not only increase the number of individuals who will be diagnosed sooner and therefore avoid the physical or mental consequences of advanced lipedema, but also improve their overall health and well-being.

References

1. Puhl RM, Heuer CA. The stigma of obesity: a review and update. *Obesity*. 2009;17(5):941–64. DOI: https://doi.org/10.1038/oby.2008.636
2. Puhl RM, Heuer CA. Obesity stigma: important considerations for public health. *Am J Public Health*. 2010 Jun 1;100(6):1019–28. DOI: https://doi.org/10.2105/ajph.2009.159491
3. Brown A, Flint SW, Batterham RL. Pervasiveness, impact and implications of weight stigma. *eClinicalMedicine*. 2022 May 1;47. Available from: https://www.thelancet.com/journals/eclinm/article/PIIS2589-5370(22)00138-9/fulltext?dm_i=1M7S%2C7XVUJ%2C9LQ0BB%2CWGA9P%2C1
4. Meadows A, Daníelsdóttir S, Goldberg D, Mercedes M. Fighting for a (wide enough) seat at the table: weight stigma in law and policy. Fat Stud. 2021 May 4;10(2):101–24. DOI: https://doi.org/10.1080/21604851.2020.1835295
5. Clark O, Lee MM, Jingree ML, O'Dwyer E, Yue Y, Marrero A, et al. Weight stigma and social media: evidence and public health solutions. *Front Nutr*. 2021 Nov 12;8. Available from: https://www.frontiersin.org/journals/nutrition/articles/10.3389/fnut.2021.739056/full
6. Wanniarachchi VU, Mathrani A, Susnjak T, Scogings C. A systematic literature review: what is the current stance towards weight stigmatization in social media platforms? *Int J Hum-Comput Stud*. 2020 Mar 1;135:102371. DOI: https://doi.org/10.1016/j.ijhcs.2019.102371
7. Nutter S, Ireland A, Alberga AS, Brun I, Lefebvre D, Hayden KA, et al. Weight bias in educational settings: a systematic review. Curr Obes Rep. 2019 Jun 1;8(2):185–200. DOI: https://doi.org/10.1007/s13679-019-00330-8
8. Gaines R, Vincent V. Weight discrimination: implications to the workplace. *Strateg HR Rev*. 2022 Feb 22;21(2):54–8. DOI: https://doi.org/10.1108/SHR-01-2022-0002
9. Giel KE, Thiel A, Teufel M, Mayer J, Zipfel S. Weight bias in work settings – a qualitative review. *Obes Facts*. 2010 Mar;3(1):33–40. DOI: https://doi.org/10.1159/000276992
10. Panza GA, Armstrong LE, Taylor BA, Puhl RM, Livingston J, Pescatello LS. Weight bias among exercise and nutrition professionals: a systematic review. *Obes Rev*. 2018;19(11):1492–503. DOI: https://doi.org/10.1111/obr.12743
11. Schvey NA, Sbrocco T, Bakalar JL, Ress R, Barmine M, Gorlick J, et al. The experience of weight stigma among gym members with overweight and obesity. *Stigma Health*. 2017;2(4):292–306. DOI: https://doi.org/10.1037/sah0000062
12. Thedinga HK, Zehl R, Thiel A. Weight stigma experiences and self-exclusion from sport and exercise settings among people with obesity. *BMC Public Health*. 2021 Mar 22;21(1):565. DOI: https://doi.org/10.1186/s12889-021-10565-7
13. Lawrence BJ, Kerr D, Pollard CM, Theophilus M, Alexander E, Haywood D, et al. Weight bias among health care professionals: a systematic review and meta-analysis. Obesity. 2021;29(11):1802–12. DOI: https://doi.org/10.1002/oby.23266
14. Lawrence SE, Puhl RM, Schwartz MB, Watson RJ, Foster GD. 'The most hurtful thing I've ever experienced': a qualitative examination of the

nature of experiences of weight stigma by family members. *SSM - Qual Res Health*. 2022 Dec 1;2:100073. DOI: https://doi.org/10.1016/j.ssmqr.2022.100073
15. Ryan L, Coyne R, Heary C, Birney S, Crotty M, Dunne R, et al. Weight stigma experienced by patients with obesity in healthcare settings: a qualitative evidence synthesis. *Obes Rev*. 2023;24(10):e13606. DOI: https://doi.org/10.1111/obr.13606
16. Talumaa B, Brown A, Batterham RL, Kalea AZ. Effective strategies in ending weight stigma in healthcare. *Obes Rev*. 2022;23(10):e13494. DOI: https://doi.org/10.1111/obr.13494
17. Puhl RM, Brownell KD. Confronting and coping with weight stigma: an investigation of overweight and obese adults. *Obesity*. 2006;14(10):1802–15. DOI: https://doi.org/10.1038/oby.2006.208
18. Phelan SM, Burgess DJ, Yeazel MW, Hellerstedt WL, Griffin JM, van Ryn M. Impact of weight bias and stigma on quality of care and outcomes for patients with obesity. *Obes Rev*. 2015;16(4):319–26. DOI: https://doi.org/10.1111/obr.12266
19. Puhl RM, Lessard LM, Pearl RL, Himmelstein MS, Foster GD. International comparisons of weight stigma: addressing a void in the field. *Int J Obes*. 2021 Sep;45(9):1976–85. DOI: https://doi.org/10.1038/s41366-021-00860-z
20. Puhl RM, Himmelstein MS, Pearl RL. Weight stigma as a psychosocial contributor to obesity. *Am Psychol*. 2020;75(2):274–89. DOI: https://doi.org/10.1037/amp0000538
21. Nutter S, Eggerichs LA, Nagpal TS, Ramos Salas X, Chin Chea C, Saiful S, et al. Changing the global obesity narrative to recognize and reduce weight stigma: a position statement from the World Obesity Federation. *Obes Rev*. 2024;25(1):e13642. DOI: https://doi.org/10.1111/obr.13642
22. Himmelstein MS, Incollingo Belsky AC, Tomiyama AJ. The weight of stigma: cortisol reactivity to manipulated weight stigma. *Obesity*. 2015;23(2):368–74. DOI: https://doi.org/10.1002/oby.20959
23. Schvey NA, Puhl RM, Brownell KD. The stress of stigma: exploring the effect of weight stigma on cortisol reactivity. *Biopsychosoc Sci Med*. 2014 Mar;76(2):156. DOI: https://doi.org/10.1097/PSY.0000000000000031
24. Wu YK, Berry DC. Impact of weight stigma on physiological and psychological health outcomes for overweight and obese adults: a systematic review. *J Adv Nurs*. 2018;74(5):1030–42. DOI: https://doi.org/10.1111/jan.13511
25. Pearl RL, Puhl RM. Weight bias internalization and health: a systematic review. *Obes Rev*. 2018;19(8):1141–63. DOI: https://doi.org/10.1111/obr.12701
26. Tiwari A, Myint F, Hamilton G. Management of lower limb lymphoedema in the United Kingdom. *Eur J Vasc Endovasc Surg*. 2006 Mar 1;31(3):311–5. DOI: https://doi.org/10.1016/j.ejvs.2005.09.017
27. Buck DW, Herbst KL. Lipedema: a relatively common disease with extremely common misconceptions. *Plast Reconstr Surg – Glob Open*. 2016 Sep;4(9):e1043. DOI: https://doi.org/10.1097/GOX.0000000000001043
28. Ghods M, Georgiou I, Schmidt J, Kruppa P. Disease progression and comorbidities in lipedema patients: a 10-year retrospective analysis. *Dermatol Ther*. 2020;33(6):e14534. DOI: https://doi.org/10.1111/dth.14534
29. Christoffersen V, Tennfjord MK. Younger women with lipedema, their experiences with healthcare providers, and the importance of social support and belonging: a qualitative study. *Int J Environ Res Public Health*. 2023 Jan;20(3):1925. DOI: https://doi.org/10.3390/ijerph20031925
30. Melander C, Juuso,Päivi, and Olsson M. Women's experiences of living with lipedema. *Health Care Women Int*. 2022 Mar 4;43(1–3):54–69. DOI: https://doi.org/10.1080/07399332.2021.1932894
31. Falck J, Herbst K, Rolander B, Nygårdh A, Jonasson LL, Mårtensson J. Health-related stigma, perceived social support, and their role in quality of life among women with lipedema. *Health Care Women Int*. 2025 May 8;1–19. DOI: https://doi.org/10.1080/07399332.2025.2499487
32. Kruppa P, Georgiou I, Biermann N, Prantl L, Klein-Weigel P, Ghods M. Lipedema – pathogenesis, diagnosis, and treatment options. *Dtsch Ärztebl Int*. 2020 Jun;117(22–23):396. DOI: https://doi.org/10.3238/arztebl.2020.0396
33. van la Parra RFD, Deconinck C, Pirson G, Servaes M, Fosseprez P. Lipedema: what we don't know.

J Plast Reconstr Aesthetic Surg JPRAS. 2023 Sep;84:302–12. DOI: https://doi.org/10.1016/j.bjps.2023.05.056
34. Persky S, Eccleston CP. Medical student bias and care recommendations for an obese versus non-obese virtual patient. *Int J Obes* 2005. 2011 May;35(5):728–35. DOI: https://doi.org/10.1038/ijo.2010.173
35. Hoffmann DE, Tarzian AJ. The girl who cried pain: a bias against women in the treatment of pain. *J Law Med Ethics J Am Soc Law Med Ethics*. 2001;29(1):13–27. DOI: https://doi.org/10.1111/j.1748-720x.2001.tb00037.x
36. Samulowitz A, Gremyr I, Eriksson E, Hensing G. 'Brave men' and 'emotional women': a theory-guided literature review on gender bias in health care and gendered norms towards patients with chronic pain. *Pain Res Manag*. 2018;6358624. DOI: https://doi.org/10.1155/2018/6358624
37. Schäfer G, Prkachin KM, Kaseweter KA, Williams AC de C. Health care providers' judgments in chronic pain: the influence of gender and trustworthiness. *Pain*. 2016 Aug;157(8):1618–25. DOI: https://doi.org/10.1097/j.pain.0000000000000536
38. Zhang L, Losin EAR, Ashar YK, Koban L, Wager TD. Gender biases in estimation of others' pain. *J Pain*. 2021 Sep;22(9):1048–59. DOI: https://doi.org/10.1016/j.jpain.2021.03.001
39. Aksoy H, Karadag AS, Wollina U. Cause and management of lipedema-associated pain. *Dermatol Ther*. 2021 Jan;34(1):e14364. DOI: https://doi.org/10.1111/dth.14364
40. Hucho T. [Lipedema pain-the neglected symptom]. *Dermatol Heidelb Ger*. 2023 Aug;74(8):575–9. DOI: https://doi.org/10.1007/s00105-023-05189-4
41. Sun TY, Hardin J, Nieva HR, Natarajan K, Cheng R fong, Ryan P, et al. Large-scale characterization of gender differences in diagnosis prevalence and time to diagnosis. *medRxiv*. 2023 Oct 16;2023.10.12.23296976. DOI: https://doi.org/2023.10.12.23296976
42. Westergaard D, Moseley P, Sørup FKH, Baldi P, Brunak S. Population-wide analysis of differences in disease progression patterns in men and women. *Nat Commun*. 2019 Feb 8;10(1):666. DOI: https://doi.org/10.1038/s41467-019-08475-9
43. Merone L, Tsey K, Russell D, Daltry A, Nagle C. Self-reported time to diagnosis and proportions of rediagnosis in female patients with chronic conditions in Australia: a cross-sectional survey. *Womens Health Rep*. 2022 Sep 12;3(1):749–58. DOI: https://doi.org/10.1089/whr.2022.0040
44. Cleghorn E. *Unwell Women: Misdiagnosis and Myth in a Man-Made World*. New York: Dutton; 2021. 400 pp. Available from: https://www.penguinrandomhouse.com/books/646468/unwell-women-by-elinor-cleghorn/
45. Tomiyama AJ, Carr D, Granberg EM, Major B, Robinson E, Sutin AR, et al. How and why weight stigma drives the obesity 'epidemic' and harms health. *BMC Med*. 2018 Aug 15;16(1):123. DOI: https://doi.org/10.1186/s12916-018-1116-5
46. Huizinga MM, Cooper LA, Bleich SN, Clark JM, Beach MC. Physician respect for patients with obesity. *J Gen Intern Med*. 2009 Nov;24(11):1236–9. DOI: https://doi.org/10.1007/s11606-009-1104-8
47. Gudzune KA, Beach MC, Roter DL, Cooper LA. Physicians build less rapport with obese patients. *Obes Silver Spring Md*. 2013 Oct;21(10):2146–52. DOI: https://doi.org/10.1002/oby.20384
48. Puhl R, Suh Y. Health consequences of weight stigma: implications for obesity prevention and treatment. *Curr Obes Rep*. 2015 Jun;4(2):182–90. DOI: https://doi.org/10.1007/s13679-015-0153-z
49. Davies AE, Burnette CB, Ravyts SG, Mazzeo SE. A randomized control trial of Expand Your Horizon: an intervention for women with weight bias internalization. *Body Image*. 2022 Mar;40:138–45. DOI: https://doi.org/10.1016/j.bodyim.2021.12.006
50. Haley EN, Dolbier CL, Campbell LC, Carels RA, Braciszewski JM. Brief Self-compassion intervention for women of higher weight and internalized weight bias: a randomized pilot study. *Int J Behav Med*. 2025 Apr;32(2):293–307. DOI: https://doi.org/10.1007/s12529-024-10297-z
51. Pearl RL, Wadden TA, Bach C, LaFata EM, Gautam S, Leonard S, et al. Long-term effects of an internalized weight stigma intervention: a randomized controlled trial. *J Consult Clin Psychol*. 2023 Jul;91(7):398–410. DOI: https://doi.org/10.1037/ccp0000819

Chapter Nine
Common lipedema co-morbidities

Angelika Chachaj and Andrzej Szuba

Introduction

Lipedema is a complex disease often associated with a variety of co-morbidities. Among these, obesity is the most frequently cited in medical literature.[1, 2, 3] Other well-documented co-morbidities include lymphatic dysfunction leading to lymphedema, hypothyroidism, physiological problems, migraine, and menstrual irregularities,[1, 2, 3] chronic venous disease, and joint hypermobility.[3] Addressing these co-morbidities is crucial for enhancing treatment effectiveness. A multidisciplinary approach involving medical professionals, nutritionists, physiotherapists, and mental health specialists is essential to provide comprehensive care tailored to the unique needs of each individual with lipedema.

Prevalence and etiology of co-morbidities

The exact prevalence of co-morbidities in individuals with lipedema remains unclear. Only a limited number of studies have investigated these co-morbidities, and most were conducted with relatively small patient samples. Larger, long-term studies are needed to accurately assess the frequency and nature of these co-morbidities. It is also still uncertain which co-morbidities are incidental, which may contribute to the onset or progression of lipedema, and which are a result of the disease itself. Additionally, distinguishing the effects of commonly coexisting obesity from those directly related to lipedema remains a significant challenge. Further pathophysiological research will be crucial in this area, as a deeper understanding of lipedema's underlying causes will improve our ability to determine the significance of its associated co-morbidities.

Another important consideration is that while lipedema frequently coexists with obesity, the cardiovascular risk, measured by the prevalence of metabolic syndrome components such as diabetes or hyperlipidemia, is lower than in the general obese population. Additionally, some co-morbidities, such as lymphedema and psychological issues, appear to result from lipedema itself and/or its association with obesity. In contrast, other diseases like hypothyroidism, joint hypermobility, and increased skin elasticity seem to genuinely co-occur with lipedema, although these conditions may also influence its onset or severity.

Co-occurrence of lipedema and obesity

Obesity is the most common comorbidity associated with lipedema, as demonstrated in numerous studies.[1, 2, 3] Although the two diseases are distinct, their overlap is significant. Lipedema is characterized by a specific pattern of fat distribution; however, many individuals with lipedema are also classified as obese, particularly in its advanced stages.[3] In a study by Ghods et al.,[1] obesity was present in 37.5% of 106 women with lipedema who underwent liposuction procedures. Similarly, a study by Patton et al.[3] involving 360 Italian patients with lipedema found that 38.9% were diagnosed with obesity. See Chapters 2 and 7 for more on this topic.

The exact pathophysiological relationship between lipedema and obesity remains unclear. It is uncertain whether a higher body mass index (BMI) contributes to the progression of lipedema or if the causal relationship also operates in reverse. It is likely that obesity and lipedema can exacerbate each other, creating a vicious cycle. Additionally, the interaction between obesity-related psychological stress and the physical symptoms of lipedema may further accelerate the progression of both diseases.

Patients with lipedema often report that their condition appeared following a significant increase in body weight. Additionally, higher disease stages are generally associated with higher BMI levels. In a study by Ghods et al.,[1] only 15% of women with stage 3 lipedema had a BMI below 35 kg/m^2. Similarly, in the Patton et al. study,[3] just 8.2% of women in the late stage of lipedema had a BMI below this threshold.

Conversely, lipedema, which has been linked to pressure-induced or spontaneous pain in adipose tissue and a feeling of heaviness in the lower extremities, can limit physical activity and contribute to emotional distress, potentially promoting further weight gain. Obesity can also have psychological consequences, such as low self-esteem and depression, which may reduce motivation to adopt healthy behaviors. These challenges are particularly significant for individuals with lipedema, as emotional well-being plays a key role in managing both diseases.

Somewhat paradoxically, despite the higher BMI in patients with lipedema, lipedema seems to be associated with a lower cardiovascular risk profile compared to those associated with lifestyle-induced obesity. Numerous studies have demonstrated that the frequency of components of metabolic syndrome, including insulin resistance, diabetes, and hyperlipidemia, is lower in lipedema than in non-lipedema obesity.[1, 2, 3, 4] To date, this observation has not been explained. Further research is needed to better understand this complex, potentially cyclical relationship and its impact on the progression of both lipedema and obesity.

Lymphatic dysfunction in lipedema

Impaired lymphatic transport in lipedema has been demonstrated in numerous imaging studies, including lymphoscintigraphy,[5, 6, 7, 8] indocyanine green (ICG) lymphography,[9, 10] and magnetic resonance (MR) lymphography.[11] In cases of lipedema without clinically visible lymphedema, abnormalities are typically of low to moderate grade,[5, 6, 8] suggesting lymphatic overload rather than complete insufficiency.

Lymphoscintigraphy performed in patients with lipedema before the onset of lymphedema often reveals additional lymphatic vessels and popliteal lymph nodes.[9] As lipedema progresses, lymphatic efficiency tends to decline.[7, 8] In its most advanced stage, lipedema is associated with lymphatic insufficiency, sometimes clinically referred to as lipolymphedema, or lipedema with secondary lymphedema.[12, 13]

Clinically, both lipedema and lifestyle-induced

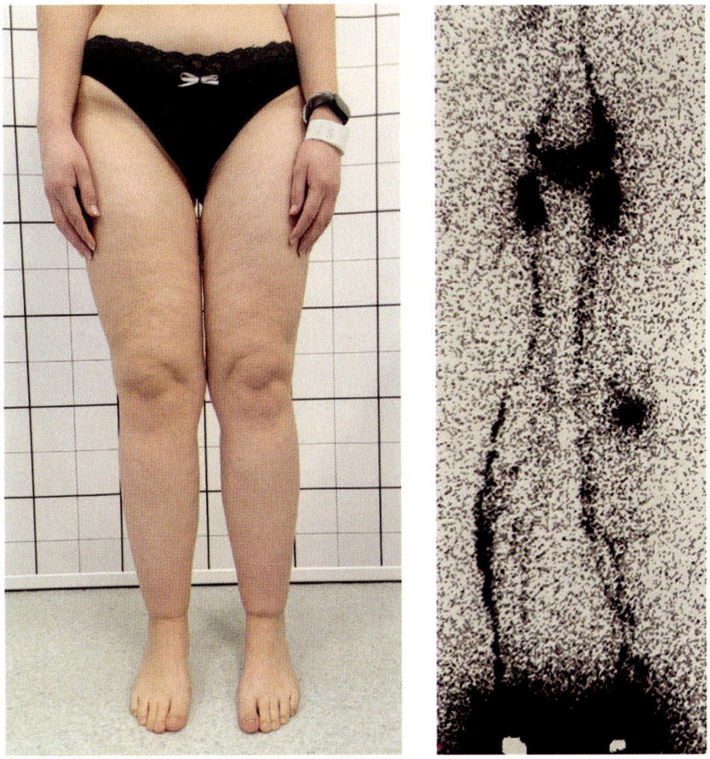

Figure 9.1: Lymphatic imaging of the lower extremities in a patient with lipedema. Courtesy of Dr. Szuba's Lab.

obesity can progress to secondary lymphedema.[14, 15] Notably, lifestyle-induced obesity can also produce lymphoscintigraphic changes in the lower extremities similar to those seen in lipedema. Moreover, research has shown a correlation between the degree of obesity and the severity of these lymphoscintigraphic alterations.[8, 15] Consequently, it cannot be ruled out that impaired lymphatic transport in lipedema may be at least partially influenced by coexisting obesity.

Thyroid dysfunction

Thyroid hormones, including thyroxine (T4) and triiodothyronine (T3), play a vital role in regulating metabolic processes, fat distribution, and overall body homeostasis. These hormones influence key functions such as lipolysis, thermogenesis, and basal metabolic rate. An imbalance in thyroid hormone levels can disrupt these processes, potentially worsening both lipedema and obesity.

Several studies have shown a higher prevalence of hypothyroidism among patients with lipedema. For example, two German studies involving 206 and 106 women with lipedema who underwent liposuction procedures found that 35.9% and 31%, respectively, were diagnosed with hypothyroidism.[1, 2] These rates were significantly higher than those observed in the general population, where hypothyroidism affects only 0.5–2%.[1] In a study of 360 Italian women with lipedema, 22.5% were diagnosed with hypothyroidism, with higher prevalence rates observed in patients with stage 3 lipedema (34.2%) compared to those in stage 1 (16.1%).[3]

Hypothyroidism is more prevalent in individuals with obesity; however, no correlation was found between BMI and the prevalence of hypothyroidism in patients with both lipedema and obesity.[3] Additionally, autoimmune thyroiditis was found in 35.5% of patients with lipedema, regardless of the disease stage.[3] In comparison, the prevalence of anti-TG and anti-TPO antibodies in the general population is 10.4% and 11.3%, respectively.[3] These findings highlight the need for further research to better understand thyroid dysfunction in lipedema.

Psychological issues

Lipedema is linked to a range of mental health issues, including a higher prevalence of depression.[1, 2, 3, 16] Estimates suggest that 23% to 45.2% of patients with lipedema experience depression, with the highest rates occurring among women in the later stages of the disease (61.2%).[3] Furthermore, the psychological stress related to obesity, when a comorbidity, may contribute to additional emotional struggles.[17]

The physical manifestations of lipedema often cause significant psychological distress. Many patients experience body image disturbances and report feelings of shame, embarrassment, and frustration due to noticeable changes in their body shape.[18] Pain associated with lipedema has been shown to worsen psychological well-being and negatively impact quality of life.[19] The resulting feelings of helplessness can further intensify mental health challenges.

Other co-morbidities

Several studies have shown a higher prevalence of migraines or headaches in women with lipedema, with significant improvement following liposuction.[1, 2, 3] However, the underlying mechanisms linking lipedema to a higher incidence of migraines still require further research. Additionally, menstrual irregularities appear to coexist with lipedema, possibly due to shared risk factors such as obesity and hypothyroidism.[1, 2, 3] Interestingly, menstrual irregularities improved after liposuction.[1]

Women with lipedema often report orthostatic edema[10] and leg swelling in hot weather,[20] which can be partially explained by concomitant chronic venous disease (see Figure 9.2). One study found that chronic venous disease was present in 71.9% of women with lipedema,[3] while another study estimated the prevalence of varicose veins at 11.29%.[20] However, studies assessing venous insufficiency in the lower limbs of patients with lipedema have been limited.

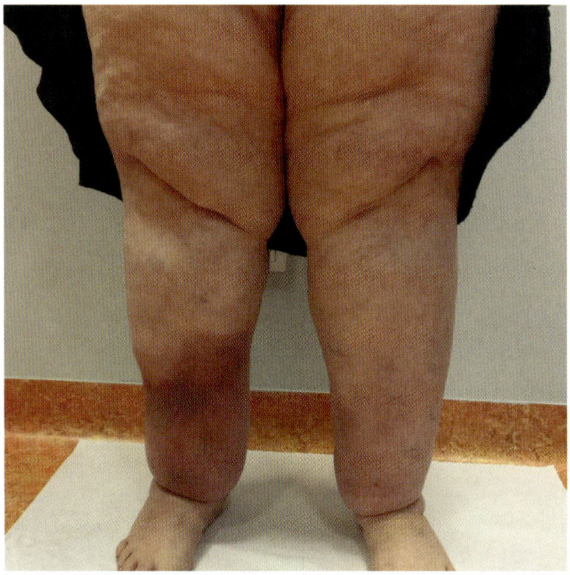

Figure 9.2: Venous disease commonly co-exists with lipedema. Courtesy of Dr. Szuba's lab.

Several less commonly reported co-morbidities, such as hypermobile joints (see Figure 9.3), reduced elasticity of skin and aorta, may support the hypothesis that lipedema is not only an adipose tissue disease but also a connective tissue disease.[13] In two studies, hypermobile joints

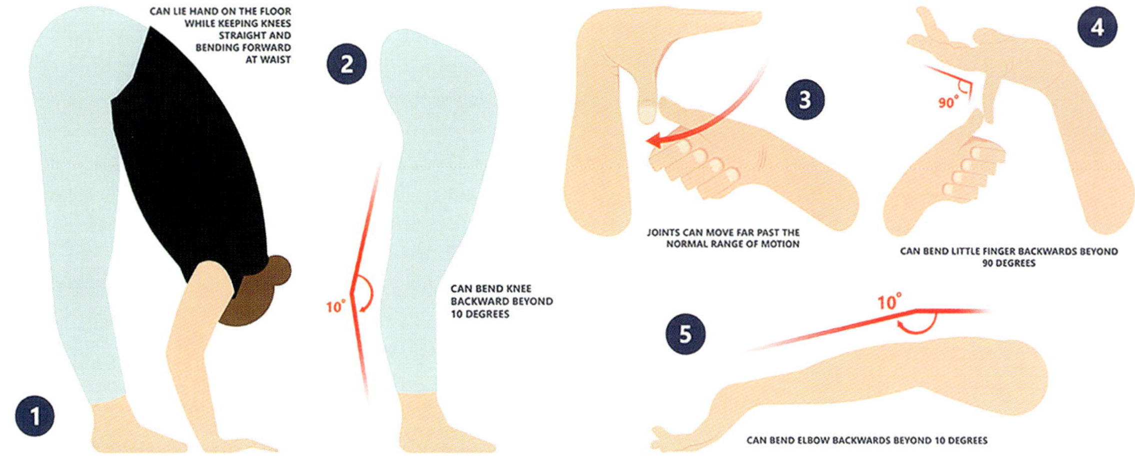

Figure 9.3: Joint hypermobility can be a co-morbidity of lipedema. © Pepermpron – stock.adobe.com.

were observed in 32.5% to 50% of women with lipedema.[3, 13] Reduced elasticity of the skin and aorta was observed in women with lipedema by Szolnoky et al.,[21] although this finding has not been confirmed by other studies.[22]

Conclusion

Lipedema is not just a localized fat disease but is associated with a range of co-morbidities that can complicate its course, diagnosis, and management. Understanding these coexisting diseases is crucial for effective management and treatment. Co-morbidities should be treated in parallel with the treatment of lipedema. A multidisciplinary approach is essential for improving outcomes for patients with lipedema.

References

1. Ghods M, Georgiou I, Schmidt J, Kruppa P. Disease progression and comorbidities in lipedema patients: a 10-year retrospective analysis. *Dermatol Ther.* 2020;33(6):e14534. DOI: https://doi.org/10.1111/dth.14534
2. Bauer AT, von Lukowicz D, Lossagk K, Aitzetmueller M, Moog P, Cerny M, et al. New insights on lipedema: the enigmatic disease of the peripheral fat. *Plast Reconstr Surg.* 2019 Dec;144(6):1475–84. DOI: https://doi.org/10.1097/PRS.0000000000006280
3. Patton L, Ricolfi L, Bortolon M, Gabriele G, Zolesio P, Cione E, et al. Observational study on a large Italian population with lipedema: biochemical and hormonal profile, anatomical and clinical evaluation, self-reported history. *Int J Mol Sci.* 2024 Jan;25(3):1599. DOI: https://doi.org/10.3390/ijms25031599
4. Milaneschi Y, Simmons WK, van Rossum EFC, Penninx BW. Depression and obesity: evidence of shared biological mechanisms. *Mol Psychiatry.* 2019 Jan;24(1):18–33. DOI: https://doi.org/10.1038/s41380-018-0017-5
5. Forner-Cordero I, Oliván-Sasot P, Ruiz-Llorca C, Muñoz-Langa J. Lymphoscintigraphic findings in patients with lipedema. *Rev Esp Med Nucl E Imagen Mol Engl Ed.* 2018 Nov 1;37(6):341–8. DOI: https://doi.org/10.1016/j.remnie.2018.10.013
6. Harwood CA, Bull RH, Evans J, Mortimer PS. Lymphatic and venous function in lipoedema. *Br*

J Dermatol. 1996 Jan;134(1):1–6. DOI: https://doi.org/10.1046/j.1365-2133.1996.d01-741.x
7. Gould DJ, El-Sabawi B, Goel P, Badash I, Colletti P, Patel KM. Uncovering lymphatic transport abnormalities in patients with primary lipedema. *J Reconstr Microsurg*. 2019 Sep 23; DOI: https://doi.org/10.1055/s-0039-1697904
8. Chachaj A, Dudka I, Jeziorek M, Sowicz M, Adaszyńska A, Szuba A. Lymphoscintigraphic alterations in lower limbs in women with lipedema in comparison to women with overweight/obesity. *Front Physiol*. 2023 Apr 10;14. Available from: https://www.frontiersin.org/journals/physiology/articles/10.3389/fphys.2023.1099555/full
9. Rasmussen JC, Aldrich MB, Fife CE, Herbst KL, Sevick-Muraca EM. Lymphatic function and anatomy in early stages of lipedema. *Obesity*. 2022;30(7):1391–400. DOI: https://doi.org/10.1002/oby.23458
10. Buso G, Favre L, Maufus M, Honorati M, Lessert C, Depairon M, et al. Indocyanine green lymphography as novel tool to assess lymphatics in patients with lipedema. *Microvasc Res*. 2022 Mar 1;140:104298. DOI: https://doi.org/10.1016/j.mvr.2021.104298
11. Lohrmann C, Foeldi E, Langer M. MR imaging of the lymphatic system in patients with lipedema and lipo-lymphedema. *Microvasc Res*. 2009 May 1;77(3):335–9. DOI: https://doi.org/10.1016/j.mvr.2009.01.005
12. Kruppa P, Georgiou I, Biermann N, Prantl L, Klein-Weigel P, Ghods M. Lipedema – pathogenesis, diagnosis, and treatment options. *Dtsch Ärztebl Int*. 2020 Jun;117(22–23):396. DOI: https://doi.org/10.3238/arztebl.2020.0396
13. Herbst KL, Kahn LA, Iker E, Ehrlich C, Wright T, McHutchison L, et al. Standard of care for lipedema in the United States. *Phlebology*. 2021 Dec 1;36(10):779–96. DOI: https://doi.org/10.1177/02683555211015887
14. Mehrara BJ, Greene AK. Lymphedema and obesity: is there a link? *Plast Reconstr Surg*. 2014 Jul;134(1):154e. DOI: https://doi.org/10.1097/PRS.0000000000000268
15. Greene AK, Sudduth CL. Lower extremity lymphatic function predicted by body mass index: a lymphoscintigraphic study of obesity and lipedema. *Int J Obes*. 2021 Feb;45(2):369–73. DOI: https://doi.org/10.1038/s41366-020-00681-6
16. Dudek JE, Białaszek W, Gabriel M. Quality of life, its factors, and sociodemographic characteristics of Polish women with lipedema. *BMC Womens Health*. 2021 Jan 15;21(1):27. DOI: https://doi.org/10.1186/s12905-021-01174-y
17. Luppino FS, de Wit LM, Bouvy PF, Stijnen T, Cuijpers P, Penninx BWJH, et al. Overweight, obesity, and depression: a systematic review and meta-analysis of longitudinal studies. *Arch Gen Psychiatry*. 2010 Mar 1;67(3):220–9. DOI: https://doi.org/10.1001/archgenpsychiatry.2010.2
18. Melander C, Juuso, Päivi, and Olsson M. Women's experiences of living with lipedema. *Health Care Women Int*. 2022 Mar 4;43(1–3):54–69. DOI: https://doi.org/10.1080/07399332.2021.1932894
19. Chachaj A, Jeziorek M, Dudka I, Sowicz M, Adaszyńska A, Truszyński A, et al. Disability and emotional symptoms in women with lipedema : a comparison with overweight/obese women. *Adv Clin Exp Med*. 2024;33(12):1367–77. DOI: https://doi.org/10.17219/acem/181146
20. Aday AW, Donahue PM, Garza M, Crain VN, Patel NJ, Beasley JA, et al. National survey of patient symptoms and therapies among 707 women with a lipedema phenotype in the United States. *Vasc Med*. 2024 Feb 1;29(1):36–41. DOI: https://doi.org/10.1177/1358863X231202769
21. Szolnoky G, Nemes A, Gavallér H, Forster T, Kemény L. Lipedema is associated with increased aortic stiffness. *Lymphology*. 2012 Jun;45(2):71–9. Available from: https://journals.librarypublishing.arizona.edu/lymph/article/id/3733/
22. Mahlmann A, Khorzom Y, Behrendt CA, Leip JL, Bachler M, Wassertheurer S, et al. Screening for peripheral vascular stiffness in lipedema patients by automatic electrocardiogram-based oscillometric detection. *Sensors*. 2024 Jan;24(5):1673. DOI: https://doi.org/10.3390/s24051673

IV
Imaging

Chapter Ten
Conventional imaging modalities to evaluate lipedema

Juan Vázquez Díez, Luz M. Herrero Manley and Isabel Forner Cordero

Introduction

Lipedema is a common disease characterized by abnormal fat accumulation in the lower and sometimes upper extremities, resulting in a disproportionate body shape between the upper and lower regions. It is often accompanied by symptoms such as swelling, pain, fibrosis, and easy bruising.[1] Diagnosis is based primarily on clinical features, but lipedema is frequently misdiagnosed as lymphedema or obesity. Because there is no definitive diagnostic marker or pathognomonic sign, a conclusive diagnosis is not currently possible. The presence of co-morbid diseases such as obesity, venous insufficiency, and lymphatic dysfunction further complicates the diagnostic process.

At present, there is no consensus on the most effective imaging technique for evaluating lipedema. Existing imaging methods mainly provide quantitative data and visual assessments of subcutaneous fat and the lymphatic system. However, they do not capture key elements of lipedema pathogenesis, such as extracellular matrix remodeling, inflammation, or fibrosis. While current guidelines recognize the value of imaging and laboratory tests for differential diagnosis, they also acknowledge that these tools are insufficient for definitive diagnosis.[2]

Ultrasound imaging

Ultrasound is probably the most readily available and the lowest cost of all imaging techniques used in lipedema. It has proven utility in both the diagnosis and management of patients with lipedema.

How does ultrasound help with diagnosis?

Ultrasound provides the opportunity to assess subcutaneous fat tissue structure. Interestingly, it has been proposed as an alternative imaging technique to MRI for this purpose.[3] Table 10.1 compares lipedema, obesity, and lymphedema regarding ultrasound examination.[4] Figure 10.1 illustrates some of these differential characteristics.

However, Hirsch et al.[5] found no consistent sonomorphological properties that could reliably differentiate lipedema from other diseases or healthy individuals. The compressibility of the cutis-subcutis complex was found to be nonspecific and did not allow any conclusions to be drawn about lipedema. Its thickness appeared to be somewhat lower in healthy individuals and greater in obesity than in lipedema and lipohypertrophy. Furthermore, no fluid retention was detected in patients with 'painful lipohypertrophy' when using this technique.[5]

Table 10.1: Ultrasound imaging.

Fat tissue characteristics	**Lipedema**	**Obesity**	**Lymphedema**
Echogenicity	Hypoechogenic areas due to enlarged fat lobules	Hyperechogenic homogeneous tissue due to denser fat	Hypoechogenic areas due to fluid accumulation
Thickness and distribution	Thicker and more irregular, especially in lower limbs	Uniform	Thicker with irregular distribution
Fibrosis	Present as hyperechoic bands within the fat tissue, especially with disease progression (utility in disease staging)	Usually absent in uncomplicated obesity	Present in advanced stages as hyperechoic bands
Fluid retention	If edema is present, visible as hypoechoic areas between fat lobules	Less prominent	Visible as hypoechoic areas between fat lobules

When palpating areas affected by lipedema, the skin tends to feel coarser (mattress phenomenon). Yet, no correlation was found between this sign and consistent identification of a septa-rich subcutis. The same applies to the 'enhanced diffuse echogenicity,' which has also been reported in cases of lipedema.

Utility of ultrasound in lipedema management

This imaging technique can be used to measure the thickness of both the skin and adipose tissue at various sites on the lower limbs. It has been suggested that the thickness of these tissues can increase with the severity of lipedema.[6, 7] This can help us to distinguish lipedema from other diseases, such as lymphedema and obesity,[7] aid in staging,[6] and help to determine the extent to which conservative treatments are effective.[7] Additionally, since lipedema may coexist to some extent with edema, ultrasound will be able to visualize if edema is diminishing. Ultrasound has also been proposed as a method to guide liposuction, potentially enabling precise fat removal while minimizing damage to surrounding areas, therefore improving procedure outcomes.

To improve the accuracy of lipedema diagnosis using ultrasound, specific cutoff values for dermal and subcutaneous tissue thickness have been suggested (see Figure 10.2), indicating the presence of lipedema when exceeded, particularly when combined with other clinical symptoms such as pain or easy bruising.[7]

Some of these cutoff values are:

1. Thigh region (good accuracy): 17.9 mm.
2. Pre-tibial region (high accuracy): 11.7 mm.
3. Lateral leg region (good accuracy): 8.4 mm.
4. Medial supramalleolar region (lower accuracy): 7.1 mm.

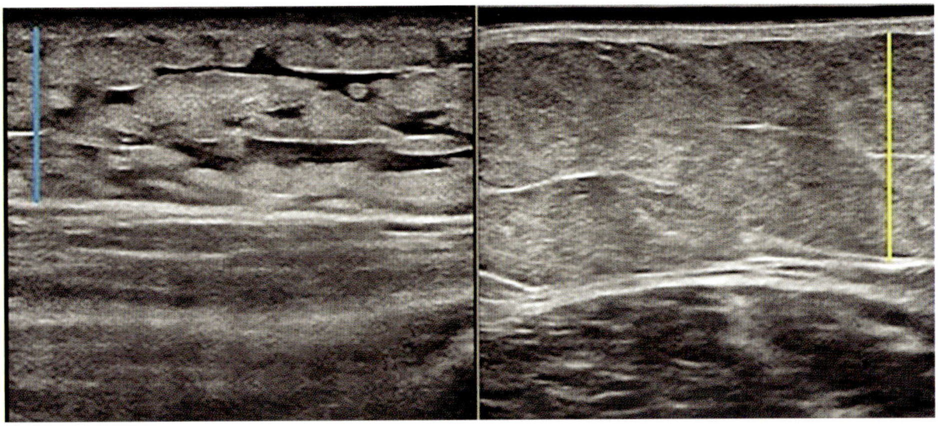

Figure 10.1: Differential diagnosis between lymphedema and lipedema. Left picture shows typical findings of lymphedema, such as hypoechogenic areas between fat lobules due to fluid accumulation. Right image shows typical findings of lipedema, such as hypoechogenic areas due to enlarged fat lobules and increased thickness of the subcutaneous tissue. Courtesy of Dr. Forner Cordero.

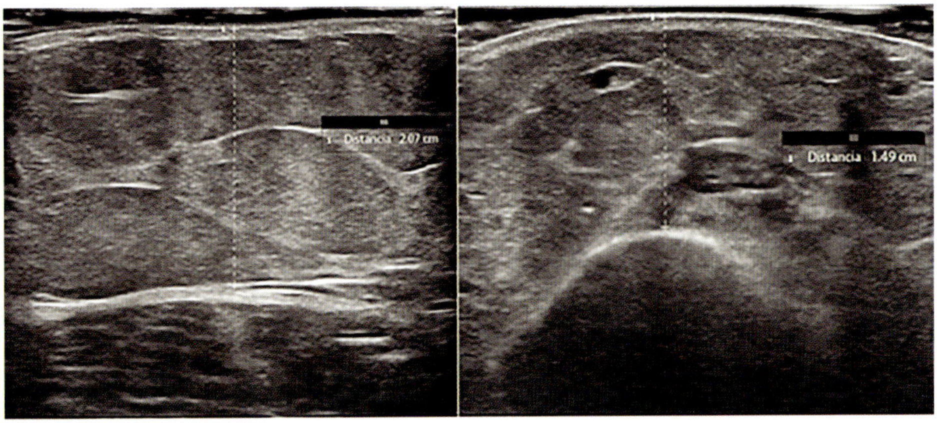

Figure 10.2: Diagnosis of lipedema with ultrasound using cutoff values for dermal and subcutaneous tissue thickness suggested by Amato et al.[8] Left image: thigh region >17.9 mm; right image: pretibial region >11.7 mm. Courtesy of Dr. Forner Cordero.

Amato et al.,[8] who first described these measurement locations, also included the anteromedial proximal region of the leg, where typical fat deposition is present. Another significant ultrasound finding in lipedema is the presence of hypoechogenicity, which refers to regions within the subcutaneous fat layer that appear darker on an ultrasound image. This tissue structure is different from that of healthy individuals or those with diseases such as obesity or lymphedema.[7] Moreover, in contrast to other imaging techniques such as MRI, ultrasound examination is not constrained by patient size or weight, making it especially suitable for use in patients with obesity.[7]

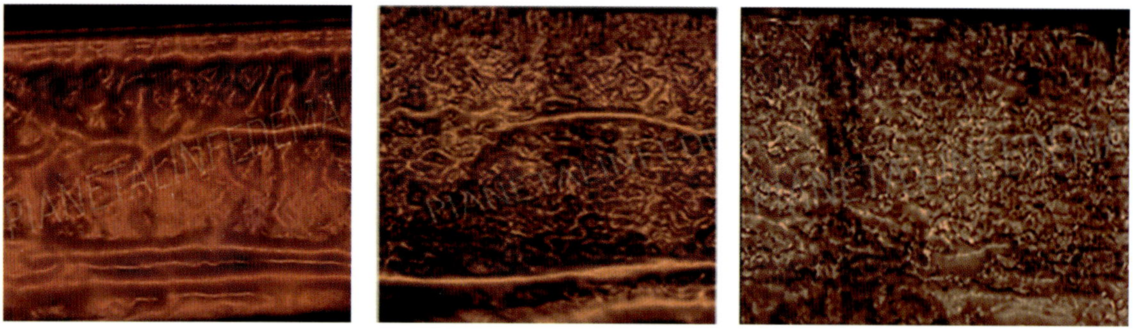

Figure 10.3: Stages 1, 2, and 3 of lipedema, with 3D ultrasound. Courtesy of Dr. Marina Cestari.

3D Ultrasound

According to Cestari et al.,[9] 3D ultrasound (17 MHz probe) has revealed normal epidermis-dermis structure in lipedema, with increased thickness in both superficial and deep fascia as well as fibrotic connective areas in the connective septa corresponding to palpable nodules. A notable finding across all stages was fluid accumulation along the superficial fascia. Lipohypertrophy showed structural similarities to early-stage lipedema. The study concluded that 3D ultrasound revealed previously unnoticed features of adipo-fascia in lipedema (Figure 10.3).

Computed tomography (CT)

The limitations of computed tomography in assessing soft tissue, compared to MRI or ultrasound, have historically restricted its use in lipedema. Although it has limited utility in the diagnosis of lipedema, it may be used in conjunction with other imaging techniques, such as lymphoscintigraphy, to assess the possible coexistence of lymphedema.

However, CT could be useful in the differential diagnosis of lipedema, lymphedema, and deep venous thrombosis. In patients with lipedema, CT scans typically do not show evidence of edema. This absence of edema is a distinguishing feature when compared to lymphedema, where CT imaging frequently reveals significant fluid retention within the subcutaneous tissue.[10] According to Monnin-Delhom et al.,[11] CT showed a sensitivity of 95% and specificity of 100% when studying 20 patients with lipedema. Key findings used for differential diagnosis with lymphedema and DVT were skin thickening (16% of patients) and the absence of subcutaneous edema (typical of lymphedema and DVT), honeycombed pattern (limited to lymphedema), and muscle enlargement (typical of DVT).[11]

In addition, CT can reveal structural changes and provide volume measurements in affected areas. It can detect the bilateral and symmetrical accumulation of subcutaneous fat characteristic of lipedema, predominantly affecting the lower extremities while sparing the feet, hands, and trunk.[7] This imaging technique can be particularly useful in complex cases where differential diagnosis is challenging or when other imaging methods yield inconclusive results.[7] In summary, while CT can be useful in differentiating lipedema from other diseases, it is not typically the first-line diagnostic tool for lipedema, as other modalities are less invasive and do not involve radiation exposure.[7]

Magnetic resonance imaging (MRI)

MRI can be a useful tool for diagnosing and distinguishing between lymphedema and lipedema. MRI provides anatomical and functional insights, including the detection of lymphatic abnormalities, assessment of tissue alterations in the extremities, and quantification of lymphedema. These capabilities render MRI especially valuable for early diagnosis and treatment planning.[6, 7] Another distinguishing feature observed in MRI is the absence of edema in patients with lipedema, which contrasts with its presence in those with lymphedema or deep venous thrombosis.[10]

MRI techniques

Various MRI techniques, such as traditional two-dimensional (2D) MRI, three-dimensional (3D) MRI, and magnetic resonance lymphography (MRL), are employed to visualize the lymphatic system and assess tissue changes.[7] Clinically, MRI, and especially MRL, is crucial for differentiating between lipedema and lymphedema. It enhances diagnostic precision by providing detailed visualization of lymphatic vessel abnormalities

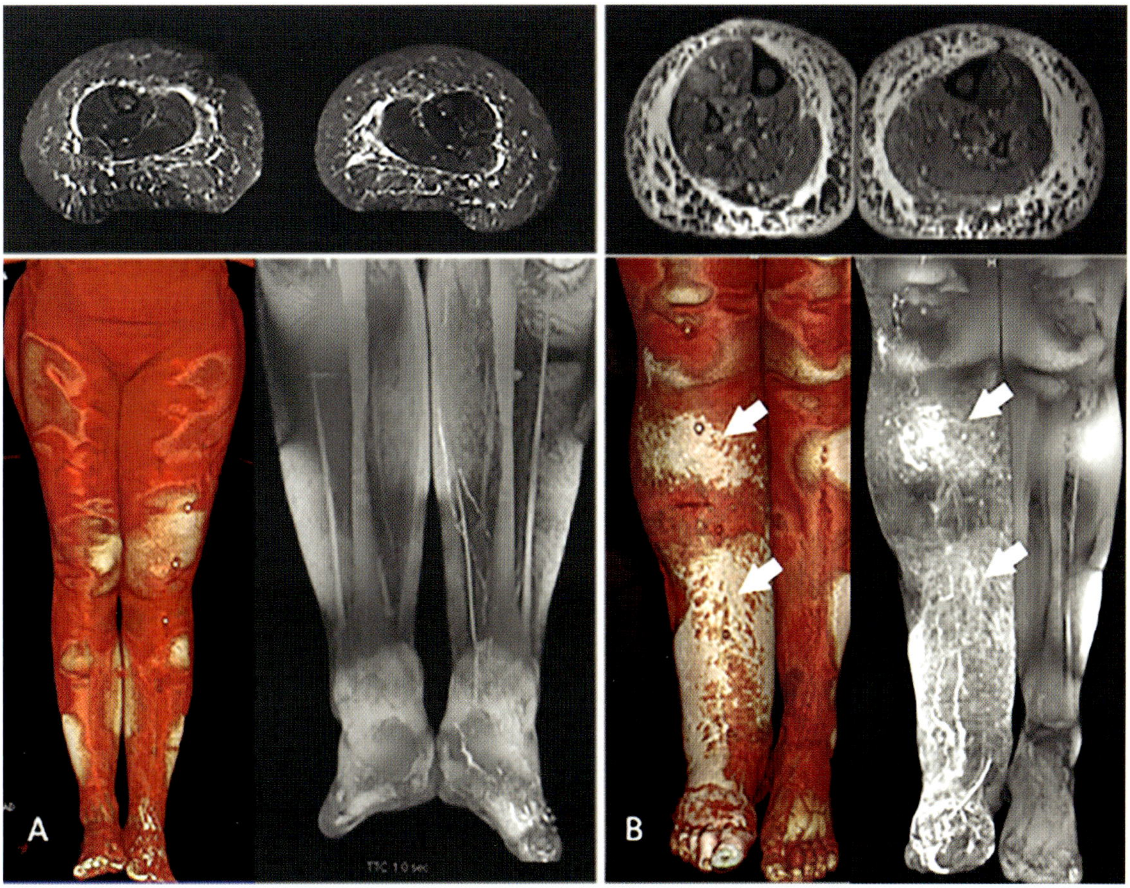

Figure 10.4: (A) shows a patient with lipedema: visible permeable lymphatics and trabeculation of subcutaneous fat without lymphatic stasis; (B) shows a lymphedema patient with dilated lymphatics and dermal backflow (arrows). Courtesy of Dr. Alberto Alonso-Burgos.

and subcutaneous tissue alterations specific to lipedema (Figure 10.4).[1]

Moreover, contrast-enhanced MRL uses gadolinium-based agents to highlight lymphatic pathways. It has identified dilated distal lymphatic vessels (exceeding 2mm in diameter) in approximately 40% of lipedema cases. Additionally, it aids in identifying increased subcutaneous fat and fluid collections, which are characteristic of lipedema with secondary lymphedema.[1, 7]

Key findings and utility

In a 1992 study, Duewell et al.[12] examined the use of MRI to distinguish between lipedema, lymphedema, and phlebedema in the lower limbs. Patients with lipedema showed a consistent enlargement of the subcutaneous fat layer without any noticeable changes in signal intensity, either in T2-weighted images or after the administration of contrast agents. In contrast, patients with lymphedema exhibited a distinctive 'honeycomb' pattern between the muscle and subcutaneous tissue, with a notable increase in signal intensity on T2-weighted images. Phlebedema, characterized by fluid accumulation within the muscles and subcutaneous fat, showed increased fluid in both areas.

Building on this, Dimakakos et al.[13] investigated the diagnostic potential of both MRI and ultrasonography in evaluating patients with lipedema and lymphedema. They noted that lipedema presented with significant thickening of the skin and subcutaneous tissue, while lymphedema showed not only skin and fat thickening but also an increase in muscle mass. Importantly, their findings showed that patient factors like age, weight, or the duration of the disease did not significantly alter the imaging results.

Lohrmann et al.[14] used MR lymphangiography (MRL) to assess lymphatic system changes in patients with lipedema and secondary lymphedema. They found that all patients with these co-occurring diseases showed typical signs of lymphedema, including high signal intensity areas and enlarged lymphatic vessels, with some revealing lymphatic obstruction. Patients with lipedema also showed enlarged lymphatic vessels, indicating potential subclinical lymphedema. MRL proved to be a safe, minimally invasive technique that provides both functional and detailed anatomical information, making it a useful tool for diagnosis and treatment planning.

More recently, in 2020, Cellina et al.[15] explored the use of non-contrast MR lymphography (NCMRL) to assess lipedema and its variant, lipedema with co-occurring lymphedema (sometimes referred to as lipolymphedema). In all cases of lipedema, the patients displayed symmetrical enlargement of the lower limbs, with uniform fat deposits and no signs of edema. However, in cases of lipedema with co-occurring lymphedema, there were additional findings, including mild fluid collections in the epifascial region and occasional dilation of the peripheral lymphatics. Interestingly, some patients with lipedema showed early signs of subclinical lymphedema, suggesting an overlap between the two diseases.

MRI can also provide important information before surgery to evaluate the extent of subcutaneous fat accumulation and to distinguish lipedema from lymphedema. Accurate differentiation is essential, as the surgical strategy may need to be adjusted based on whether lymphatic involvement is present.[7] MRI is especially valuable in this context, providing detailed anatomical and functional insights into the affected tissues, which facilitates precise surgical planning. It helps identify any lymphatic abnormalities or fluid accumulations that might influence the choice of surgical techniques.[7]

Lymphoscintigraphy

Lymphoscintigraphy is a nuclear medicine imaging technique that represents the current gold standard for evaluating lymphatic pathways. It involves the injection of a radioactive tracer into the lymphatic system, allowing clinicians to visualize and evaluate lymphatic drainage and detect any dysfunctions. In our hospital, we use 99mTc-albumin nanocolloids tracer, which is one of the most widely used agents in Europe.[16]

Procedure and interpretation of results

Lymphoscintigraphy is initiated with the subcutaneous injection of 22.2 MBq of 99mTc-albumin nanocolloids, in a small volume of physiological saline solution (<0.2 ml). Four injections are performed in total in the first and third interdigital spaces of both feet.[17] After the injection, patients are asked to perform a slight exercise (10-minute walk) to activate lymphatic function and promote maximum drainage. Subsequently, a total body scan is obtained at 15 and 180 minutes after injection.

The deep lymphatic system of the lower limbs can be evaluated in cases with dermal backflow or lymphatic stasis (1–2 subfascial administrations in the retro-malleolar or plantar region). SPECT/CT is recommended to study the thoracic, abdominal, and pelvic territories.[17]

Two independent nuclear medicine physicians described the findings in lymphoscintigraphy and classified them into different degrees[18, 19] (Table 10.2).

Is it really useful?

When examining current literature, a lack of consensus was found between authors regarding the clinical applicability of lymphoscintigraphy in lipedema:

On the one hand, some authors state that lymphoscintigraphy can aid in distinguishing between lipedema and lymphedema. In the context of lymphedema, lymphoscintigraphy typically reveals significant abnormalities in lymphatic drainage, such as delayed or absent tracer movement through the lymphatic vessels. These findings are indicative of impaired lymphatic function. In contrast, patients with lipedema generally have normal lymphatic function on lymphoscintigraphy.[10, 20]

Table 10.2: Determination of lymphatic dysfunction severity using lymphoscintigraphy findings.

Score	Degree	Findings	Interpretation
0	Normal	Normal migration and distribution of radiopharmaceutical	No lymphatic dysfunction
1	Low	Delayed migration or discrete asymmetry in distribution	Minimal lymphatic impairment
2	Low–Moderate	Migration and lymph node filling with slightly altered characteristics	Suggestive of mild lymphatic hypoplasia
3	Moderate	Migration and lymph node filling with moderately altered characteristics	Suggestive of moderate lymphatic hypoplasia
4	Moderate–Severe	Migration and lymph node filling with markedly altered characteristics	Indicative of severe lymphatic hypoplasia
5	Severe	No migration and no lymph node filling	Suggestive of lymphatic aplasia

Note: Add 1 point to the score if dermal backflow or radiopharmaceutical retention at the popliteal fossa is observed.

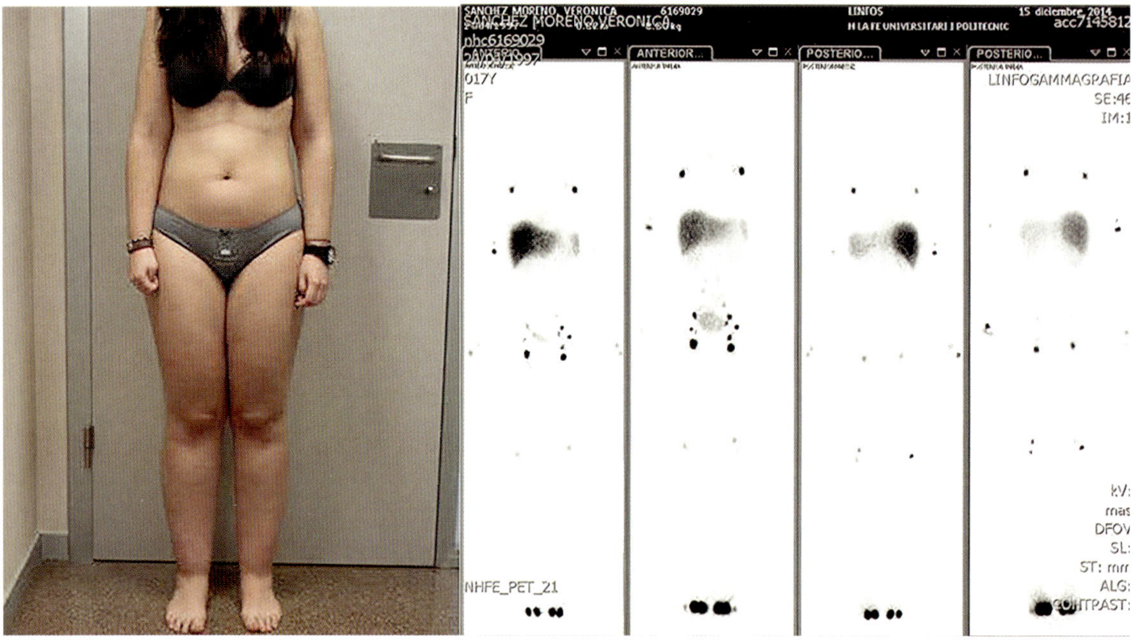

Figure 10.5: Patient with stage 1 lipedema and moderate findings in lymphoscintigraphy. Courtesy of Dr. Forner Cordero's Lab.

However, a prospective study involving 83 women with lipedema reported the presence of abnormal lymphoscintigraphy findings in 47% of the sample (low degree in 35.9%, 48.7% low-moderate, and 15.4% moderate delay in transportation and asymmetric distribution).[21] These findings lacked association with the lipedema stage and were present even in stage 1 patients (Figure 10.5).

On the other hand, Markarian et al.[7] state that lymphoscintigraphy is not particularly effective in distinguishing between lipedema and lymphedema, as both diseases can exhibit analogous lymphatic alterations. Consequently, the detection of changes in the lymphatic system does not preclude lipedema, nor does their absence confirm it.[7] Additionally, lymphoscintigraphy is unable to assess the clinical stage and severity of lipedema. Neither does it differentiate between lipedema and obesity, as the detection of collateral lymph vessels indicating lymphatic overload was common in both cases.[22]

Expert representatives from 11 professional societies researched and developed appropriate use criteria for lymphoscintigraphy in sentinel lymph node mapping and lymphedema. Their document includes the statement that lymphoscintigraphy may be appropriate when studying lipedema.[23]

Differential diagnosis with lymphedema

Lipedema is typically well differentiated from lymphedema in most cases. However, this can become particularly challenging in cases of lower-limb bilateral lymphedema, for example. Lymphoscintigraphy helps differentiate between the two by showing whether there is normal or abnormal lymphatic drainage.

- In lymphedema, lymphoscintigraphy typically shows impaired lymphatic flow or a complete blockage in the lymphatic vessels.

- In lipedema, the lymphatic system is usually functioning normally, though in some advanced stages of lipedema, there may be secondary lymphatic involvement.

Evaluating the extent of secondary lymphatic compromise

In advanced lipedema, some patients may develop secondary lymphedema, where lymphatic function becomes compromised due to increased tissue pressure from excessive fat deposition. Lymphoscintigraphy can detect this secondary lymphatic dysfunction, helping clinicians tailor treatment strategies for the patient. If lymphedema is detected, adequate compression therapy will not only provide symptom relief but also reduce limb volume. Moreover, subsequent evaluations may discover changes in lymphatic flow or function that can guide adjustments in therapy.

Pre-surgical assessment

For patients undergoing surgery such as liposuction for lipedema, lymphoscintigraphy can provide information about the condition of the lymphatic system, helping surgeons avoid damaging healthy lymphatics during the procedure.

Dual energy X-ray absorptiometry (DEXA)

DEXA is commonly used for assessing body composition, including fat and lean mass distribution. In the context of lipedema, a chronic disease characterized by the abnormal accumulation of fat in the lower extremities, DEXA plays a vital role in diagnosis and management.

However, while DEXA can measure fat distribution, it does not offer insights into the lymphatic system or the functional abnormalities associated with lipedema, thereby limiting its diagnostic capabilities to structural analysis rather than functional evaluation.[7]

In addition, DEXA has limitations in differentiating between extracellular and intracellular fluid compartments (an important distinction in the diagnosis of lymphedema). Since DEXA does not provide direct measurements of fluid compartments, it may be less effective in distinguishing lipedema from lymphedema, where fluid accumulation plays a critical role.[10]

To overcome this challenge, DEXA is often used with bioimpedance spectroscopy. Bioimpedance spectroscopy provides information on fluid distribution within the body, complementing the fat mass data obtained from DEXA. The combination of these methods enables a more comprehensive evaluation, thereby enhancing the accuracy of diagnosis and management of lipedema.[10]

Fat distribution analysis

DEXA provides a detailed breakdown of fat distribution, differentiating between fat, lean tissue, and bone density. DEXA can help confirm the disproportionate fat deposition that is characteristic of lipedema compared to obesity, where fat associated with obesity is more uniformly distributed.

Fat mass quantification

One of the significant utilities of DEXA in lipedema is the ability to quantify the amount of fat mass in different regions of the body (Figure 10.6). It can determine the ratio of fat in affected areas versus non-affected areas. This precise measurement is useful for distinguishing lipedema from other forms of fat disease, such as obesity or lymphedema. Over time, DEXA can be used to monitor changes in fat distribution, help track the progression of lipedema, and evaluate the effectiveness of treatments.

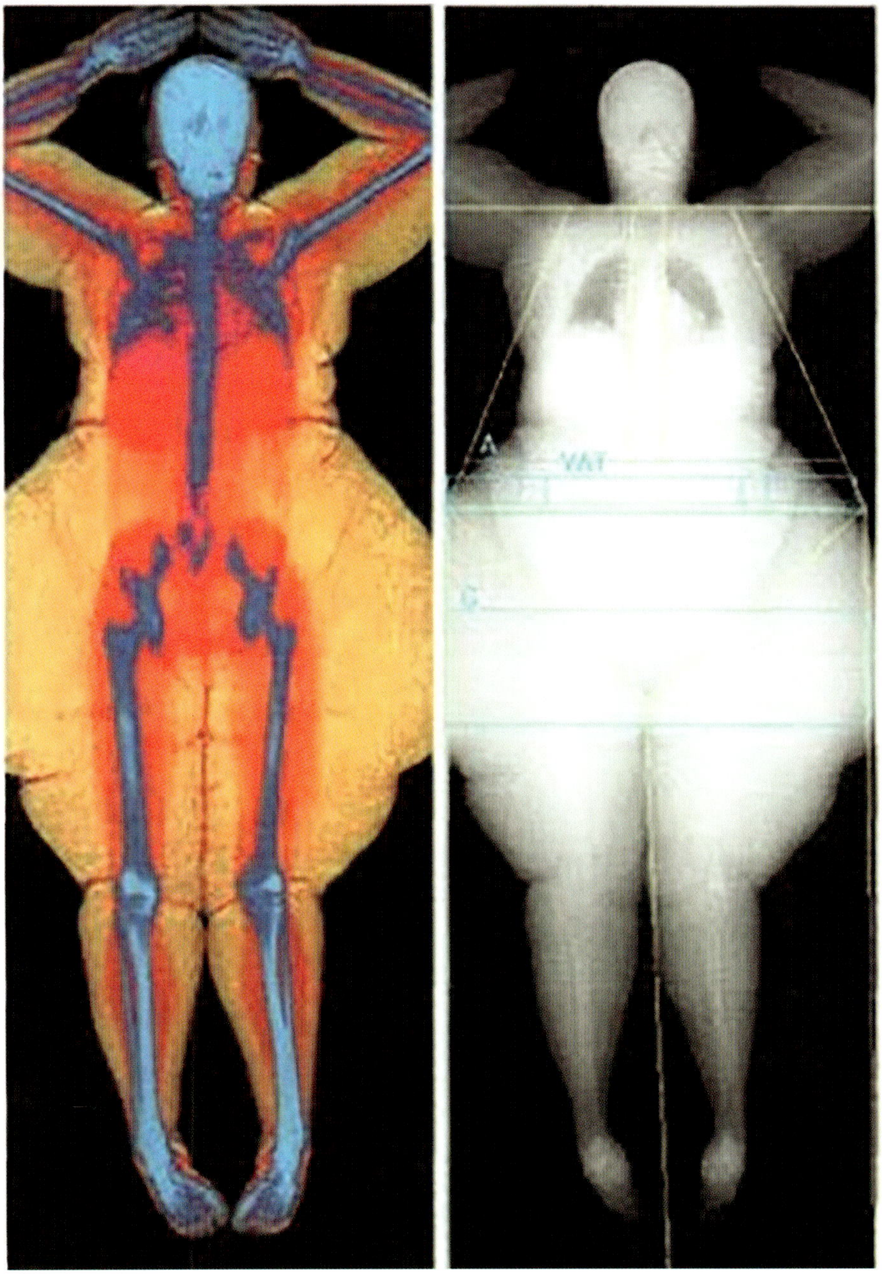

Figure 10.6: DEXA of a patient with lipedema and obesity. Courtesy of Dr. Eraci Drehmer.

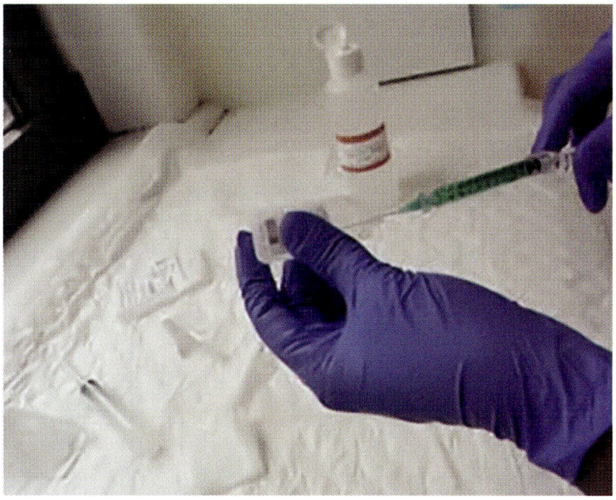

Figure 10.7: ICG lymphography. Courtesy of Dr. Forner Cordero.

Bone density assessment

Patients with lipedema may also be at risk for osteoporosis or other bone density issues due to limited mobility and other factors. DEXA's ability to assess bone mineral density is an added benefit in managing overall health in these patients. When comparing body composition measurements for lipedema, device-specific variations were found to affect lipedema diagnosis; however, applying standardization equations improved the agreement between measurements.[24]

Indocyanine green (ICG) lymphography

Indocyanine green (ICG) lymphography has become a valuable diagnostic tool for evaluating lymphatic system abnormalities in patients with lipedema (Figure 10.7). This imaging technique effectively detects disruptions in superficial lymphatic flow, which are marked by slower lymphatic movement, an increased number of abnormal lymphatic vessels, and heightened fluorescent intensity in the skin. It can also reveal dilated lymphatic vessels, intravascular pooling, and elevated propulsion rates, all of which point to underlying lymphatic dysfunction associated with lipedema. By offering detailed visualization of these specific lymphatic alterations, ICG lymphography deepens our understanding of the disease's pathophysiology and helps distinguish lipedema from other similar diseases.[1]

Ultra micro angiography technology

When using ultra micro angiography in lipedema, which can detect small, slow-flowing vessels, Kempa et al.[25] found it to be superior to traditional color Doppler flow imaging in visualizing microvascular structures. In patients with lipedema, increased subcutaneous vascularization and angiogenesis were observed, particularly in advanced stages, suggesting heightened inflammation.

Although microaneurysms, vessel fragility, and caliber variations were observed sporadically, they were not associated with advanced stages.[26] The increased angiogenesis, driven by vascular endothelial growth factor (VEGF), plays a central role in the inflammation seen in lipedema, as new blood vessels form through processes like vasodilation and endothelial cell activation.

Conclusion

While no single imaging modality can definitively diagnose lipedema, a range of tools offer valuable insights into its structural and, in some cases, functional features. Ultrasound stands out for its accessibility and utility in assessing subcutaneous tissue characteristics. At the same time, MRI provides high-resolution detail that is especially helpful in distinguishing lipedema from lymphedema or guiding surgical planning. Lymphoscintigraphy and ICG lymphography are instrumental in evaluating lymphatic involvement, particularly in differentiating lipedema from overlapping diseases. DEXA and bioimpedance spectroscopy enhance understanding of fat and fluid distribution, and emerging techniques such as ultra micro angiography provide a window into the microvascular changes associated with disease progression. Together, these imaging strategies support more accurate diagnosis, individualized treatment planning, and a deeper understanding of lipedema's pathophysiology.

References

1. van la Parra RFD, Deconinck C, Krug B. Diagnostic imaging in lipedema: a systematic review. *Obes Rev*. 2024;25(1):e13648. DOI: https://doi.org/10.1111/obr.13648
2. Faerber G, Cornely M, Daubert C, Erbacher G, Fink J, Hirsch T, et al. S2k guideline lipedema. *JDDG J Dtsch Dermatol Ges*. 2024;22(9):1303–15. DOI: https://doi.org/10.1111/ddg.15513
3. Poojari A, Dev K, Rabiee A. Lipedema: insights into morphology, pathophysiology, and challenges. *Biomedicines*. 2022 Dec;10(12):3081. DOI: https://doi.org/10.3390/biomedicines10123081
4. Tuğral A, Bakar Y. An approach to lipedema: a literature review of current knowledge of an underestimated health problem. *Eur J Plast Surg*. 2019 Dec 1;42(6):549–58. DOI: https://doi.org/10.1007/s00238-019-01519-9
5. Hirsch T, Schleinitz J, Marshall M, Faerber G. [Is differential diagnosis of lipedema possible using high-resolution sonography?]. *Phlebologie*. 2018 Aug 22;47:182–7. DOI: https://doi.org/10.12687/phleb2431-4-2018
6. Patton L, Ricolfi L, Bortolon M, Gabriele G, Zolesio P, Cione E, et al. Observational study on a large Italian population with lipedema: biochemical and hormonal profile, anatomical and clinical evaluation, self-reported history. *Int J Mol Sci*. 2024 Jan;25(3):1599. DOI: https://doi.org/10.3390/ijms25031599
7. Markarian B, Toro C, Moreira K, Polam S, Mathew N, Mayrovitz HN. Assessment modalities for lower extremity edema, lymphedema, and lipedema: a scoping review. *Cureus*. 2024 Mar;16(3):e55906. DOI: https://doi.org/10.7759/cureus.55906
8. Amato ACM, Saucedo DZ, Santos K da S, Benitti DA. Ultrasound criteria for lipedema diagnosis. *Phlebology*. 2021 Sep 1;36(8):651–8. DOI: https://doi.org/10.1177/02683555211002340
9. Cestari M. Lipedema: Usefulness of 3D ultrasound diagnostics. *Lymphat Res Biol*. 2023 Oct;21(5):485–7. DOI: https://doi.org/10.1089/lrb.2022.0082
10. Stellmaker R, Thompson B, Mackie H, Koelmeyer L. Comparison of fluid and body composition measures in women with lipoedema, lymphoedema, and control participants. *Clin Obes*. 2024 Aug;14(4):e12658. DOI: https://doi.org/10.1111/cob.12658
11. Monnin-Delhom ED, Gallix BP, Achard C, Bruel JM, Janbon C. High resolution unenhanced computed tomography in patients with swollen legs. *Lymphology*. 2002 Sep;35(3):121–8. Available from: https://journals.librarypublishing.arizona.edu/lymph/article/id/3459/
12. Duewell S, Hagspiel KD, Zuber J, von Schulthess GK, Bollinger A, Fuchs WA. Swollen lower extremity: role of MR imaging. *Radiology*. 1992 Jul;184(1):227–31. DOI: https://doi.org/10.1148/radiology.184.1.1609085
13. Dimakakos PB, Stefanopoulos T, Antoniades P, Antoniou A, Gouliamos A, Rizos D. MRI and ultrasonographic findings in the investigation of lymphedema and lipedema. *Int Surg*. 1997;82(4):411–6. Available from: https://pubmed.ncbi.nlm.nih.gov/9412843/
14. Lohrmann C, Foeldi E, Langer M. MR imaging of the lymphatic system in patients with lipedema and lipo-lymphedema. *Microvasc Res*. 2009 May 1;77(3):335–9. DOI: https://doi.org/10.1016/j.mvr.2009.01.005
15. Cellina M, Gibelli D, Soresina M, Menozzi A, Martinenghi C, Panzeri M, et al. Non-contrast MR lymphography of lipedema of the lower extremities. *Magn Reson Imaging*. 2020 Sep 1;71:115–24. DOI: https://doi.org/10.1016/j.mri.2020.06.010
16. Giammarile F, Alazraki N, Aarsvold JN, Audisio RA, Glass E, Grant SF, et al. The EANM and SNMMI practice guideline for lymphoscintigraphy and sentinel node localization in breast

cancer. *Eur J Nucl Med Mol Imaging*. 2013 Dec 1;40(12):1932–47. DOI: https://doi.org/10.1007/s00259-013-2544-2

17. Bourgeois P. Critical analysis of the literature on the lymphoscintigraphic investigations of the limb edemas. *Eur J Lymphology Relat Probl.* 1996;6:1–9.
18. Sampathirao N, Indirani M, Manokaran G, Jaykanth A, Patel A, Simon S. Assessment of lymphedema with lymphoscintigraphy: can nodal quantification help? *Lymphology*. 2021;54(2):92–105. Available from: https://journals.librarypublishing.arizona.edu/lymph/article/id/4730/
19. Keeley V. The use of lymphoscintigraphy in the management of chronic oedema. *J Lymphoedema*. 2006;1(1):42–57. Available from: https://woundsinternational.com/wp-content/uploads/2023/02/content_11075.pdf
20. Bräutigam P, Földi E, Schaiper I, Krause T, Vanscheidt W, Moser E. Analysis of lymphatic drainage in various forms of leg edema using two compartment lymphoscintigraphy. *Lymphology*. 1998 Jun;31(2):43–55. Available from: https://journals.librarypublishing.arizona.edu/lymph/article/id/3343/
21. Forner-Cordero I, Oliván-Sasot P, Ruiz-Llorca C, Muñoz-Langa J. Lymphoscintigraphic findings in patients with lipedema. *Rev Esp Med Nucl E Imagen Mol Engl Ed*. 2018 Nov 1;37(6):341–8. DOI: https://doi.org/10.1016/j.remnie.2018.10.013
22. Chachaj A, Dudka I, Jeziorek M, Sowicz M, Adaszyńska A, Szuba A. Lymphoscintigraphic alterations in lower limbs in women with lipedema in comparison to women with overweight/obesity. *Front Physiol*. 2023 Apr 10;14. Available from: https://www.frontiersin.org/journals/physiology/articles/10.3389/fphys.2023.1099555/full
23. Donohoe KJ, Carroll BJ, Chung DKV, Dibble EH, Diego E, Giammarile F, et al. Summary: appropriate use criteria for lymphoscintigraphy in sentinel node mapping and lymphedema/lipedema. *J Nucl Med Off Publ Soc Nucl Med*. 2023 Apr;64(4):525–8. DOI: https://doi.org/10.2967/jnumed.123.265560
24. Vendrami C, Gatineau G, Gonzalez Rodriguez E, Lamy O, Hans D, Shevroja E. Standardization of body composition parameters between GE Lunar iDXA and Hologic Horizon A and their clinical impact. *JBMR Plus*. 2024 Jul 10;8(9):ziae088. DOI: https://doi.org/10.1093/jbmrpl/ziae088
25. Kempa S, Gross M, Oliinyk D, Siegmund A, Müller M, Prantl L, et al. Health implications of lipedema: analysis of patient questionnaires and population-based matched controls. *Life*. 2024 Mar;14(3):295. DOI: https://doi.org/10.3390/life14030295
26. Al-Ghadban S, Cromer W, Allen M, Ussery C, Badowski M, Harris D, et al. Dilated blood and lymphatic microvessels, angiogenesis, increased macrophages, and adipocyte hypertrophy in lipedema thigh skin and fat tissue. *J Obes*. 2019 Mar 3;2019:1–10. DOI: https://doi.org/10.1155/2019/8747461

Chapter Eleven
Novel approaches to lipedema diagnosis through magnetic resonance imaging

Rachelle Crescenzi, Shannon Taylor, Michael Pridmore, Vanessa Crain, Allison O'Brien Scott and Sara Al-Ghadban

Introduction

Novel questions need novel approaches. Lipedema is novel, not because it is newly discovered, but because it is being brought to new light. Highly skilled clinicians have developed systematic characterizations of lipedema symptoms. Instructive materials are available for fellow clinicians to learn more about how to diagnose lipedema.[1, 2, 3]

This raises the question: What remains uncertain about the diagnosis of lipedema? The key challenge lies in distinguishing it more clearly and earlier from other similar diseases. Lipedema is commonly misdiagnosed as either obesity or lymphedema due to overlapping clinical features. One major diagnostic challenge is that lipedema shares characteristics with both diseases. Like obesity, lipedema involves excess fat accumulation, but in lipedema, this growth is disproportionately concentrated in the lower extremities. Similarly, lipedema and lymphedema both present with limb swelling; however, lipedema typically spares the feet, while lymphedema often includes swelling of the feet. Unlike either, lipedema is also associated with distinct symptoms such as pain and easy bruising in the affected areas. Diagnosis is further complicated by the heterogeneity of patient presentations, which range from mild to severe, and by frequent co-morbidities, including obesity and lymphedema.

The clinical diagnosis of lipedema requires specialized training to identify the subtle differences between lipedema, obesity, and lymphedema. In order to become comfortable with the diagnosis of lipedema, clinicians undergo years of training. Patients often travel to academic medical centers to obtain an expert diagnosis. The fact remains that people with lipedema are being diagnosed roughly 20 years after their symptoms onset.[4, 5]

Beyond diagnosis, questions remain about the cause of certain symptoms of lipedema. One question is whether edema, and thereby lymphatic involvement, is present in lipedema. Could edema be only a result of obesity, causing secondary edema in lipedema? This is important to identify in order to treat the cause of the disease more directly. Should lipedema be treated similarly to lymphedema, using compression therapy? Or, similarly to obesity, using metabolic treatments?

A second challenging symptom of lipedema is pain. This is a dynamic symptom that often comes and goes with various influences, both from disease within and external stimuli. What a challenge we are handed, to diagnose a disease where pain is the second most common symptom.[6] Should pain be required in the diagnosis of lipedema, and how should pain be evaluated?

What type of measurement would help identify the onset of lipedema symptoms? Or in advanced stages of disease, when obesity and/or lymphedema often coincide, how might lipedema be confirmed? How can we reduce the time to diagnosis for the millions of people living with lipedema? How will clinical trials be designed without objective, reproducible diagnostic criteria?

These are central questions that remain unanswered surrounding the diagnosis of lipedema. The novel question of how to diagnose lipedema as distinct from obesity or lymphedema will require novel approaches. This chapter will report on some novel approaches to diagnosing lipedema through imaging and objective measurement tools, aiming to address significant questions from patients, healthcare providers, and researchers.

Researchers are systematically evaluating tools that could aid the clinical diagnosis of lipedema. Candidate tools should have specificity for aspects of disease pathophysiology. They should also be sensitive to the anticipated clinical scenario. This requires knowing how the measured value differs in lipedema, obesity, or lymphedema, compared to unaffected areas in an individual, or in response to treatment. Finally, candidate tools should be feasible to acquire in the setting of interest, whether in a community clinic or a state-of-the-art research facility.

Pathophysiology of lipedema

To introduce the various tools being trialed for lipedema diagnosis, we'll begin by discussing the pathophysiology of lipedema. Lipedema derives its name from the co-occurrence of fat ('lipid') and fluid ('edema'). Therefore, common research approaches aim to measure the amount of fat and fluid in affected areas of the body with lipedema. Tools that measure aspects of fat include MRI, DEXA, and ultrasound. Tools that measure aspects of fluid include water-weighted MRI methods such as MR lymphangiography and bioimpedance. We propose measuring a third element of lipedema tissue composition, which is tissue sodium. Tools for measuring tissue sodium non-invasively include sodium[23] Na-MRI. Tissue sodium may be relevant to lipedema because it is sensitive to tissue fibrosis, which is present in adipose tissue biopsies of patients with lipedema.[7, 8, 9] The pathophysiology of lipedema in terms of fat, fluid, and fibrosis has been discussed in a recent review article.[10] These approaches are summarized in Table 11.1.

Evaluating diagnostic tools for lipedema

Next, we present the current knowns, unknowns, and conjectures regarding the ability of objective measurement tools to aid the diagnosis of lipedema. First, we will discuss the measurement of the fat in lipedema, as this is a known feature of the disease. Next, we will address the measurement of fluid and edema in lipedema, as this represents an area of uncertainty in the field. Finally, we will present observations of adipose tissue sodium in lipedema, revealed by sodium MRI. We conjecture tissue sodium will be additionally necessary to diagnose and develop treatments specifically for lipedema.

Known: subcutaneous adipose tissue is thick in lipedema and can be measured by multiple imaging modalities

Lipedema manifests as bilateral swelling of the legs. Imaging shows which part of the legs is affected by swelling in lipedema. One of the first imaging reports in a case of lipedema used MRI. Radiologists described the enlargement of subcutaneous adipose tissue (SAT) in the legs with

Table 11.1: Body composition measures relevant to lipedema research. The various modalities and observables presented are being explored to aid in the diagnosis of lipedema.

Type of measure	Modality	Observable	Reference
Fat-sensitive measure	Fat-weighted MRI	Calf SAT area (mm^2)	Crescenzi et al.[11]
	Fat-weighted MRI	Thigh SAT volume (mL)	Taylor et al.[12]
	DEXA	Leg fat mass / total fat mass (ratio)	Buso et al.[13]
	Ultrasound	Calf, thigh SAT thickness (cm)	Iker et al.[14]
Water-sensitive measure	Water-weighted MR lymphangiography	Leg tissue edema (radiologist score)	Crescenzi et al.[15]
	Bioimpedance	Leg/arm impedance (ratio)†	Crescenzi et al.[16]
Sodium-sensitive measure	Sodium ^{23}Na-MRI	Calf tissue sodium content (mmol/L)	Crescenzi et al.[7, 11]

†Impedance is inversely proportional to extracellular water content.

lipedema.[17] Nearly three decades later, the first MRI study in a group of patients with lipedema was reported. This work was supported by a research grant from the Lipedema Foundation. In this study, we applied conventional MRI to measure SAT area in the calf (in units of millimeters squared, mm^2). We demonstrated significantly greater calf SAT area (42% difference, $p<0.001$) in patients with lipedema ($n=15$) compared to female controls ($n=14$) who were of similar age, and had similar body mass index (BMI), and calf circumference.[13] This finding was confirmed in an independent cohort of patients and controls, in which MRI of the SAT area was significantly elevated in the lower extremities but not the upper extremities of patients with lipedema.[7]

Next, imaging was used to answer the question: where is the most diagnostic region to evaluate the SAT area in legs with lipedema? To answer this, we performed whole-leg fat-weighted imaging by MRI.[8] We developed a semi-automated image segmentation method to measure SAT volume (in units of milliliters, mL) in each MRI slice. MRI slices were grouped into 10 segments, ranging from the ankles to the thighs, for each person to account for differences in height. This analysis was performed in people with lipedema ($n=15$) and female controls without lipedema ($n=13$) who had similar BMIs and were without prior liposuction. We found that SAT volume was greater in every segment of the leg in individuals with lipedema ($p<0.01$), whereas leg muscle volume was not significantly different in any segment. SAT volume was most differential in the upper thigh segment (68% difference, $p=0.002$). Together, these data provide objective evidence using noninvasive MRI that lipedema is distinct from obesity based on higher SAT in the legs.

Other imaging modalities have confirmed that SAT deposition is increased in the legs affected by lipedema. DEXA is an imaging modality that utilizes X-ray technology to measure the percentage of tissue composed of fat. DEXA imaging is acquired in a whole-body manner, and fat content can be quantified from each segment of the body, including arms and legs. A study by Dr. G. Buso and colleagues performed the most extensive DEXA study to date in 74 patients with lipedema compared to a control cohort of 148 females with similar age and BMI.[18] One of the most distinguishing metrics was leg fat mass per total body fat mass, which was 27% higher in patients with lipedema (p <0.001).

Bedside modalities that can measure fat in legs with lipedema are also of interest because they could provide clinically feasible, high-throughput diagnostics for lipedema. Ultrasound may be useful as an accessible alternative to MRI or DEXA for measuring SAT deposition in lipedema. In a study by Dr. E. Iker and colleagues,[10] clinically standard diagnostic ultrasound was performed in 12 patients with lipedema, 10 patients with leg lymphedema, and eight control legs without lipedema or lymphedema with similar BMI. Ultrasound images were used to measure SAT thickness (in units of centimeters, cm) from the skin down to the muscle. Results showed that SAT thickness was 107% larger in the calves and 125% larger in the thighs of patients with lipedema compared to those in the control group. SAT thickness was more similar in patients with lipedema compared to those with lymphedema.

Conclusion

Leg SAT amount has high potential to serve as a diagnostic biomarker of lipedema. The amount of SAT in lipedema-affected areas, whether measured by volume or thickness, has a strong capacity to distinguish lipedema from females with similar BMI but without lipedema. Leg SAT amount can be measured by multiple modalities and is simple to calculate and reproduce. In particular, the thighs may be the most diagnostic region to distinguish lipedema based on SAT amount. Future applications of SAT measurements will require clinical trials to test and validate their diagnostic value and response to interventions.

Unknown: is edema present in lipedema? How can it be measured?

Edema is an elusive symptom in lipedema, partly because traditional methods for detecting edema have proven inconclusive. Lymphoscintigraphy, for instance, is the clinical gold standard imaging modality to test for lymphatic transport insufficiency in lymphedema. However, lymphoscintigraphy reports mixed findings in lipedema, summarized by Dr. van la Parra and colleagues in their recent review of diagnostic imaging.[19] Lymphoscintigraphy in lipedema reports delayed uptake of the injected tracer, or delayed transport in some, but not the majority of cases, with lipedema.[20, 21] Delayed transport appears to worsen with lipedema stage in some cohorts,[20] but not in the larger, well-characterized cohort studied by Dr. Forner Cordero and colleagues.[21] Other alterations were observed in lipedema, including distal collateral flow, dilated or tortuous vessels, and additional lymphatic vessels.[22, 23, 24, 25] Additional lymphatic vessels are also observed in obesity, as noted in a study by Dr. Chachaj and colleagues,[23] who concluded that lymphoscintigraphy may not be useful for differentiating lipedema from obesity. Lymphoscintigraphy may also not be conclusive enough to distinguish lipedema from lymphedema, given the frequent presence of abnormalities in both diseases.[21]

Modern imaging technology utilizes optical imaging and an injected tracer to visualize lymphatics and their clearance function, known as indocyanine green near-infrared (ICG-NIR) lymphography. In a study by Dr. Zaleska and colleagues,[26] a larger number of lymphatic vessels were reported in lipedema. Yet, these appear to be pumping faster than normal in two independent cohorts, reported by Dr. Zaleska, Dr. Rasmussen and colleagues.[26, 27] Faster lymphatic vascular pumping is not inconsistent with the slow transport rate observed by lymphoscintigraphy. Instead, faster pumping could indicate the vessels are compensating for a larger lymphatic load or impaired function in the ability to transport fluid upstream.

Still, neither lymphoscintigraphy nor ICG-NIR lymphography consistently reports edema or dermal back flow in their observations of lipedema. One technical point is that ICG lymphography is limited to observing the superficial lymphatics. Is it possible that edema occurs deeper in lipedema fat? If the SAT thickness is greater than 2 cm in some cases, perhaps the imaging modality was not appropriate for the pathophysiology of lipedema.

MRI can be tailored to visualize slow-moving fluid in tissue and vasculature, using a technique called MR lymphangiography. MR lymphangiography is a clinically feasible imaging modality that enables the visualization of lymph stasis in a 3D manner. It does not require the injection of a contrast agent, making this technique completely noninvasive. It can be performed in the lower extremities to resolve superficial and deep leg tissues, including the skin, subcutaneous adipose tissue, and muscle. Because it does not require a contrast agent, it can be acquired in healthy individuals to better understand the normal physiology of tissue edema. In studies of lymphedema where the source of lymphatic disease is known, MR lymphangiography quantified tissue edema in unilateral upper-extremity lymphedema[28] and lower-extremity lymphedema.[29] Tissue edema on MR lymphangiography also mobilizes in response to therapeutic manual lymphatic drainage.[28] These studies helped demonstrate the specificity of MR lymphangiography for imaging lymphatic disease and treatments.

In lipedema, MR lymphangiography revealed the presence of deep, subcutaneous adipose tissue edema in the legs. We thought these patterns might be distinct from those associated with lymphedema and obesity. To test this hypothesis, the National Heart, Lung and Blood Institute (NHLBI) and Lipedema Foundation are supporting further research about MR lymphangiography in lipedema compared to obesity and lymphedema.[29, 30] Thus far, initial observations from MR lymphangiography have been reported in 14 patients with lipedema, 14 females without lipedema but with similar age and BMI (controls), and 8 with leg lymphedema secondary to cancer therapies.[31] Diffuse edema and dilated lymphatic vessels in the SAT are most prevalent in cases with leg lymphedema, as expected. In lipedema, diffuse edema in the SAT was 20 times more likely to occur than in controls; dilated vessels were 1.9 times more likely ($p<0.05$). Patterns of edema in leg lymphedema due to cancer therapy were more often focal rather than diffuse, like lipedema. These observations are consistent with imaging features reported from related MR lymphangiography techniques by investigators Dr. Cellina, Dr. Lohrman, and their colleagues.[32, 33] To date, these observations are reported in limited group sizes of heterogeneous patients. MR lymphangiography is beginning to reveal distinct patterns of edema, which could be useful in differentiating lipedema from obesity or lymphedema, and locating areas of edematous adipose tissue in patients with lipedema that could be targeted for therapy.

It may be possible to detect tissue edema in lipedema using a bedside tool, such as bioimpedance spectroscopy (BIS). BIS measures the tissue's resistance to an electrical signal. BIS works on the principle that fluid is a conductor and fat is an insulator; therefore, lower resistance values indicate greater tissue fluid content, such as in edema. BIS is typically applied in a segmental manner, allowing for the measurement of total tissue water and extracellular water in each arm and leg. BIS is already used as an early indicator of lymphedema development in people at risk for lymphedema due to cancer therapies.

In lipedema, might BIS be sensitive to edema in affected areas? In a study published in 2019, patients with lipedema were assessed using BIS at the annual conference of the Fat Disorders Resource Society (FDRS) over a 3-year period.[16] This study assessed a total of 110 women with lipedema stage

1–3. Leg bioimpedance decreases with increasing lipedema stage (p=0.03), indicating that extracellular fluid volume increases as lipedema worsens.

Useful BIS metrics in lipedema are still being determined for different clinical use cases. The BIS metric, which is best able to distinguish lipedema from non-lipedema, should exploit the disproportionate nature of lipedema. Edema in lipedema typically affects the lower extremities, often symmetrically, more so than the upper extremities. In this case, the ratio of fluid in the lower compared to the upper body segments could effectively distinguish lipedema from non-lipedema body water retention. In a small pilot study, the ratio of bioimpedance in the legs compared to arms was 9% lower in 10 patients with early-stage 1 lipedema compared to 21 women without lipedema matched for age and BMI.[16] This finding highlights the disproportionate nature of lipedema and how it might be exploited for diagnostic purposes. If such a metric is validated for lipedema, it would be clinically valuable in a bedside screening exam.

Conclusion

MR lymphangiography observations are visualizing deep tissue edema in lipedema, where traditional lymphatic imaging modalities are not optimized to probe. Bedside modalities, such as bioimpedance spectroscopy, are also being investigated for their sensitivity to fluid accumulation in lipedema and their utility at the bedside. Further research is needed to understand the cause of edema in lipedema, its relationship to various disease stages, and to exploit this observation to aid in the diagnosis and treatment of lipedema.

Current research is asking to what extent blood and lymphatic vascular mechanisms are involved in lipedema pathogenesis. How could vascular disease mechanisms lead to edema and SAT accumulation? More broadly, lipedema is potentially a model disease of vascular mechanisms of fat dysregulation. Discovering disease mechanisms of lipedema could have broad implications for treating fluid and fat accumulation in other diseases such as hypertension, peripheral vascular disease, renal disease, and other fat diseases.

Conjecture: measuring tissue sodium in lipedema by ^{23}Na-MRI could aid diagnosis, discovery of disease mechanisms, and development of treatments

Thus far, we have described ways to measure fat and fluid in lipedema and how these relate to diagnosis. There is a third component of the tissue's composition that may reveal a significant aspect of adipose tissue pathology in lipedema. This is tissue sodium content.

Tissue sodium storage is an emerging indicator of cardiovascular disease. It is known to be elevated in the legs of people with diseases of the kidney, heart, and peripheral vascular system.[32] Tissue sodium levels can be elevated partly due to poor circulation or the inadequate clearance of sodium from the tissue. Another way sodium is stored in tissue is through tissue fibrosis, where a matrix of proteins builds up outside cells that are undergoing inflammation, injury, or disease. This matrix is called the extracellular matrix, and it is composed of negatively charged proteins called glycosaminoglycans that attract positively charged sodium ions.

Both poor circulation and tissue fibrosis could be occurring in lipedema adipose tissue, which would contribute to tissue sodium storage. In tissue, two independent studies by Dr. Al-Ghadban and Dr. Felmerer, along with their colleagues, revealed angiogenesis and fibrosis in the skin and subcutaneous tissue biopsies from patients with lipedema.[8, 9, 35] Circulating blood markers in lipedema are beginning to reveal altered platelet biology, including increased platelet factor 4, as discovered by Ma et al.,[36] and decreased glycosaminoglycan synthesis, discovered by Scalise et al.[37] Platelet factor 4 binds to glycosaminoglycans to perform its function in coagulation, inflammation, and angiogenesis. Because sodium is highly concentrated in the blood, and when bound to glycosaminoglycans in tissue, it could be an interesting indicator of these biological processes in lipedema.

Tissue sodium content can be measured by sodium ^{23}Na-MRI. Sodium ^{23}Na-MRI is a noninvasive imaging method being trialed in translational research to support the diagnosis, discovery of disease mechanisms, and development of treatments for lipedema. The first study using this technique applied[23] Na-MRI in the calf of patients with lipedema compared to controls without lipedema who had similar age, BMI, sex, race, and calf circumference.[7] Tissue sodium was significantly elevated in the calf of patients with lipedema compared to controls, in the skin (14.9±2.9 vs. 11.9±2.0 mmol/L, p=0.01), and SAT (11.9±3.1 vs. 9.4±1.6 mmol/L; p=0.04). This finding was confirmed in an independent cohort. In this follow-up study, tissue sodium by sodium ^{23}Na-MRI was significantly elevated in the lower extremities, but not upper extremities, of patients with lipedema compared to controls.[8, 9, 35]

Both studies of tissue sodium ^{23}Na-MRI in lipedema also measured the amount of SAT in the calf by conventional fat-weighted ^{1}H-MRI. Together, comprehensive ^{23}Na^{1}H-MRI studies concluded that swollen limbs with lipedema are not only full of adipose tissue but also contain high tissue sodium. This provided objective evidence, using non-invasive MRI, that lipedema is distinct from obesity based on a profile of adiposity and sodium retention in the lower extremities. These pilot studies remain to be replicated at other institutions and in larger cohorts for validation. Further studies are ongoing to compare how tissue sodium storage may be similar or different between patients with lipedema and/or lymphedema. This data motivated a larger study supported by the NHLBI to observe tissue sodium in lipedema, which is ongoing.[29]

Tissue sodium appears to have relevance not only in distinguishing lipedema from obesity, but also in indicating the severity of the disease. For instance, tissue sodium significantly increases with lipedema stage (Spearman's *rho*=0.82, $p<0.001$) and with the experience of pain in the legs related to lipedema (Spearman's *rho*=0.55, p=0.03).[11] These analyses do not yet show the cause of tissue sodium or pain in lipedema, but indicate at least a common mechanism, which is an active area of research.

How might excess sodium be removed or mobilized from lipedema tissue? Complete decongestive therapy (CDT) is a standard-of-care lymphatic therapy that can be readily applied to patients with lipedema, provided it demonstrates improvement in disease symptoms. As discussed in Chapter 12, CDT utilizes compression garments, exercise, education, and manual lymphatic drainage (MLD) treatments applied by a trained therapist. In a preliminary study of 5 patients with early-stage 1 or 2 lipedema, sodium ^{23}Na-MRI was acquired before and after 6 weeks of CDT.[38] Tissue sodium was reduced in the legs following CDT compared to baseline. On average, skin sodium content was 14.2±1.7 mmol/L pre-treatment, compared to 13.0±2.2 mmol/L post-treatment (8.5% mean difference, p=0.05), and a similar amount of tissue sodium was reduced in the leg SAT by 8%. All five patients reported reduced leg pain and improved daily functioning, confirming a clinically significant response. Although results are preliminary, this study demonstrates the proof of principle that tissue sodium can be reduced in lipedema legs using standard-of-care lymphatic therapy, which is clinically accessible.

Conclusion

Tissue sodium content measured by standardized sodium MRI helped demonstrate the distinct nature of adipose tissue in lipedema, compared to females without lipedema with similar BMI. Sodium levels in lipedema tissue could be a helpful biomarker to aid in the differential diagnosis of lipedema, indicate disease severity, and potentially predict the response to lymphatic therapy. Promising translational applications of sodium MRI in lipedema include studying disease mechanisms of edema and fibrosis formation, as well as quantifying therapeutic responses in affected tissues.

Conclusion

This chapter surveyed the novel technologies being applied to aid in the diagnosis of lipedema, with a focus on MRI and related imaging and bedside modalities. Tools were presented that are sensitive to fat, fluid, and fibrosis, which we propose are three important aspects of characterizing lipedema that will help to distinguish the disease from obesity or lymphedema. As new aspects of the pathophysiology of lipedema come to light, the list of candidate diagnostic tools will grow. This is an exciting area of lipedema research!

In the coming years, progress is anticipated in developing candidate therapies to address the full range of symptoms and stages of patients with lipedema. Candidate therapies are being developed in four categories: manual techniques, nutrition, pharmaceuticals, and surgical procedures. The MRI tools presented, which are sensitive to fat, fluid, and fibrosis in lipedema, could serve as indicators of hypothesized therapeutic response. For instance, in a recent study of the ketogenic diet in patients with lipedema, fat-weighted MRI was used to demonstrate reduced calf SAT area and pain.[39] Numerous studies are ongoing to determine promising diagnostics and therapeutics for lipedema worldwide. Imaging and objective measurement tools provide essential translational technologies to ensure that research questions about lipedema are answered, in a way that impacts the lives of patients with lipedema.

References

1. Herbst KL, Kahn LA, Iker E, Ehrlich C, Wright T, McHutchison L, et al. Standard of care for lipedema in the United States. *Phlebology.* 2021 Dec 1;36(10):779–96. DOI: https://doi.org/10.1177/02683555211015887
2. Kruppa P, Georgiou I, Biermann N, Prantl L, Klein-Weigel P, Ghods M. Lipedema – pathogenesis, diagnosis, and treatment options. *Dtsch Ärztebl Int.* 2020 Jun;117(22–23):396. DOI: https://doi.org/10.3238/arztebl.2020.0396
3. Halk AB, Damstra RJ. First Dutch guidelines on lipedema using the international classification of functioning, disability and health. *Phlebol J Venous Dis.* 2017 Apr;32(3):152–9. DOI: https://doi.org/10.1177/0268355516639421
4. Fetzer A, Fetzer, S. *Lipoedema UK Big Survey 2014 Research Report.* Chichester, UK: Lipoedema UK; 2016 Jul p. 1–8. Available from: https://lipoedema.co.uk/wp-content/uploads/2024/05/LATEST-LUK000-UK-Big-Survey16-Mar24-web.pdf
5. Lipedema Foundation. *Lipedema Foundation registry: first look report.* Lipedema Foundation; 2022 p. 12. Available from: https://www.lipedema.org/registry-first-look-report
6. Aday AW, Donahue PM, Garza M, Crain VN, Patel NJ, Beasley JA, et al. National survey of patient symptoms and therapies among 707 women with a lipedema phenotype in the United States. *Vasc Med.* 2024 Feb 1;29(1):36–41. DOI: https://doi.org/10.1177/1358863X231202769
7. Crescenzi R, Marton A, Donahue PMC, Mahany HB, Lants SK, Wang P, et al. Tissue sodium content is elevated in the skin and subcutaneous adipose tissue in women with lipedema. *Obesity.* 2018;26(2):310–7. DOI: https://doi.org/10.1002/oby.22090
8. Al-Ghadban S, Cromer W, Allen M, Ussery C, Badowski M, Harris D, et al. Dilated blood and lymphatic microvessels, angiogenesis, increased macrophages, and adipocyte hypertrophy in lipedema thigh skin and fat tissue. *J Obes.* 2019 Mar 3;2019:1–10. DOI: https://doi.org/10.1155/2019/8747461
9. Felmerer G, Stylianaki A, Hollmén M, Ströbel P, Stepniewski A, Wang A, et al. Increased levels of

VEGF-C and macrophage infiltration in lipedema patients without changes in lymphatic vascular morphology. *Sci Rep*. 2020 Jul 2;10(1):10947. DOI: https://doi.org/10.1038/s41598-020-67987-3
10. Duhon BH, Phan TT, Taylor SL, Crescenzi RL, Rutkowski JM. Current mechanistic understandings of lymphedema and lipedema: tales of fluid, fat, and fibrosis. *Int J Mol Sci*. 2022 Jan;23(12):6621. DOI: https://doi.org/10.3390/ijms23126621
11. Crescenzi R, Donahue PMC, Petersen KJ, Garza M, Patel N, Lee C, et al. Upper and lower extremity measurement of tissue sodium and fat content in patients with lipedema. *Obesity*. 2020 May;28(5):907–15. DOI: https://doi.org/10.1002/oby.22778
12. Taylor SL, Donahue PMC, Pridmore MD, Garza ME, Patel NJ, Custer CA, et al. Semiautomated segmentation of lower extremity MRI reveals distinctive subcutaneous adipose tissue in lipedema: a pilot study. *J Med Imaging*. 2023 May;10(3):036001. DOI: https://doi.org/10.1117/1.JMI.10.3.036001
13. Buso G, Favre L, Maufus M, Honorati M, Lessert C, Depairon M, et al. Indocyanine green lymphography as novel tool to assess lymphatics in patients with lipedema. *Microvasc Res*. 2022 Mar 1;140:104298. DOI: https://doi.org/10.1016/j.mvr.2021.104298
14. Iker E, Mayfield CK, Gould DJ, Patel KM. Characterizing lower extremity lymphedema and lipedema with cutaneous ultrasonography and an objective computer-assisted measurement of dermal echogenicity. *Lymphat Res Biol*. 2019 Oct;17(5):525–30. DOI: https://doi.org/10.1089/lrb.2017.0090
15. Crescenzi R, Donahue PMC, Garza M, Patel NJ, Lee C, Guerreso K, et al. Subcutaneous adipose tissue edema in lipedema revealed by noninvasive 3T MR lymphangiography. *J Magn Reson Imaging*. 2022. Available from: https://onlinelibrary.wiley.com/doi/abs/10.1002/jmri.28281
16. Crescenzi R, Donahue PMC, Weakley S, Garza M, Donahue MJ, Herbst KL. Lipedema and Dercum's disease: a new application of bioimpedance. *Lymphat Res Biol*. 2019 Dec;17(6):671–9. DOI: https://doi.org/10.1089/lrb.2019.0011
17. Duewell S, Hagspiel KD, Zuber J, von Schulthess GK, Bollinger A, Fuchs WA. Swollen lower extremity: role of MR imaging. *Radiology*. 1992 Jul;184(1):227–31. DOI: https://doi.org/10.1148/radiology.184.1.1609085
18. Buso G, Favre L, Vionnet N, Gonzalez-Rodriguez E, Hans D, Puder JJ, et al. Body composition assessment by dual-energy X-ray absorptiometry: a useful tool for the diagnosis of lipedema. *Obes Facts*. 2022 Oct 28;15(6):762–73. DOI: https://doi.org/10.1159/000527138
19. van la Parra RFD, Deconinck C, Krug B. Diagnostic imaging in lipedema: a systematic review. *Obes Rev*. 2024;25(1):e13648. DOI: https://doi.org/10.1111/obr.13648
20. Gould DJ, El-Sabawi B, Goel P, Badash I, Colletti P, Patel KM. Uncovering lymphatic transport abnormalities in patients with primary lipedema. *J Reconstr Microsurg*. 2019 Sep 23; DOI: https://doi.org/10.1055/s-0039-1697904
21. Forner-Cordero I, Oliván-Sasot P, Ruiz-Llorca C, Muñoz-Langa J. Lymphoscintigraphic findings in patients with lipedema. *Rev Esp Med Nucl E Imagen Mol Engl Ed*. 2018 Nov 1;37(6):341–8. DOI: https://doi.org/10.1016/j.remnie.2018.10.013
22. Ceylan S, Yilmaz N. Evaluation of Interstitium by lymphatic uptake method in chronic bilateral lower extremity edema. *Curr Med Imaging*. 20(1):1–6. DOI: https://doi.org/10.2174/1573405620666230328091624
23. Chachaj A, Dudka I, Jeziorek M, Sowicz M, Adaszyńska A, Szuba A. Lymphoscintigraphic alterations in lower limbs in women with lipedema in comparison to women with overweight/obesity. *Front Physiol*. 2023 Apr 10;14. Available from: www.frontiersin.org/journals/physiology/articles/10.3389/fphys.2023.1099555/full
24. Tartaglione G, Visconti G, Bartoletti R, Ieria FP, Salgarello M. Rest/stress intradermal lymphoscintigraphy in diagnosis of lipedema. *World J Nucl Med*. 2020;19(4):376–81. DOI: https://doi.org/10.4103/wjnm.WJNM_5_20
25. Van De Pas CB, Boonen RS, Stevens S, Willemsen S, Valkema R, Neumann M. Does tumescent liposuction damage the lymph vessels in lipoedema patients? *Phlebol J Venous Dis*. 2020 May;35(4):231–6. DOI: https://doi.org/10.1177/0268355519885217

26. Zaleska MT, Olszewski WL, Krzesniak NE. Lower limb lipedema – superficial lymph flow, skin water concentration, skin and subcutaneous tissue elasticity. *Lymphat Res Biol*. 2023 Feb;21(1):60–9.
DOI: https://doi.org/10.1089/lrb.2022.0010
27. Rasmussen JC, Aldrich MB, Fife CE, Herbst KL, Sevick-Muraca EM. Lymphatic function and anatomy in early stages of lipedema. *Obesity*. 2022;30(7):1391–400.
DOI: https://doi.org/10.1002/oby.23458
28. Crescenzi R, Donahue PMC, Hartley KG, Desai AA, Scott AO, Braxton V, et al. Lymphedema evaluation using noninvasive 3T MR lymphangiography. *J Magn Reson Imaging*. 2017;46(5):1349–60.
DOI: https://doi.org/10.1002/jmri.25670
29. ClinicalTrials.gov. Identifier: NCT05464927. *Visualizing vascular mechanisms of lipedema (VMP)*. [Ongoing]. Available from: https://clinicaltrials.gov/study/NCT05464927
30. ClinicalTrials.gov. Identifier: NCT05242900. *Imaging sodium and lymphatics in lymphedema*. [Ongoing]. Available from: https://reporter.nih.gov/search/EaC3BhVN6USBfOMuTswDVQ/project-details/11264103
31. Crescenzi R, Donahue PMC, Garza M, Patel NJ, Lee C, Guerreso K, et al. Subcutaneous adipose tissue edema in lipedema revealed by noninvasive 3T MR lymphangiography. *J Magn Reson Imaging*. 2023;57(2):598–608.
DOI: https://doi.org/10.1002/jmri.28281
32. Cellina M, Gibelli D, Soresina M, Menozzi A, Martinenghi C, Panzeri M, et al. Non-contrast MR lymphography of lipedema of the lower extremities. *Magn Reson Imaging*. 2020 Sep 1;71:115–24.
DOI: https://doi.org/10.1016/j.mri.2020.06.010
33. Lohrmann C, Foeldi E, Langer M. MR imaging of the lymphatic system in patients with lipedema and lipo-lymphedema. *Microvasc Res*. 2009 May 1;77(3):335–9.
DOI: https://doi.org/10.1016/j.mvr.2009.01.005
34. Gast LV, Platt T, Nagel AM, Gerhalter T. Recent technical developments and clinical research applications of sodium (23Na) MRI. *Prog Nucl Magn Reson Spectrosc*. 2023 Nov 1;138–139:1–51.
DOI: https://doi.org/10.1016/j.pnmrs.2023.04.002
35. Felmerer G, Stylianaki A, Hägerling R, Wang A, Ströbel P, Hollmén M, et al. Adipose tissue hypertrophy, an aberrant biochemical profile and distinct gene expression in lipedema. *J Surg Res*. 2020 Sep 1;253:294–303.
DOI: https://doi.org/10.1016/j.jss.2020.03.055
36. Ma W, Gil HJ, Escobedo N, Benito-Martín A, Ximénez-Embún P, Muñoz J, et al. Platelet factor 4 is a biomarker for lymphatic-promoted diseases. *JCI Insight*. 2020;5(13). Available from: https://www.ncbi.nlm.nih.gov/pmc/articles/PMC7406300/
37. Scalise A, Aggarwal A, Sangwan N, Hamer A, Guntupalli S, Park HE, et al. A divergent platelet transcriptome in patients with lipedema and lymphedema. *Genes*. 2024 Jun;15(6):737.
DOI: https://doi.org/10.3390/genes15060737
38. Donahue PMC, Crescenzi R, Petersen KJ, Garza M, Patel N, Lee C, et al. Physical therapy in women with early stage lipedema: potential impact of multimodal manual therapy, compression, exercise, and education interventions. *Lymphat Res Biol*. 2022 Aug;20(4):382–90.
DOI: https://doi.org/10.1089/lrb.2021.0039
39. Lundanes J, Gårseth M, Taylor S, Crescenzi R, Pridmore M, Wagnild R, et al. The effect of a low-carbohydrate diet on subcutaneous adipose tissue in females with lipedema. *Front Nutr*. 2024 Nov 7;11. Available from: https://www.frontiersin.org/journals/nutrition/articles/10.3389/fnut.2024.1484612/full

V
Summary of conservative treatment methodologies

Chapter Twelve
Complete decongestive therapy in lipedema

Franz-Josef Schingale

Introduction

Lipedema is a chronic disease characterized by abnormal, symmetrical fat accumulation primarily in the lower body, accompanied by pain, swelling, and tissue changes. Inflammation plays a central role in its pathophysiology.[1, 2] The exact cause of lipedema is not fully understood, but in many cases, a genetic component is suggested and may be influenced by hormonal changes. [3, 4, 5, 6, 7, 8] As no causal treatment is currently known, symptom-relieving measures are the first line of treatment.[9]

Although there is currently no known cure for lipedema, both conservative and surgical treatments can help prevent complications. One conservative approach is physiotherapy and rehabilitation (PR). However, a review of the literature reveals that few studies have specifically examined the efficacy of PR in this patient population. A review was published by the author in 2024 to enhance understanding of PR's effectiveness by compiling and analyzing existing research.[10] A bibliographic search identified studies on PR in the management of lipedema, covering 68 years from 1951 to 2019. Articles were selected based on a review of their abstracts, followed by full-text analysis of those that met the inclusion criteria. A total of 15 studies were included in this analysis.

The results highlight the benefits of PR for individuals with lipedema and illustrate the effectiveness of various rehabilitation methods. Interventions such as complex decongestive physiotherapy, gait training, hydrotherapy, aerobic exercise, and resistance training were all found to offer value in lipedema management. While the reported effects of PR varied across studies, the overall evidence suggests that it is a beneficial component of treatment. Nonetheless, physiotherapy should be integrated with other treatment modalities for optimal outcomes. Further high-quality research is needed to better establish the efficacy and role of PR in treating lipedema.

Complete decongestive therapy

Complete decongestive therapy (CDT) is a comprehensive, multimodal approach grounded in PR principles for managing symptoms associated with lipedema. It aims to reduce swelling, improve lymphatic flow, and enhance quality of life through a combination of therapeutic strategies. CDT consists of two phases: an initial reduction phase followed by an optimization and maintenance phase.[11] A targeted therapy aimed at the cause of lipedema is not yet known, as the exact etiology remains unexplained. Therapy has essentially two objectives: (1) resolve or improve symptoms (edema, pain, and disproportion); and (2) prevent disease progression and the development of complications (lymphatic, dermatologic, and orthopedic problems).

The main components of each phase of CDT include:

- manual lymphatic drainage (MLD)
- skin care
- compression therapy
- exercise
- self-management.

Manual lymphatic drainage (MLD)

Manual lymphatic drainage (MLD) is a specialized massage technique designed to stimulate the lymphatic system and promote the movement of lymph fluid. In individuals with lipedema (see Figure 12.1), MLD can help reduce inflammation and alleviate symptoms such as pain, tenderness, and heaviness. The technique involves gentle, rhythmic strokes performed by trained therapists and is tailored to the individual's specific needs. Beyond physical benefits, MLD often provides a sense of relaxation and emotional relief.

Historically, lipedema was thought to be primarily associated with edema,[12] but current research has suggested it as a disease of adipose tissue rather than the lymphatic system. The swelling observed in lipedema may be the result of orthostatic (gravity-induced) edema[13] and may not be true fluid retention. As such, initiating treatment with decongestive techniques aimed at shifting fluid may not be considered essential in pure lipedema cases.

Although there is no consensus on a standardized treatment protocol, management generally focuses on symptom relief, preventing disease progression, and minimizing disability.[14] In this context, MLD remains valuable, not solely to mobilize excess fluid, but also to reduce inflammation and pain, particularly pain on palpation or pressure.[15] Effective MLD can significantly improve patient comfort and make it more tolerable to wear custom-fitted compression garments.

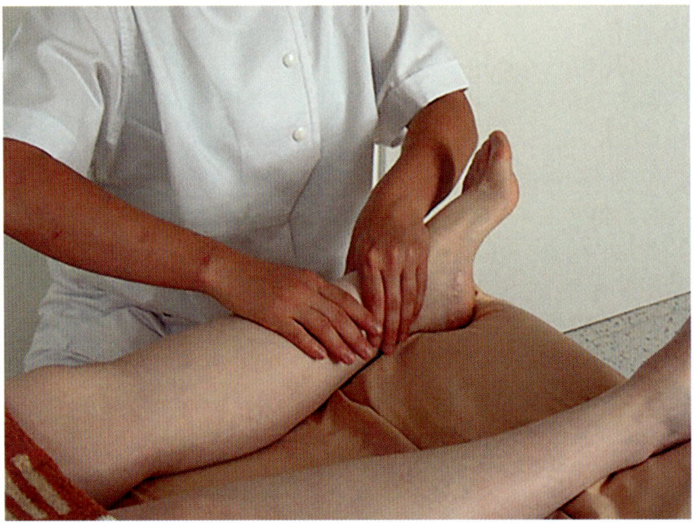

Figure 12.1: Manual lymphatic drainage (MLD). Used with permission from the clinic of Dr. med. Franz-Josef Schingale.

Skin care

Proper skin care is vital in preventing infections and maintaining the health of the skin, which can be compromised by swelling and inflammation (Figure 12.2). CDT includes guidelines for daily skin hygiene, moisturizing, and the treatment of any skin issues that may arise. Keeping the skin clean and hydrated helps to prevent complications and supports overall well-being.

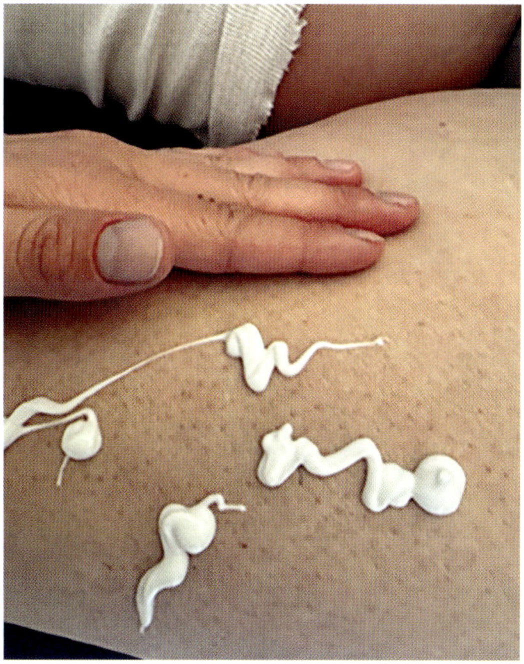

Figure 12.2: Skincare. Used with permission from the clinic of Dr. med. Franz-Josef Schingale.

Compression therapy

Compression therapy includes the use of bandages, stockings, or sleeves that are specifically designed to fit the contours of the body (see Figure 12.3). The basis for prescribing compression therapy might not be the edema reduction anymore, but rather the reduction of pain by the frequently demonstrated anti-inflammatory effects of compression therapy on the subcutaneous tissue. The etiology of pain in lipedema is unclear, though histological findings of inflammation and hypoxia may be contributing elements.[16] Recent findings that identify a chronic low-grade state of inflammation and tissue hypoxia as the most plausible explanations for the pain in patients with lipedema support this hypothesis.[17]

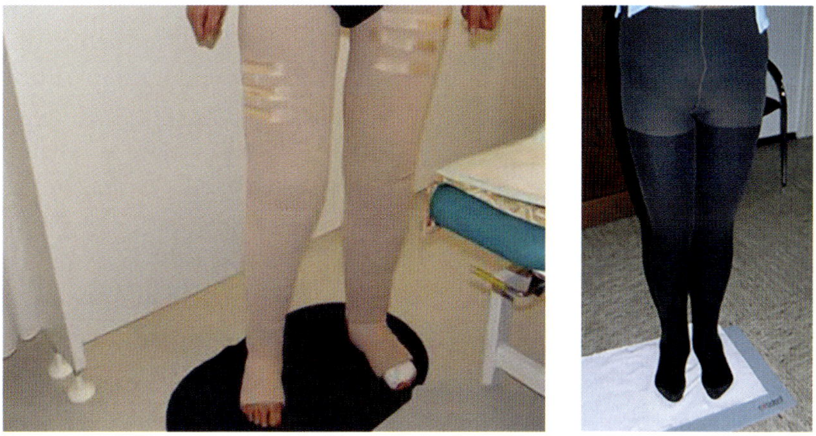

Figure 12.3: (Left) compression bandages; (right) compression hosiery. Used with permission from the clinic of Dr. med. Franz-Josef Schingale.

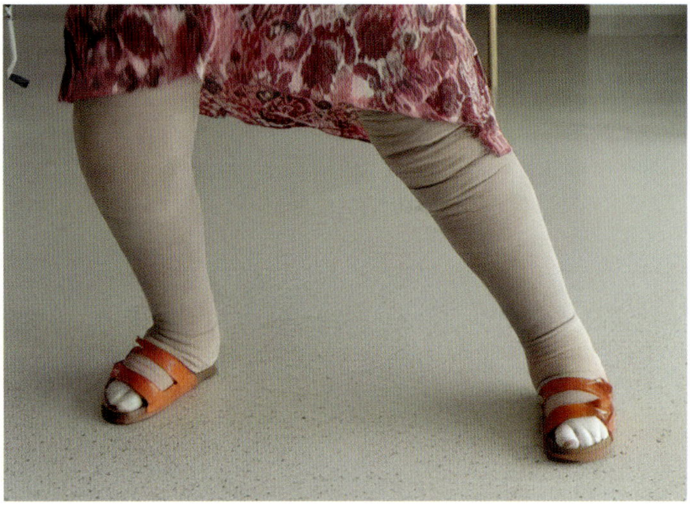

Figure 12.4: Exercise is performed while wearing compression bandages. Used with permission from the clinic of Dr. med. Franz-Josef Schingale.

Compression garments are essential in managing lipedema. These garments apply consistent pressure to the affected areas, reducing pain and inflammation. Regular use of compression garments can significantly improve mobility and reduce discomfort and pain. Since fluid displacement is not the primary goal, compression therapy often begins directly with the application of compression stockings rather than bandaging. The choice between round-knit and flat-knit garments depends on the patient's limb shape and degree of sensitivity.

A pilot study examining the effects of compression therapy in individuals with lipedema found a significant reduction in self-reported bruising tendency and pain upon palpation among participants who received the intervention. Preliminary findings suggest that when combined with exercise, compression therapy may contribute to improved quality of life and a reduction in the severity of lipedema-related symptoms.[18] Further studies on a large clinical group are advisable.

An online survey of 250 women with self-described lipedema[19] reported that the top three reasons for wearing compression garments were to feel supported (73%), reduce lipedema pain (67%), and improve mobility (54%). Most respondents who wore compression garments found compression helpful in managing their symptoms, but overall satisfaction was low. Problems with existing compression garments were so severe in some cases that the garments were used less often or not worn at all. The information collected might be useful for the design and development of compression garments specifically for lipedema.

Exercise

Physical activity plays a crucial role in CDT. Exercise helps to stimulate lymphatic flow, strengthen muscles, and enhance overall cardiovascular health (Figure 12.4). Low-impact exercises such as swimming, walking, and cycling are particularly beneficial for individuals with lipedema. These activities are gentle on the joints while promoting movement and circulation. Exercise programs are often customized to accommodate the individual's physical capabilities and limitations.[20]

Self-management

Self-care is a crucial part of managing lipedema and is expanded upon in Chapter 18 of this text. Facilitating and enhancing the patient's ability to perform self-care and cope with the physical and psychosocial impact of the disease is important.

Self-care for individuals with lipedema often includes skin care and, in some cases, self-administered MLD. However, the cornerstone of self-management is the consistent use of compression therapy. Recognizing this need, the medical garment industry has developed a wide range of compression hosiery in various colors, patterns, and materials to promote patient acceptance and adherence.

An increasingly popular compression alternative is the use of adjustable Velcro wrap garments. These provide firm, customizable support that can be easily readjusted within minutes, offering a more practical and comfortable solution, especially during physical activity, compared to traditional bandages, which can shift or slip during movement.

Self-care for individuals with lipedema also involves regular engagement in low-impact physical activities such as walking, swimming, cycling, yoga, Pilates, or water aerobics. Water-based exercises are particularly beneficial, as the natural hydrostatic pressure provides gentle compression and support, helping to reduce discomfort and promote circulation. In addition to physical activity, maintaining a healthy, balanced diet is essential. A nutrition plan rich in fruits, vegetables, and antioxidants may help reduce systemic inflammation and support overall health. Adequate hydration further aids in metabolic function and tissue health. This topic is further discussed in Chapter 14. Finally, incorporating stress-reduction practices, such as deep breathing, mindfulness, meditation, or yoga, can contribute to symptom relief and enhance overall well-being.

Intermittent pneumatic compression

In addition to MLD and compression therapy, intermittent pneumatic compression (IPC) can be used as an adjunct or alternative treatment option.[9, 21] The intensity and frequency of IPC use should be tailored to the severity of symptoms and the stage of lipedema. To monitor treatment progress, objective assessment methods, such as limb circumference measurements or volumetry, should be employed. It is important to note that IPC does not directly reduce adipocyte size or number.[1]

Benefits of complete decongestive therapy

The comprehensive nature of CDT offers numerous benefits for individuals with lipedema, including improvements in pain management, functional mobility, and quality of life.[21, 22, 23] In cases where surgical treatment (e.g. liposuction) is being considered, CDT may be used pre- and post-operatively to optimize outcomes and reduce swelling or inflammation. Additionally, proper skin care, along with compression therapy, is important for preventing complications, such as post-surgical infections.[24]

Evaluation and assessment

Setting realistic expectations is crucial for both the patient and the medical care provider. The primary aims of management are multimodal, aiming to improve quality of life, reduce heaviness and pain, reshape the affected limbs, promote weight control, and enhance mobility. For this reason, compression garments, physical therapy, exercise regimens, nutrition, and psychological counseling are essential.[25]

The tools currently used in evaluating the effectiveness of conservative treatment in women with lipedema are: volume and circumference measurement, waist-to-hip ratio, body fat percentage, ultrasonography, pain intensity (Visual Analog Scale), quality of life scales (SF-36, RAND-36), symptom severity questionnaire (QuASiL), lower extremity functional scale and 6-minute walk test. Choosing a proper tool to measure the treatment outcome is essential to objectively rate the effectiveness of the therapeutic method.[18]

What is known about CDT for lipedema?

The Lipedema World Alliance (LWA) is a leading non-profit organization dedicated to advancing the understanding and management of lipedema. By bringing together global experts, the LWA has critically reviewed existing clinical guidelines and strongly advocates for a multidisciplinary approach as the standard of care. This comprehensive model typically involves collaboration with lymphedema therapists, nutritional counseling, and personalized compression garment education and fitting.

While conservative therapies remain the first-line and gold-standard interventions for managing lipedema, LWA experts acknowledge their limitations. The outcomes of conservative treatments can vary significantly between individuals and may not fully address all aspects of the disease. For instance, conservative measures often have little impact on mobility impairments caused by disproportionate fat accumulation around the knees or thighs. Furthermore, they are not equipped to address the psychological or social challenges many patients face due to the visible and distressing changes in body shape. Perhaps most concerning, current evidence suggests that conservative therapies alone may not be sufficient to halt the progression of lipedema. These limitations highlight the urgent need for ongoing research, patient-centered care, and the development of more effective, individualized treatment strategies.

It is essential to consider psychological stress in diseases such as lipedema to improve quality of life and treat chronic pain. Psychosocial therapy approaches and self-management are important components of holistic treatment that need to be further developed in practice. For instance, it is known that MLD not only has a physical effect, but also influences the patient's nervous system and mental state through neurophysiological reflexes and psychosocial factors.[26] The shift from a sympathetic to a parasympathetic state promotes relaxation and pain reduction. It is also acknowledged that CDT has a positive effect on pain and inflammation.[18, 24, 27, 28]

What is unknown about CDT in lipedema?

In my opinion, there is no scientific evidence that lipedema is an 'edema problem' or that MLD reduces patients' symptoms due to its drainage effects on the lymphatic system. Neither the clinical examination nor the diagnosis has shown that there is a significant accumulation of fluid in the tissue of patients with lipedema, which makes 'decongestion of the tissue' by manual or automated lymphatic drainage techniques superfluous, in my experience. The term 'lipedema' may be outdated and should be reconsidered.[13]

What are the conjectures of CDT in lipedema?

The psychological influence of MLD plays an important role in the overall therapeutic concept, especially in the treatment of pain and chronic diseases such as lipedema. MLD is carried out with even, rhythmic movements and warm hands to trigger a so-called 'tender reflex,' which is controlled by the spinal cord. This reflex causes a shift from the sympathetic (excited) state to the parasympathetic phase, which leads to relaxation of the patient.[26] In addition to the manual technique, external factors such as room temperature, lighting, and background noise also influence the parasympathetic effect of MLD. A relieving conversation between therapist and patient can also contribute to relaxation, with the therapist taking on the role of an active listener.

Conclusion

Complete decongestive therapy is a cornerstone in the management of lipedema, offering a holistic approach that addresses both the physical and emotional aspects of the disease. By combining MLD, compression therapy, exercise, and skincare, CDT provides a comprehensive treatment plan that can significantly improve the quality of life for individuals with lipedema. Despite challenges such as accessibility and cost, the benefits of CDT make it an invaluable tool in the ongoing effort to manage and alleviate the symptoms of lipedema.

References

1. Kruppa P, Gohlke S, Łapiński K, Garcia-Carrizo F, Soultoukis GA, Infanger M, et al. Lipedema stage affects adipocyte hypertrophy, subcutaneous adipose tissue inflammation and interstitial fibrosis. *Front Immunol.* 2023 Jul 28;14. Available from: www.frontiersin.org/journals/immunology/articles/10.3389/fimmu.2023.1223264/full
2. Grewal T, Kempa S, Buechler C. Lipedema: A disease triggered by M2 polarized macrophages? *Biomedicines.* 2025 Mar;13(3):561. DOI: https://doi.org/10.3390/biomedicines13030561
3. Kaftalli J, Bonetti G, Marceddu G, Dhuli K, E Maltese P, Donato K, et al. AKR1C1 and hormone metabolism in lipedema pathogenesis: a computational biology approach. *Eur Rev Med Pharmacol Sci.* 2023; 27(6 Suppl): 137-147. Available from: https://usiena-air.unisi.it/handle/11365/1261114
4. Michelini S, Chiurazzi P, Marino V, Dell'Orco D, Manara E, Baglivo M, et al. Aldo-keto reductase 1C1 (AKR1C1) as the first mutated gene in a family with nonsyndromic primary lipedema. *Int J Mol Sci.* 2020 Jan;21(17):6264. DOI: https://doi.org/10.3390/ijms21176264
5. Kaftalli J, Donato K, Bonetti G, Dhuli K, Macchia A, Maltese PE, et al. Aldo-keto reductase 1C2 (AKR1C2) as the second gene associated to non-syndromic primary lipedema: investigating activating mutation or overexpression as causative factors. *Eur Rev Med Pharmacol Sci.* 2023;27(6 Suppl.):127-36. 2023; Available from: https://usiena-air.unisi.it/handle/11365/1281494
6. Bonetti G, Dhuli K, Kaftalli J, Micheletti C, Michelini S, Ricci M, et al. Characterization of somatic mutations in the pathogenesis of lipedema. *Clin Ter.* 2023 Nov 23;174(6). DOI: 10.7417/CT.2023.2495 Available from: https://www.clinicaterapeutica.it/ojs/index.php/1/article/view/843
7. Paolacci S, Precone V, Acquaviva F, Chiurazzi P, Fulcheri E, Pinelli M, et al. Genetics of lipedema: new perspectives on genetic research and molecular diagnoses. *Eur Rev Med Pharmacol Sci.* 2019 Jul;23(13):5581–94. DOI: https://doi.org/10.26355/eurrev_201907_18292
8. Michelini S, Herbst KL, Precone V, Manara E, Marceddu G, Dautaj A, et al. A multi-gene panel to identify lipedema-predisposing genetic variants by a next-generation sequencing strategy. *J Pers Med.* 2022 Feb 11;12(2):268. DOI: https://doi.org/10.3390/jpm12020268
9. Aust M, Aliu A, Leuthner P, von Lukowicz D. Lipödem erkennen und effektiv behandeln. *Ästhetische Dermatol Kosmetol.* 2020 Feb 1;12(1):32–42. DOI: https://doi.org/10.1007/s12634-019-0609-3
10. Esmer M, Schingale FJ, Unal D, Yazıcı MV, Güzel NA. Physiotherapy and rehabilitation applications in lipedema management: a literature review. *Lymphology.* 2020;53(2):88–95. Available from: https://journals.librarypublishing.arizona.edu/lymph/article/id/4659/
11. Consensus 2023. The diagnosis and treatment of peripheral lymphedema: 2023 Consensus document of the International Society of Lymphology. *Lymphology.* 2024 Aug 27;56(4). Available from: http://journals.librarypublishing.arizona.edu/lymph/article/id/6372/
12. Foeldi M, Foeldi E. *Földi's Textbook of Lymphology: for Physicians and Lymphedema Therapists.* 3rd ed. München: Elsevier Urban & Fischer; 2012. Available from: https://search.worldcat.org/title/Foldi's-textbook-of-lymphology-:-for-

physicians-and-lymphedema-therapists/oclc/792987093

13. Bertsch T, Erbacher G, Elwell R, Partsch H. Lipoedema: a paradigm shift and consensus. *J Wound Care*. 2020 Nov;29(Sup11b):1–51. DOI: https://doi.org/10.12968/jowc.2020.29.Sup11b.1
14. Redondo Galán C, García Bascones M, Marquina Valero MA. [Lipoedema: symptoms, diagnosis and treatment: a literature review]. *Rehabilitacion*. 2019 Apr 1;53(2):104–10. DOI: https://doi.org/10.1016/j.rh.2018.04.007
15. Schingale FJ, Esmer M, Küpeli B, Ünal D. Investigation of the less known effects of manual lymphatic drainage: a narrative review. *Lymphat Res Biol*. 2022 Feb;20(1):7–10. DOI: https://doi.org/10.1089/lrb.2019.0091
16. Herbst KL, Kahn LA, Iker E, Ehrlich C, Wright T, McHutchison L, et al. Standard of care for lipedema in the United States. *Phlebology*. 2021 Dec 1;36(10):779–96. DOI: https://doi.org/10.1177/02683555211015887
17. Szolnoky G, Varga E, Varga M, Tuczai M, Dosa-Racz E, Kemeny L. Lymphedema treatment decreases pain intensity in lipedema. *Lymphology*. 2011 Aug 20;44(4):178–82. Available from: https://journals.uair.arizona.edu/index.php/lymph/article/view/17067
18. Czerwińska M, Teodorczyk J, Spychała D, Hansdorfer-Korzon R. The usefulness of the application of compression therapy among lipedema patients-pilot study. *Int J Environ Res Public Health*. 2023 Jan 4;20(2):914. DOI: https://doi.org/10.3390/ijerph20020914
19. Fetzer A, Fetzer, Sharie. *Lipoedema UK Big Survey 2014 Research Report*. Lipoedema UK; 2016 Jul p. 1–8. Available from: https://lipoedema.co.uk/wp-content/uploads/2024/05/LATEST-LUK000-UK-Big-Survey16-Mar24-web.pdf
20. Annunziata G, Paoli A, Manzi V, Camajani E, Laterza F, Verde L, et al. The role of physical exercise as a therapeutic tool to improve lipedema: a consensus statement from the Italian Society of Motor and Sports Sciences (Società Italiana di Scienze Motorie e Sportive, SISMeS) and the Italian Society of Phlebology (Società Italiana di Flebologia, SIF). *Curr Obes Rep*. 2024 Dec;13(4):667–79. DOI: https://doi.org/10.1007/s13679-024-00579-8
21. Szolnoky G, Borsos B, Bársony K, Balogh M, Kemény L. Complete decongestive physiotherapy with and without pneumatic compression for treatment of lipedema: a pilot study. *Lymphology*. 2008 Mar;41(1):40–4. Available from: https://journals.librarypublishing.arizona.edu/lymph/article/id/3645/
22. Atan T, Bahar-Özdemir Y. The effects of complete decongestive therapy or intermittent pneumatic compression therapy or exercise only in the treatment of severe lipedema: a randomized controlled trial. *Lymphat Res Biol*. 2021 Feb;19(1):86–95. DOI: https://doi.org/10.1089/lrb.2020.0019
23. Szolnoky G, Nagy N, Kovács RK, Dósa-Rácz E, Szabó A, Bársony K, et al. Complex decongestive physiotherapy decreases capillary fragility in lipedema. *Lymphology*. 2008 Dec 1;41(4):161–6. Available from: https://journals.librarypublishing.arizona.edu/lymph/article/id/3624/
24. Villefrance M, Høgh A, Kristensen LH. [Compression is important in erysipelas treatment]. *Ugeskr Laeger*. 2017 Oct 9;179(41):V04170284. Available from: https://ugeskriftet.dk/videnskab/kompression-er-et-vigtigt-element-i-behandling-af-erysipelas
25. Forner-Cordero I, Forner-Cordero A, Szolnoky G. Update in the management of lipedema. *Int Angiol J Int Union Angiol*. 2021 Aug;40(4):345–57. DOI: https://doi.org/10.23736/S0392-9590.21.04604-6
26. Hutzschenreuter P, Ehlers R. [Effect of manual lymph drainage on the autonomic nervous system]. *Z Lymphol*. 1986 Dec;10(2):58–60. Available from: https://pubmed.ncbi.nlm.nih.gov/3825241/
27. Honigman L, Bar-Bachar O, Yarnitsky D, Sprecher E, Granovsky Y. Nonpainful wide-area compression inhibits experimental pain. *Pain*. 2016 Sep;157(9):2000. DOI: https://doi.org/10.1097/j.pain.0000000000000604
28. Macciò A. Compression in dermato-lymphangio-adenits. *Veins Lymphat*. 2016 Jun 14;5(1). Available from: https://www.pagepressjournals.org/vl/article/view/5982

Chapter Thirteen
Complementary therapies in lipedema

Ayça Utkan Karasu and Pınar Borman

Introduction

Lipedema, first described by Allen and Hines in 1940, is a chronic, progressive disease characterized by pathological, disproportionate accumulation of subcutaneous adipose tissue (SAT), primarily in the thighs, buttocks, lower legs, and occasionally the arms. Affecting nearly exclusively women, this disease leads to pain, swelling, and increased tissue volume, significantly impairing mobility, daily function, and psychosocial well-being.[1, 2, 3]

Unlike obesity, lipedema is symmetrical and spares the hands, feet, head, and trunk. The structural abnormalities in SAT include nodular and fibrotic changes, which progress through three stages. Early stages feature smooth but enlarged subdermal tissue with nodular formations. In contrast, advanced stages are characterized by thickened fascia and reduced skin elasticity, resulting in tissue folding and impaired lymphatic and blood flow (Figure 13.1). This can exacerbate inflammation, fibrosis, and lymphedema in later stages due to impaired fluid drainage.[1, 2, 4]

Although lipedema is not caused by obesity and cannot be reversed with diet or exercise, coexisting obesity may aggravate the disease, increasing the risk of secondary lymphedema. Dysregulated vascular function within SAT leads to capillary leaks and interstitial fluid accumulation, rendering fat lobules palpable as nodules and often causing significant pain. Inflammatory mediators and poor lymphatic flow perpetuate a cycle of swelling, fibrosis, and discomfort.[2, 5]

Clinical features and associated complications

Lipedema is characterized by bilateral, symmetrical hypertrophy of fatty tissue that disproportionately affects the limbs. Patients commonly report heaviness, tension, and pain in the affected areas, alongside a tendency for hematoma formation. Despite weight loss or caloric restriction, limb circumference remains unchanged, distinguishing it from other diseases.[6]

In advanced stages, particularly with weight gain, secondary complications such as lymphedema may develop. Mechanical irritation from large fatty deposits near joints can impair mobility, cause skin maceration, and contribute to the development of arthritis. Additionally, the psychosocial impact of the disease, including reduced self-esteem and emotional distress due to deviation from societal beauty norms, is significant.[7] These challenges highlight the need for a comprehensive treatment approach that addresses both the physical and emotional burdens of lipedema.

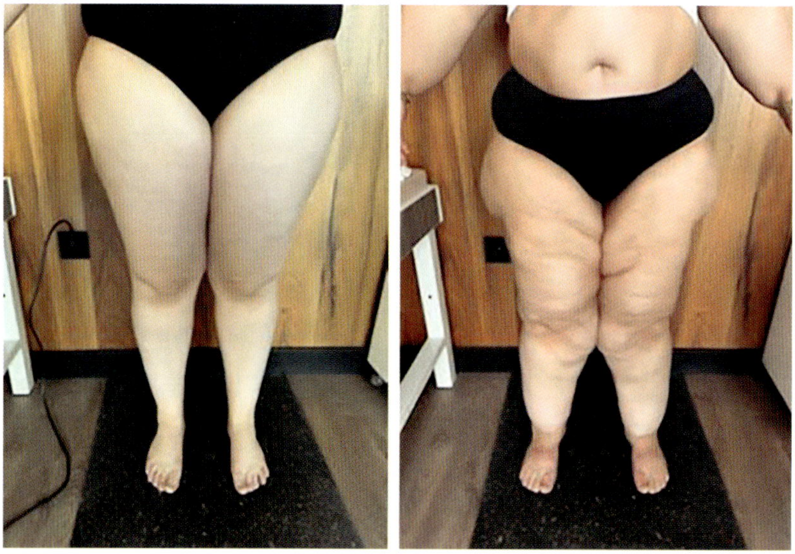

Figure 13.1: (Left) early and (right) late-stage lipedema. Photo courtesy of Prof. Dr. Pınar Borman.

Treatment of lipedema

Lipedema is a chronic and progressive disease for which no causally directed treatment has been identified. Conservative management strategies, including manual lymphatic drainage (MLD), compression therapy, physiotherapy, exercise, dietary counseling, and psychosocial support, are primarily designed to alleviate symptoms and prevent further SAT accumulation rather than addressing the underlying pathology or improving limb appearance.[6] While these interventions may offer modest reductions in tissue volume and relieve symptoms such as tenderness and tightness,[6] they remain palliative, with limited efficacy in halting disease progression.[8]

Given the chronic nature of lipedema and the limited impact of existing treatments, there is a pressing need for innovative approaches that can more effectively address both the physical and psychosocial burdens of the disease.[9, 10] As a result, healthcare providers and patients are increasingly turning their attention to alternative and adjunctive therapeutic options. This chapter aims to explore the scientific evidence supporting complementary, alternative, and non-conventional treatment modalities in the management of lipedema.

Complementary treatment modalities

Intermittent pneumatic compression

Intermittent pneumatic compression (IPC) therapy is a mechanical intervention designed to support lymphatic drainage and alleviate symptoms associated with lipedema, such as pain and edema. The method utilizes multi-chamber devices that apply graduated pressure to affected limbs, facilitating the movement of fluid through the lymphatic system. While IPC is not a replacement for MLD or compression garments, it complements complete decongestive therapy (CDT) regimens, especially for managing lower extremity symptoms in patients with lipedema[1, 11] (Figure 13.2).

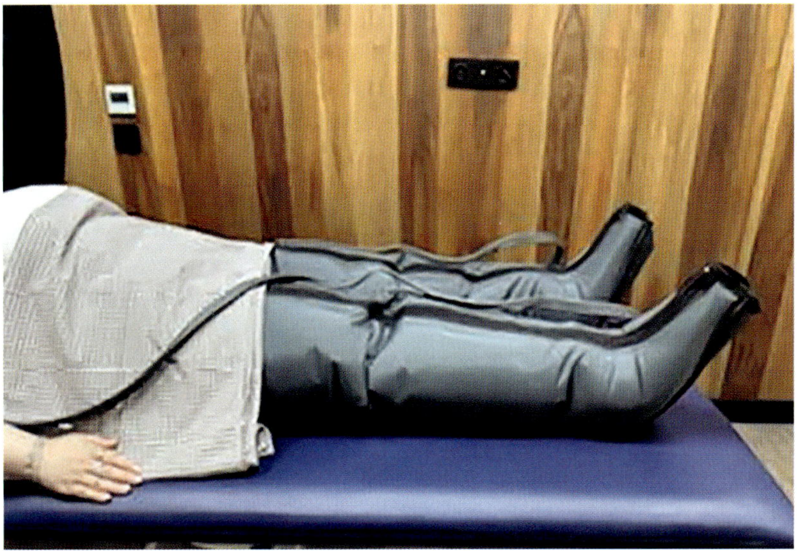

Figure 13.2: Intermittent pneumatic compression therapy. Photo courtesy of Prof. Dr. Pınar Borman.

Research indicates that IPC devices may offer additional benefits, such as reducing capillary fragility and enhancing lymphatic flow. However, while clinical reports and case studies document symptom relief, high-quality evidence remains limited.[12, 13] A prospective randomized trial compared the effectiveness of complete decongestive physiotherapy (CDP) alone to CDP combined with IPC in treating lipedema.[13] In this study, 11 participants underwent 60-minute CDP sessions, while 13 received 30 minutes of CDP followed by 30 minutes of IPC over a 5-day course. All participants also received multilayered compression bandaging, physical exercise, and skin care. Both groups demonstrated significant reductions in lower extremity volume, confirming the efficacy of CDP. However, IPC did not provide additional limb volume reduction under the study conditions, although it was considered safe. These results suggest that IPC may serve as a supplementary option, but it does not enhance primary outcomes when combined with CDP. To mitigate discomfort during IPC use, pressure levels should be customized, and cotton padding can be added between the device and the skin.[1]

Another randomized controlled trial explored the efficacy of conservative treatment methods for severe lipedema.[14] Participants were randomized into three groups: (1) CDT with exercise, (2) IPC with exercise, and (3) exercise alone (control). Over a 6-week, 30-session program, all groups participated in aerobic, strengthening, and stretching exercises, with CDT or IPC administered five times weekly in each respective group. Results showed improvements across all groups. However, the CDT-plus-exercise group achieved significantly greater reductions in limb volume, pain, and physical function scores. While the IPC-plus-exercise group did not surpass the CDT group, it provided notable benefits in limb volume and pain reduction, highlighting its value as an adjunctive therapy, particularly when CDT access is limited.

A study by Wright, Scarfino, and O'Malley assessed the short-term effects of IPC combined with conservative care (CC) versus CC alone in women with bilateral lipedema and secondary lymphedema.[15] The IPC+CC group exhibited greater improvements in leg circumference, bioimpedance, and pain scores as measured by the SF-36 and numerical rating scales, compared to the CC group. While trends toward improvement were observed in both groups, the IPC+CC group consistently achieved superior outcomes. This study highlights the potential of IPC as a beneficial adjunct for managing lipedema and lymphedema symptoms, as well as improving quality of life.

Although data remain limited, IPC is increasingly recognized as a viable option for home-based management of lipedema and lymphedema when monitored appropriately. Guidelines recommend IPC to reduce swelling and pain and to prevent complications such as deep vein thrombosis after lipedema surgery.[1, 16] Future research involving larger cohorts is essential to validate the effectiveness of IPC and establish standardized treatment protocols for clinical practice.

Whole body vibration plate

Engaging in exercise is widely recognized for its numerous health benefits, including a reduced risk of chronic illnesses. Recently, whole-body vibration (WBV) has emerged as a promising alternative or adjunct to conventional exercise, attributed to its exercise-mimetic properties. The vibrations generated by WBV trigger reactive contractions in skeletal muscles, stimulate sensory and motor neurons, and increase both cardiovascular load and oxygen uptake. Consequently, WBV has been applied in acute and long-term therapeutic settings across both healthy and clinical populations.[24]

Whole-body vibration therapy (WBVT) has been shown to have positive effects on body composition, muscle strength, and cardiovascular health.[25] Its unique advantage lies in its suitability for populations who may struggle with traditional dynamic exercises, such as those with chronic diseases or the elderly. Unlike conventional exercise methods, WBVT relies on vibration-induced oscillatory shear stress, which not only activates muscular contractions but also promotes local vasodilation and enhances microcirculation through endothelial stimulation.[25]

Although lipedema is often resistant to traditional interventions such as diet and exercise, physical activity remains critical for its management. Exercise contributes to improved mitochondrial function, enhanced lymphatic flow, and reduced inflammation, all of which are beneficial for alleviating the symptoms of lipedema. Specific modalities, such as aquatic exercises and resistance training, have shown potential for symptom relief and improving patients' quality of life. However, the absence of standardized guidelines for exercise prescriptions highlights the need for further research to establish evidence-based recommendations and optimize therapeutic outcomes.[26]

A study conducted by Schwarze in 2012[27] investigated the impact of vibration plate training (Galileo) on pain thresholds in individuals with lipedema. Over a six-week intervention involving 38 participants, the study demonstrated a significant increase in the pressure pain threshold. The randomized controlled trial consisted of two groups: one group performed leg exercises using a vibration plate, while the other group engaged in traditional leg training. Participants completed 45-minute sessions twice weekly, with the first six weeks conducted in a clinical setting and the following six weeks at home. While the vibration plate group achieved significant improvements in pain threshold after six weeks, the traditional training group required 12 weeks to achieve similar outcomes. Neither group experienced a significant reduction in leg volume throughout the study.[27]

Another study has explored the effectiveness of vibration therapy in patients with lipedema. Conducted by Schneider et al.,[28] this study included 30 participants who were evenly assigned to two groups. One group underwent MLD alone, while the other group received MLD combined with whole-body vibration therapy (15–42 Hz) for six 30-minute sessions. The findings revealed a reduction in the volume of the affected areas and an improvement in quality of life, with significantly greater benefits observed in the group receiving the combination of MLD and vibration therapy compared to MLD alone.[28]

While WBVT offers promising benefits for improving body composition, muscular strength, and cardiovascular health, its application in lipedema remains underexplored. However, initial findings suggest that it may serve as a supportive therapy to alleviate symptoms such as pain and improve patients' quality of life, particularly when integrated with comprehensive management strategies. Further research is needed to establish the long-term efficacy and optimize the use of this treatment in lipedema.

Kinesiology taping

Kinesiology taping, an intervention originally developed in Japan, involves applying elastic adhesive tape to specific areas of the skin. It is widely recognized for its role in managing sports-related and musculoskeletal injuries, with suggested mechanisms including the promotion of blood and lymphatic circulation, reduction of pain, and stabilization of tissues and joints[3, 16, 17] (Figure 13.3). While evidence specific to lipedema remains limited, initial reports suggest kinesiology taping may help alleviate symptoms such as knee pain, plantar fasciitis, and limb deformities, as well as streamline limb contour.[3, 18]

The application of kinesiology taping for lymphatic drainage is believed to enhance vascular and lymphatic flow by creating a slight lifting effect on the skin and underlying fascia, reducing local pressure, and facilitating lymph displacement.[19, 20] This effect is further supported by natural body movements and muscle contractions. Additionally, the tape's elasticity reduces compression on cutaneous mechanoreceptors, contributing to pain relief.[17, 20]

A pilot study exploring kinesiology taping in combination with shock wave therapy and mesotherapy for stage 2 lipedema reported notable improvements in pain levels, limb circumferences, and the quality of life of participants.[20] These findings were complemented by enhanced ultrasound assessments of SAT, including reductions in SAT thickness and improvements in tissue elasticity. While these preliminary results underscore the potential benefits of kinesiology taping in lipedema management, further research with larger sample sizes and multicenter trials is essential to establish its efficacy.

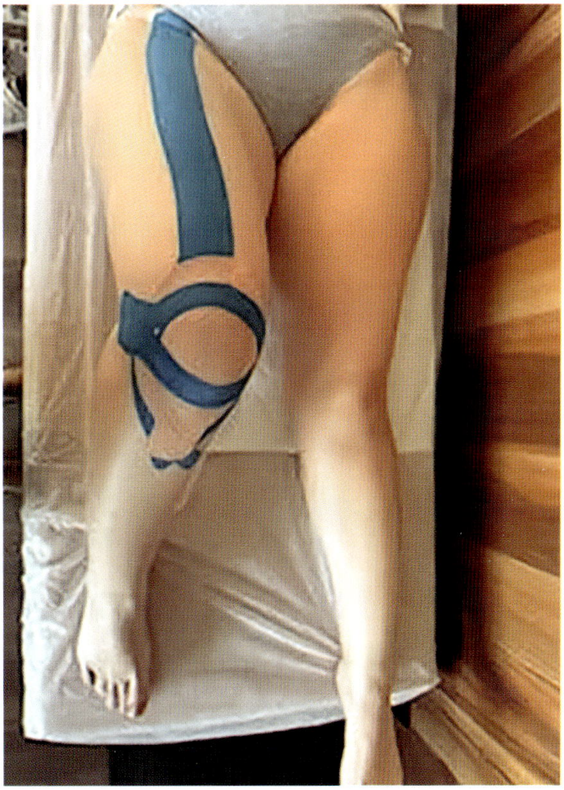

Figure 13.3: Kinesiology taping. Photo courtesy of Prof. Dr. Pınar Borman.

Alternative treatment modalities

Alternative treatment modalities for lipedema typically refer to approaches that can complement or be an alternative to conventional medical treatment.

Electrostatic massage therapy (DEEP OSCILLATION®)

Electrostatic massage therapy, such as DEEP OSCILLATION®, is proposed as a potential adjunctive treatment for managing lipedema by stimulating lymphatic drainage. Although its application in lipedema management is still under-researched, the mechanism involves the creation of an electrostatic effect within the tissues. This is achieved through a therapist using the device in a massaging motion while wearing a glove connected to the device, with the patient holding a linked electrode (Figure 13.4). It is hypothesized that this approach may alleviate pain and inflammation.[21, 22]

A pilot study investigated the use of the HIVAMAT® 200 device, which employs an intermittent electrostatic field, in combination with MLD.[23] This study included three women with lipedema and two men with lymphedema, where each participant's larger limb was treated with HIVAMAT® 200 and MLD, and the contralateral limb received MLD alone over three weeks. The outcomes were assessed through leg volume measurements and high-definition ultrasound to evaluate edema. The study reported a mean volume reduction of 902 ml (SD 793 ml) in the limbs treated with HIVAMAT® 200 plus MLD, compared to a mean reduction of 707 ml (SD 630 ml) in the MLD-only limbs. Although the volume reduction was greater in the HIVAMAT® 200 group, the difference did not reach statistical significance ($p = 0.06$). However, ultrasound analysis revealed significantly greater edema reduction in the HIVAMAT® 200 group compared to MLD alone ($p = 0.017$). These findings suggest that electrostatic massage therapy may offer additional benefits in managing lower-limb edema in lipedema and lymphedema. However, larger,

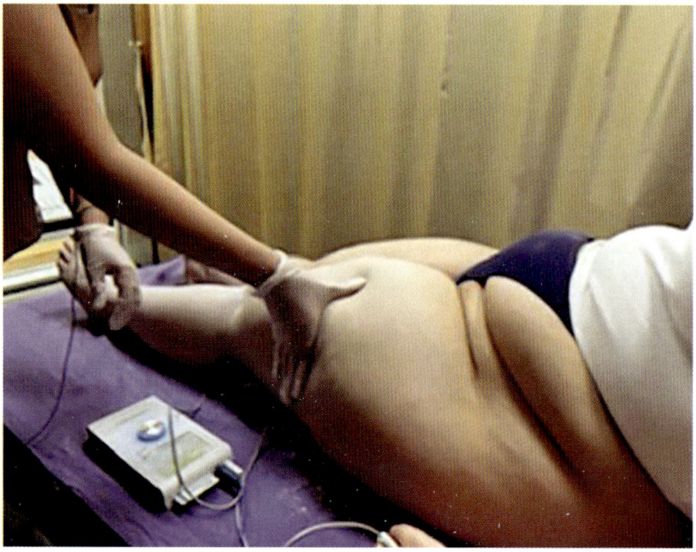

Figure 13.4: Electrostatic massage therapy with DEEP OSCILLATION®. Photo courtesy of Prof. Dr. Pınar Borman.

controlled studies are necessary to confirm its efficacy and determine its potential role in standard lipedema treatment protocols.

Manual therapies: massage and subcutaneous adipose tissue (SAT) therapy

Standard manual therapy for lipedema includes soft tissue mobilization to reduce pain, inflammation, and musculoskeletal restrictions, and MLD as part of an individualized comprehensive therapy program to stimulate lymphatic flow and reduce edema[2] (Figure 13.5). Lipedema tissue should be mobilized more deeply with myofascial release, other manual techniques, or instrument-assisted soft tissue therapy to reduce fibrotic restrictions and improve the interstitial space, considering patient tolerance and tissue integrity.

Moderate-intensity massage has been shown to improve the deep sleep phase, which in turn reduces the secretion of substance P, a neurotransmitter associated with pain. This reduction in substance P is thought to contribute to pain relief. Research on other pain-related conditions, such as burns, juvenile rheumatoid arthritis, and migraines, has revealed that moderate massage decreases cortisol levels while increasing serotonin and dopamine, as confirmed through saliva and urine analyses.[2, 29, 30]

Another manual approach, SAT therapy, targets the adipose tissue layer throughout the body, from the head to the dorsal foot, and aims to improve the nodules and masses characteristic of lipedema through its antifibrotic effects. The manual techniques include thumb-over-thumb pressure, scraping motions with flat fingers, scissor-like movements using the side of the palm, and deep sweeping pressure into the tissue.[30]

As treatment progresses and the SAT softens, the intensity of pressure is increased to address deeper structures, including fascia and muscles near the bone. Areas with SAT nodules and masses, which are rich in blood vessels, are a focus during therapy, often leading to bruising that diminishes with continued sessions.[2, 30]

A prospective pilot study examined the effects of SAT therapy on pain and tissue structure in women

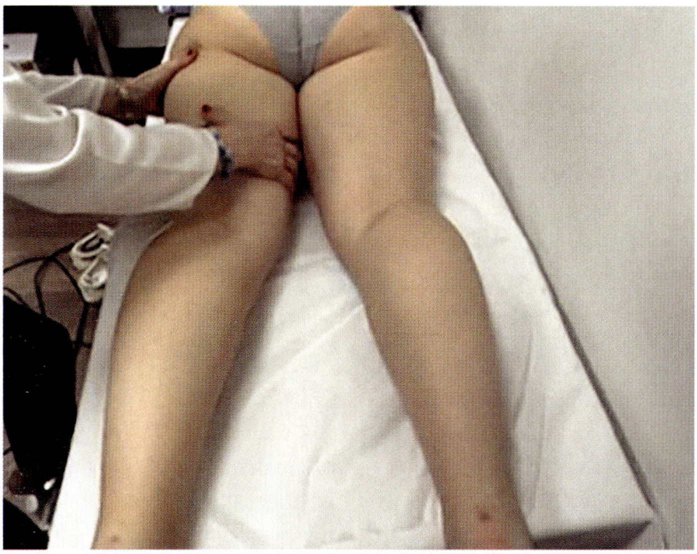

Figure 13.5: Manual therapy is performed on the affected tissue in lipedema. Photo courtesy of Prof. Dr. Pınar Borman.

with lipedema.[2] Over the course of four weeks, seven participants underwent twelve 90-minute sessions. The study evaluated outcomes, including dual-energy X-ray absorptiometry (DXA) scans, SAT ultrasound imaging, leg volume measurements, skin caliper readings, pain scores, the lower extremity functional scale (LEFS), and the body shape questionnaire (BSQ). Significant improvements were observed in leg volume, skin caliper readings, LEFS scores, and pain levels. Fibrosis decreased in nodules, hips, and groin areas, and ultrasound imaging revealed improvements in SAT structure for some participants.

Conversely, there were no significant changes in weight, resting metabolic rate, or BSQ scores, and reductions in limb and trunk fat were only marginal. Reported side effects included pain, bruising, itching, swelling, and gastroesophageal reflux. Despite these symptoms, all participants stated they would recommend the therapy to others. Although the small sample size limits the generalizability of the results, the study concluded that SAT therapy improves tissue quality, reduces pain, and enhances leg function, with minimal effects on body shape.[2] These findings underscore the potential of massage therapy as a valuable tool for managing pain. However, no comparative studies are focusing specifically on lipedema, and further research is needed to determine the relevance of these findings for this disease.

While these findings highlight the potential benefits of SAT therapy and moderate massage techniques in managing lipedema symptoms, the evidence remains limited. The lack of large-scale, comparative studies specifically addressing the efficacy of manual therapy in lipedema prevents definitive conclusions.

Physical agent modalities

Physical agent modalities (PAM) are defined as externally applied interventions that elicit biophysiological responses in tissues through the application of light, water, temperature, sound, electricity, or mechanical devices. Specifically, PAMs refer to forms of energy or materials used to target specific body regions and achieve desired biophysiological effects, such as alleviating symptoms. These modalities can be classified into different categories: thermal, mechanical, and electromagnetic.[31, 32]

In advanced stages of lipedema, musculoskeletal issues may arise due to increased BMI and joint laxity. These complications can include arthropathy, tendinosis, gait abnormalities, and ligament problems, which often manifest as foot arch pathologies, plantar fasciitis, impaired muscle pump function, gait disturbances, pain, and restricted joint motion. Such impairments can significantly affect both fine and gross motor functions, sometimes to the extent of limiting mobility to the point of being housebound or unable to perform self-care. In addressing these challenges, physical agent modalities may serve as adjunctive therapeutic strategies, offering potential benefits in managing the musculoskeletal pathologies associated with lipedema.[1, 2, 31]

Donahue et al.[29] investigated the effects of a 6-week physical therapy program, consisting of 9 sessions, in 5 patients. The sessions included manual therapy, tailored exercise guidance, and individualized compression. MLD and soft tissue mobilization were enhanced with hand and instrument-assisted techniques. A negative-graded pneumatic device was combined with hands-on techniques for broader tissue release. The study demonstrated improvements in pain and function, confirmed by objective MRI findings.[29]

Aquatherapy

Aquatic therapy, commonly referred to as hydrotherapy, involves performing exercises and movements in water to provide therapeutic benefits. This method leverages water's unique properties, including buoyancy, temperature, and hydrostatic pressure, to enhance its effectiveness. Buoyancy reduces the load on joints, making it particularly beneficial for patients with lipedema, who often experience joint strain due to increased body mass index (BMI).[26, 33] Additionally, hydrostatic pressure supports lymphatic drainage and alleviates edema, a common symptom in individuals with lipedema.[26, 34]

Exercises performed in water, including swimming, aqua jogging, and water aerobics, not only relieve joint pressure but also increase calorie expenditure due to resistance. However, while water resistance exercises contribute to calorie burning, they alone may not suffice for significant weight loss without complementary interventions.[31] Studies combining aquatic therapy with other treatments, such as dietary adjustments, lymphatic drainage, and antioxidant herbal medications, have shown promising outcomes, although further research is needed to validate these findings.[35]

The use of water-based therapies also addresses the discomfort associated with worsening lower-limb swelling, often exacerbated by orthostasis and heat at the end of the day.[34] By providing a supportive environment, water-based exercises allow patients to engage in physical activity without exacerbating joint degeneration, which can occur even in the early stages of lipedema.[26, 36] Nonetheless, the specificity and long-term efficacy of aquatic exercise protocols remain areas requiring more targeted investigation.

Overall, while the evidence supporting hydrotherapy for lipedema is limited, existing preliminary studies highlight its potential role in alleviating symptoms and improving patient outcomes. Future research focusing on larger cohorts and standardized exercise protocols is essential to establish its therapeutic benefits conclusively.

Pilates

Physical exercise (PE) is a cornerstone of lipedema management, forming a critical component of CDT, which is widely accepted as the standard conservative treatment. The available literature highlights the potential benefits of tailored PE programs, particularly water-based exercises, which can enhance lymphatic drainage, relieve joint stress, and improve weight control and functional activity. Beyond these physiological benefits, PE has a positive impact on psychological well-being, including self-esteem, mood, and overall quality of life (Figure 13.6).[26]

Among the various exercise modalities, Pilates emerges as a promising approach due to its focus on controlled movements, core strengthening, and whole-body conditioning. Developed by Joseph Pilates in the 1920s, this mind-body exercise emphasizes principles such as centering, precision, flow, and breathing, fostering both physical and mental well-being.[37] Pilates' adaptability and low-impact nature make it particularly suitable for addressing the mobility limitations and discomfort often experienced by individuals with lipedema.

Although no studies have specifically evaluated Pilates in lipedema, its benefits in enhancing flexibility, muscle strength, and body awareness

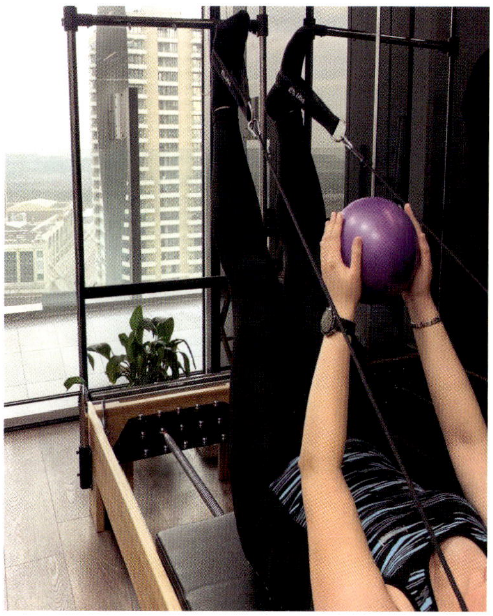

Figure 13.6: Lipedema patient performing Pilates. Photo courtesy of Prof. Dr. Pinar Borman.

suggest it could serve as an effective adjunctive therapy. However, further research is essential to validate its efficacy and to establish standardized guidelines for its use in lipedema care.

Yoga

Yoga has been investigated for its potential benefits in managing lymphedema, particularly in women with breast cancer-related lymphedema. A recent review[38] synthesized findings from three randomized controlled trials (RCTs) and several systematic reviews, highlighting improvements in quality of life and reductions in symptoms, including fatigue, pain, and insomnia. These outcomes underscore yoga's holistic approach, which integrates physical postures,[39] breathing exercises,[40] and mental relaxation.[41] However, the review noted no significant reductions in arm volume, suggesting that while yoga enhances overall well-being, its direct impact on lymphedema-related swelling might be limited.[38]

Although studies specifically investigating yoga's effects in lipedema are currently unavailable, the parallels between lipedema and lymphedema suggest that yoga may offer similar benefits to patients with lipedema. Both diseases share challenges such as pain, reduced mobility, and diminished quality of life, making yoga's gentle and integrative approach potentially valuable. Further research is necessary to establish evidence-based guidelines for the implementation of yoga in lipedema management.

Non-conventional treatment modalities

Non-conventional treatment modalities for lipedema are evidence-informed approaches that fall outside of standard medical care but are often used in conjunction with it.

Herbal therapies

Herbal medicine has been extensively explored in the treatment of vascular and lymphatic diseases due to its diverse therapeutic potential. Certain herbs have been shown to promote lymphangiogenesis, potentially aiding in fluid drainage and offering a therapeutic avenue for diseases such as lymphedema.[42] Additionally, the effects of herbal extracts on swelling, inflammation, and edema volume have been documented in various studies, highlighting their role in reducing pathological symptoms.[43, 44] Herbal interventions are also recognized for their contributions to skincare, particularly in wound healing, an essential component of lymphedema management.[45]

A study by Campisi et al.[46] investigated the role of phytotherapeutic natural products as part of a pre-surgical treatment regimen for patients with lymphedema and lipedema. The study included 150 participants who were randomly assigned to three groups: a control group following the standard complete lymphedema functional therapy (CLyFT) protocol, and two treatment groups incorporating either Linfolipase® tablets or Lipolipase® cream alongside the CLyFT program. Both products demonstrated significant benefits in improving skin conditions associated with lipedema, including reduced skin dimpling and enhanced softness. Lipolipase® cream, formulated with ingredients like *Melilotus officinalis* and caffeine, was particularly effective in softening the skin and reducing dimpling, while Linfolipase® tablets, containing components like bromelain and co-enzyme Q10, contributed to improved microcirculation.[46] The results highlight the potential of these phytotherapeutic agents as adjunctive options to enhance pre-surgical outcomes for patients with lipedema. However, further large-scale, standardized trials are needed to evaluate the comparative effectiveness of these interventions, clarify their pharmacokinetics, and elucidate their mechanisms of action.

Dietary supplementation

Lipedema is a chronic disease characterized by the abnormal accumulation of subcutaneous adipose tissue, often accompanied by reduced muscle function. In advanced stages, the coexistence of obesity can exacerbate health complications. Traditional approaches, including diet and exercise, are typically ineffective in targeting lipedema fat, making invasive procedures such as liposuction a common option. However, incorporating dietary supplements into treatment strategies may provide a less invasive alternative to support fat loss and enhance muscle mass and function. These supplements operate through mechanisms that include enhancing energy expenditure, boosting fat metabolism, and reducing fat absorption, all of which could indirectly enhance muscle performance.[47]

Fat-burning supplements can be categorized based on their mode of action. These include energy enhancers, protein and amino acid supplements, adrenergic stimulators, and lean mass enhancers. Common active ingredients, such as green tea extract, caffeine, chromium, carnitine, and conjugated linoleic acid (CLA), play key roles in promoting weight loss by increasing the metabolic rate and suppressing appetite. Additionally, some supplements contain herbal stimulants, such as ephedrine, yohimbine, pyruvate, and chitosan, which provide complementary benefits.[48]

By targeting multiple molecular pathways, these supplements not only facilitate fat loss but may also improve overall body composition, offering potential benefits for patients with lipedema.[47, 48] The use of dietary supplements represents a promising adjunct to traditional treatments for managing adipose tissue and associated complications in lipedema. However, rigorous human studies are essential to establish the safety, efficacy, and optimal use of these treatments in this patient population.

Hesperidin and diosmin are antioxidant treatments suggested for venous insufficiency and lymphedema.[45, 49] These agents can be used in patients with lipedema who have associated venous disease or lymphedema. The use of quercetin, pycnogenol, flavonoids, selenium, rutosides, and butcher's broom has been mentioned in other books in the treatment of lipedema and/or lymphedema.[45, 50]

Conclusion

Lipedema management necessitates an integrated, multidisciplinary, and patient-centered approach that involves collaboration across multiple specialties. The current body of evidence on complementary therapies for lipedema remains limited in both quantity and methodological rigor. Many areas lack research entirely, and small sample sizes and varying quality often characterize existing studies. This is particularly concerning given that lipedema is not a rare disease; it significantly impacts patients' functional abilities, psychological well-being, and overall quality of life. To address these gaps, it is imperative for the scientific community, professional organizations, and healthcare system providers, such as health ministries and governmental agencies, to prioritize and support robust research efforts in this field. By fostering high-quality, large-scale studies, these stakeholders can help guide patients and clinicians toward evidence-based practices, ultimately improving outcomes and enhancing the quality of care for individuals living with lipedema.

References

1. Faerber G, Cornely M, Daubert C, Erbacher G, Fink J, Hirsch T, et al. S2k guideline lipedema. *JDDG J Dtsch Dermatol Ges*. 2024;22(9):1303–15. DOI: https://doi.org/10.1111/ddg.15513
2. Herbst KL, Ussery C, Eekema A. Pilot study: whole body manual subcutaneous adipose tissue (SAT) therapy improved pain and SAT structure in women with lipedema. *Horm Mol Biol Clin*

Investig. 2017 Sep 20;33(2):/j/hmbci.2018.33. issue-2/hmbci-2017-0035/hmbci-2017-0035.xml. DOI: https://doi.org/10.1515/hmbci-2017-0035
3. Hardy D, Williams A. Best practice guidelines for the management of lipoedema. *Br J Community Nurs*. 2017 Oct;22(Sup10):S44–8. DOI: https://doi.org/10.12968/bjcn.2017.22.Sup10.S44
4. Buck DW, Herbst KL. Lipedema: A relatively common disease with extremely common misconceptions. *Plast Reconstr Surg – Glob Open*. 2016 Sep;4(9):e1043. DOI: https://doi.org/10.1097/GOX.0000000000001043
5. L'Hermitte F, Behar A, Pariès J, Cohen-Boulakia F, Attali JR, Valensi P. Impairment of lymphatic function in women with gynoid adiposity and swelling syndrome. *Metabolism*. 2003 Jul 1;52(7):810–4. DOI: https://doi.org/10.1016/S0026-0495(03)00093-3
6. Kruppa P, Georgiou I, Biermann N, Prantl L, Klein-Weigel P, Ghods M. Lipedema – pathogenesis, diagnosis, and treatment options. *Dtsch Ärztebl Int*. 2020 Jun;117(22–23):396. DOI: https://doi.org/10.3238/arztebl.2020.0396
7. Forner-Cordero I, Szolnoky G, Forner-Cordero A, Kemény L. Lipedema: an overview of its clinical manifestations, diagnosis and treatment of the disproportional fatty deposition syndrome – systematic review. *Clin Obes*. 2012;2(3–4):86–95. DOI: https://doi.org/10.1111/j.1758-8111.2012.00045.x
8. Child AH, Gordon KD, Sharpe P, Brice G, Ostergaard P, Jeffery S, et al. Lipedema: an inherited condition. Am J Med Genet A. 2010;152A(4):970–6. DOI: https://doi.org/10.1002/ajmg.a.33313
9. Torre YSD la, Wadeea R, Rosas V, Herbst KL. Lipedema: friend and foe. *Horm Mol Biol Clin Investig*. 2018 Jan 1;33(1). Available from: https://www.degruyterbrill.com/document/doi/10.1515/hmbci-2017-0076/html
10. Reich-Schupke S, Mohren E, Stücker M. [Survey on the diagnostics and therapy of patients with lymphedema and lipedema]. *Hautarzt Z Dermatol Venerol Verwandte Geb*. 2018 Jun;69(6):471–7. DOI: https://doi.org/10.1007/s00105-018-4151-4
11. Schwahn-Schreiber C, Breu FX, Rabe E, Buschmann I, Döller W, Lulay GR, et al. [S1 guideline on intermittent pneumatic compression (IPC)]. *Hautarzt Z Dermatol Venerol Verwandte Geb*. 2018 Aug;69(8):662–73. DOI: https://doi.org/10.1007/s00105-018-4219-1
12. Svensson BH, Frellsen MB, Basse PN, Bliddal H, Caspers J, Parby K. [Effect of pneumatic compression in connection with ergotherapeutic treatment of Colles' fracture. A clinical controlled exercise onlyrtrial]. *Ugeskr Laeger*. 1993 Feb 15;155(7):463–6. Available from: https://pubmed.ncbi.nlm.nih.gov/8465450/
13. Szolnoky G, Borsos B, Bársony K, Balogh M, Kemény L. Complete decongestive physiotherapy with and without pneumatic compression for treatment of lipedema: a pilot study. *Lymphology*. 2008 Mar;41(1):40–4. Available from: https://journals.librarypublishing.arizona.edu/lymph/article/id/3645/
14. Atan T, Bahar-Özdemir Y. The effects of complete decongestive therapy or intermittent pneumatic compression therapy or exercise only in the treatment of severe lipedema: a randomized controlled trial. *Lymphat Res Biol*. 2021 Feb;19(1):86–95. DOI: https://doi.org/10.1089/lrb.2020.0019
15. Wright T, Scarfino CD, O'Malley EM. Effect of pneumatic compression device and stocking use on symptoms and quality of life in women with lipedema: a proof-in-principle randomized trial. *Phlebology*. 2023 Feb 1;38(1):51–61. DOI: https://doi.org/10.1177/02683555221145779
16. Herbst KL, Kahn LA, Iker E, Ehrlich C, Wright T, McHutchison L, et al. Standard of care for lipedema in the United States. *Phlebology*. 2021 Dec 1;36(10):779–96. DOI: https://doi.org/10.1177/02683555211015887
17. Kurt EE, Büyükturan Ö, Erdem HR, Tuncay F, Sezgin H. Short-term effects of kinesio tape on joint position sense, isokinetic measurements, and clinical parameters in patellofemoral pain syndrome. *J Phys Ther Sci*. 2016 Jul;28(7):2034–40. DOI: https://doi.org/10.1589/jpts.28.2034
18. Fetzer A. Specialist approaches to managing lipoedema. *Br J Community Nurs*. 2016 Apr;21(Sup4):S30–5. DOI: https://doi.org/10.12968/bjcn.2016.21.Sup4.S30
19. Thomaz JP, Dias T dos SM, Rezende LF de. Effect of taping as treatment to reduce breast cancer lymphedema: literature review. *J Vasc Bras*. 2018 May 14;17:136–40. DOI: https://doi.org/https://

doi.org/10.1590/1677-5449.007217

20. Michelini S, Musa F, Vetrano M, Santoboni F, Nusca SM, Latini E, et al. Defocused and radial shock wave therapy, mesotherapy, and kinesio taping effects in patients with lipedema: a pilot study. *Lymphology*. 2023;56(1):13–26. DOI: https://doi.org/10.2458/lymph.5872
21. Boisnic S, Branchet MC. Anti-inflammatory and draining effect of the Deep Oscillation® device tested clinically and on a model of human skin maintained in survival. *Eur J Dermatol EJD*. 2013;23(1):59–63. DOI: https://doi.org/10.1684/ejd.2012.1904
22. Jahr S, Schoppe B, Reisshauer A. Effect of treatment with low-intensity and extremely low-frequency electrostatic fields (Deep Oscillation) on breast tissue and pain in patients with secondary breast lymphoedema. *J Rehabil Med*. 2008 Aug 1;40(8):645–50. DOI: https://doi.org/10.2340/16501977-0225
23. Teo I, Coulborn A, Munnoch DA. Use of the HIVAMAT(®) 200 with manual lymphatic drainage in the management of lower-limb lymphoedema and lipoedema. *J Lymphoedema*. 2016;11(1):49–53. Available from: https://woundsinternational.com/wp-content/uploads/2023/02/09888380619e160ffcb84c711f3372df.pdf
24. Betik AC, Parker L, Kaur G, Wadley GD, Keske MA. Whole-body vibration stimulates microvascular blood flow in skeletal muscle. *Med Sci Sports Exerc*. 2021 Feb 1;53(2):375–83. DOI: https://doi.org/10.1249/mss.0000000000002463
25. Park SY, Son WM, Kwon OS. Effects of whole body vibration training on body composition, skeletal muscle strength, and cardiovascular health. *J Exerc Rehabil*. 2015 Dec 31;11(6):289–95. DOI: https://doi.org/10.12965/jer.150254
26. Annunziata G, Paoli A, Manzi V, Camajani E, Laterza F, Verde L, et al. The role of physical exercise as a therapeutic tool to improve lipedema: a consensus statement from the Italian Society of Motor and Sports Sciences (Società Italiana di Scienze Motorie e Sportive, SISMeS) and the Italian Society of Phlebology (Società Italiana di Flebologia, SIF). *Curr Obes Rep*. 2024 Dec;13(4):667–79. DOI: https://doi.org/10.1007/s13679-024-00579-8
27. Schwarze D. *Vibrationstraining zur Therapie des Lipödems der Beine*. 2012. Available from: https://refubium.fu-berlin.de/handle/fub188/9361
28. Schneider R. Low-frequency vibrotherapy considerably improves the effectiveness of manual lymphatic drainage (MLD) in patients with lipedema: a two-armed, randomized, controlled pragmatic trial. *Physiother Theory Pract*. 2020 Jan;36(1):63–70. DOI: https://doi.org/10.1080/09593985.2018.1479474
29. Donahue PMC, Crescenzi R, Petersen KJ, Garza M, Patel N, Lee C, et al. Physical therapy in women with early stage lipedema: potential impact of multimodal manual therapy, compression, exercise, and education interventions. *Lymphat Res Biol*. 2022 Aug;20(4):382–90. DOI: https://doi.org/10.1089/lrb.2021.0039
30. Ibarra M, Eekema A, Ussery C, Neuhardt D, Garby K, Herbst KL. Subcutaneous adipose tissue therapy reduces fat by dual X-ray absorptiometry scan and improves tissue structure by ultrasound in women with lipoedema and Dercum disease: subcutaneous adipose tissue therapy reduces fat. *Clin Obes*. 2018 Dec;8(6):398–406. DOI: https://doi.org/10.1111/cob.12281
31. Esmer M, Schingale FJ, Unal D, Yazıcı MV, Güzel NA. Physiotherapy and rehabilitation applications in lipedema management: a literature review. *Lymphology*. 2020;53(2):88–95. Available from: https://journals.librarypublishing.arizona.edu/lymph/article/id/4659/
32. Rodrick JR, Poage E, Wanchai A, Stewart BR, Cormier JN, Armer JM. Complementary, alternative, and other noncomplete decongestive therapy treatment methods in the management of lymphedema: a systematic search and review. *PM&R*. 2014 Mar 1;6(3):250–74. DOI: https://doi.org/10.1016/j.pmrj.2013.09.008
33. Alwardat N, Di Renzo L, Alwardat M, Romano L, De Santis GL, Gualtieri P, et al. The effect of lipedema on health-related quality of life and psychological status: a narrative review of the literature. *Eat Weight Disord – Stud Anorex Bulim Obes*. 2020 Aug 1;25(4):851–6. DOI: https://doi.org/10.1007/s40519-019-00703-x
34. Gianesini S, Tessari M, Bacciglieri P, Malagoni AM, Menegatti E, Occhionorelli S, et al. A specifically designed aquatic exercise protocol to reduce chronic lower limb edema. *Phlebology*. 2017 Oct

1;32(9):594–600.
DOI: https://doi.org/10.1177/0268355516673539
35. Amato ACM, Benitti DA. Lipedema can be treated non-surgically: a report of 5 cases. *Am J Case Rep*. 2021 Dec 6;22:e934406-1-e934406-8. DOI: https://doi.org/10.12659/AJCR.934406
36. Reich-Schupke S, Schmeller W, Brauer WJ, Cornely ME, Faerber G, Ludwig M, et al. S1 guidelines: lipedema. *J Dtsch Dermatol Ges*. 2017;15(7):758–67.
DOI: https://doi.org/10.1111/ddg.13036
37. Wells C, Kolt GS, Bialocerkowski A. Defining Pilates exercise: a systematic review. Complement Ther Med. 2012 Aug 1;20(4):253–62.
DOI: https://doi.org/Defining Pilates exercise: a systematic review
38. Freguia S, Platano D, Donati D, Giorgi F, Tedeschi R. Closing the gaps: an integrative review of yoga's benefits for lymphedema in breast cancer survivors. *Life*. 2024 Aug;14(8):999.
DOI: https://doi.org/10.3390/life14080999
39. Tedeschi R. Biomechanical alterations in lower limb lymphedema: Implications for walking ability and rehabilitation. *Phlebology*. 2023 Sep 1;38(8):496–502.
DOI: https://doi.org/10.1177/02683555231188236
40. Ashwini BC, Nagarathna R, Garner C, Bilagi A, Palukuru S. Comprehensive in-patient neuro-rehabilitation: harnessing yoga's potential – a pilot study in Germany. *Adv Mind Body Med*. 2024 Fall;38(4):25–30. Available from: https://advances-journal.com/research/comprehensive-in-patient-neuro-rehabilitation-harnessing-yogas-potential-a-pilot-study-in-germany/
41. Rhoads MC, Barber ,Madison E., Grevstad ,Nels, Kirkland ,Rena A., Myers ,Shannon, Gruidel ,Katherine A., et al. Yoga as an intervention for stress: a meta-analysis. *Health Psychol Rev*. 2025 Apr 3;19(2):257–77. DOI: https://doi.org/10.1080/17437199.2024.2420974
42. Li J, Chen Y, Zhang L, Xing L, Xu H, Wang Y, et al. Total saponins of panaxnotoginseng promotes lymphangiogenesis by activation VEGF-C expression of lymphatic endothelial cells. *J Ethnopharmacol*. 2016 Dec 4;193:293–302.
DOI: https://doi.org/10.1016/j.jep.2016.08.032
43. Qin J, Wang W, Zhang R. Novel natural product therapeutics targeting both inflammation and cancer. *Chin J Nat Med*. 2017 Jun;15(6):401–16. DOI: https://doi.org/10.1016/S1875-5364(17)30062-6
44. Kirsch G, Abdelwahab AB, Chaimbault P. Natural and synthetic coumarins with effects on inflammation. *Mol Basel Switz*. 2016 Oct 2;21(10):1322. DOI: https://doi.org/10.3390/molecules21101322
45. Sheikhi-Mobarakeh Z, Yarmohammadi H, Mokhatri-Hesari P, Fahimi S, Montazeri A, Heydarirad G. Herbs as old potential treatments for lymphedema management: a systematic review. *Complement Ther Med*. 2020 Dec;55:102615. DOI: https://doi.org/10.1016/j.ctim.2020.102615
46. Campisi CC, Ryan M, di Summa P, Scarabosio A, Campisi CS, Campisi C. Inclusion of targeted skin products in the pre-surgical treatment regimen of peripheral lymphedema & lipedema. *Lymphology*. 2019;52(4):194–201.
DOI: https://doi.org/10.2458/lymph.4642
47. Bonetti G, Herbst KL, Dhuli K, Kiani AK, Michelini S, Michelini S, et al. Dietary supplements for lipedema. *J Prev Med Hyg*. 2022 Oct 17;63(2 Suppl 3):E169–73. DOI: https://doi.org/10.15167/2421-4248/jpmh2022.63.2S3.2758
48. Jeukendrup AE, Randell R. Fat burners: nutrition supplements that increase fat metabolism. *Obes Rev Off J Int Assoc Study Obes*. 2011 Oct;12(10):841–51. DOI: https://doi.org/10.1111/j.1467-789X.2011.00908.x
49. Herbst KL. Subcutaneous adipose tissue diseases: Dercum disease, lipedema, familial multiple lipomatosis, and Madelung disease. In: Feingold KR, Ahmed SF, Anawalt B, Blackman MR, Boyce A, Chrousos G, et al., editors. *Endotext*. South Dartmouth (MA): MDText.com, Inc.; 2000. Available from: http://www.ncbi.nlm.nih.gov/books/NBK552156/
50. Nourollahi S, Mondry T, Herbst K. Bucher's Broom and selenium improve lipedema: a retrospective case study. *Altern Integr Med*. 2013;02(04). Available from: http://www.esciencecentral.org/journals/buchers-broom-and-selenium-improve-lipedema-a-retrospective-case-study-2327-5162.1000119.php?aid=14337

Chapter Fourteen
Nutritional management of lipedema

Gabriele Faerber

Introduction

Until about a decade ago, it was widely believed that nutritional interventions, such as caloric restriction, had no meaningful role in the management of lipedema. This assumption extended to both symptom relief and weight reduction, and was commonly conveyed to patients, even in clinics specializing in lymphatic diseases. Scientific literature at the time reinforced this view, often dismissing the potential impact of diet on the disease. The prevailing focus was on the frequent coexistence of obesity and lipedema, particularly the apparent diet resistance of the characteristic, disproportionately distributed adipose tissue.[1, 2] As a result, the potential for nutritional strategies to alleviate symptoms or influence disease progression remained largely unexplored.

As recently as 2010, reports on nutritional interventions for lipedema were sparse and primarily limited to presentations at German lymphatic and phlebological conferences. Beginning in 2015, however, interest in this area began to grow, with emerging information from the United States, such as resources from Lipedema Simplified, and a few retrospective studies marking the start of broader exploration. By 2020, research on the role of nutrition in lipedema had expanded significantly, leading to a surge in publications in international peer-reviewed journals. In addition to a greater volume of research, the quality and scope of studies have also advanced. What began with isolated case reports and small observational studies has now evolved to include larger investigations, including randomized controlled trials with comparison groups. These studies have provided valuable insights into the effects of nutritional interventions, not only in reducing weight and limb volume but also in improving metabolic health, enhancing quality of life (QoL), and, most notably, reducing pain.

While the role of chronic, low-grade inflammation has long been recognized as a key pathogenic factor in obesity,[3] emerging evidence suggests that similar pro-inflammatory processes are also involved in lipedema.[4,5,6,7] In addition to inflammation, elevated oxidative stress has been identified as a contributing factor.[7] Supposing that inflammation is indeed a central component of lipedema pathophysiology, it can be assumed that dietary factors influencing inflammatory status, whether promoting or reducing it, may significantly affect symptom expression and disease progression. Based on this premise, nutritional interventions aimed at minimizing pro-inflammatory triggers and supporting metabolic health may be particularly beneficial for individuals with lipedema.

This chapter will review the current research

on the use of carbohydrate-reduced diets, such as a Mediterranean diet, a low-carb diet, and a ketogenic diet, for the management of symptoms associated with lipedema, including pain, excess adipose tissue, and QoL. The impact of diet on obesity, inflammation, and general health and wellness is also explored. Evidence-based recommendations for a healthy diet for individuals with lipedema are proposed, including optimizing intake of protein and healthy fats while minimizing carbohydrate consumption. Other topics discussed are disordered eating, nutritional ketosis, intermittent fasting, and satiation.

Recent research in nutritional interventions for lipedema

In recent years, a growing number of studies have explored the effects of anti-inflammatory dietary approaches, such as Mediterranean, low-carbohydrate (LCD), and ketogenic diets (KD), on outcomes including pain, fatigue, limb volume, mobility, and overall QoL. All recent publications support the therapeutic potential of these dietary strategies, not only for symptom management but also for improving body composition and reducing the need for invasive treatments.[6, 8, 9, 10, 11] The following section reviews this emerging body of literature, highlighting the clinical relevance and evolving role of nutrition in comprehensive lipedema care.

Ketogenic diet: mechanisms and theoretical benefits

Keith et al.[12] highlighted the potential of KDs to reduce lipedema symptoms through weight loss, decreased adipose tissue, pain relief, and improved QoL. Benefits were linked to the anti-inflammatory effects of the ketone body β-hydroxybutyrate and improved insulin regulation. In their paper, Cannataro and Cione[10] emphasized the diet's anti-inflammatory properties through the reduction of glycemic spikes and advanced glycation end products (AGEs). They recommended personalizing diets to address pro-inflammatory triggers and advised supplementation with omega-3s and polyphenols.

Mediterranean and anti-inflammatory diets

Di Renzo et al.[11] investigated a hypocaloric modified Mediterranean diet over a four-week period in women with lipedema. Compared to controls, the lipedema group had greater extremity fat loss and improved daily function. QoL scores improved significantly, attributed to a reduction in pain, fatigue, and anxiety. Similarly, Amato and Benitti[13] reported outcomes from four patients treated with conservative interventions, including anti-inflammatory diets. One additional patient using a ketogenic diet showed limb volume reductions of up to 10,000 ml and QoL improvement of 78%. Results suggest non-surgical interventions may relieve pain and improve mobility. Finally, Cannataro et al.[14] described a 22-month ketogenic intervention in a patient with stage 3 lipedema, leading to a 41 kg weight loss, 67% pain reduction, and 48% QoL improvement. Inflammatory markers normalized. A brief interruption in diet caused symptom flare-ups, but these were quickly reversed upon resumption.

Pilot and controlled trials: Norway

Sørlie[15] conducted a 13-week pilot study in nine patients with lipedema. A seven-week ketogenic phase reduced pain independently of weight loss. Pain increased when switching to a standard Nordic diet, suggesting ketosis, not weight loss, drove symptom relief. Lundanes et al.[16] then led a randomized controlled trial (RCT) comparing a hypocaloric LCD to a standard control diet in 70 women. Once again, pain reduction in the LCD group was significant and independent of weight loss. QoL improved in both groups, only more so in the LCD group.

Several secondary analyses of the Lundanes et al. RCTs were conducted by the same group and revealed additional important outcomes regarding the impact of an LCD on patients with lipedema. One analysis used MRI to assess changes in subcutaneous adipose tissue (SAT) after the eight-week diet intervention on the two groups.[16] Only the LCD group saw significant reductions in SAT, calf circumference, and pain. Both groups lost weight and fat mass, but muscle loss did not alter the SAT/muscle ratio.

Impacts on appetite hormones and markers of inflammation were demonstrated in two other secondary analyses. In the first study, Lundanes et al.[17] examined inflammatory markers after consuming LCD vs. low-fat diets. LCD participants showed reducing levels of TNF-α, MIP-1, and hsCRP, although these changes did not correlate with pain relief, suggesting that inflammation may not directly mediate pain reduction. The second study[18] examined appetite hormones. Postprandial ghrelin levels decreased and fullness increased in the LCD group only, which may explain the greater weight loss and satiety associated with this diet.

Polish cohort studies: comparative diet efficacy

Jeziorek et al.[19] compared a low-carbohydrate, high-fat (LCHF) and moderate-carbohydrate and fat (MCMF) diet over 16 weeks in 91 women with lipedema. While both diets improved body composition, the LCHF group had greater reductions in fat mass, pain, and edema, as well as better QoL outcomes.

The same group evaluated cardiometabolic and endocrine markers in women with lipedema and in overweight controls after 16 weeks of a personalized ketogenic diet.[20] Triglycerides decreased, HDL increased, and glucose regulation improved. LDL levels changed inconsistently; kidney and thyroid function remained stable. Outcomes were further analyzed from the same cohort and found that while weight loss was similar between lipedema and overweight groups, lipedema participants experienced greater reductions in pain and subjective symptom burden.[21] This supports the idea that ketogenic diets may offer symptom relief beyond weight loss in this population.

Nutrition as a core therapeutic strategy in lipedema

These recent studies challenge the long-held belief that dietary interventions are largely ineffective in managing lipedema. Evidence now indicates that not only can overall body weight be reduced, but limb volume and symptom burden, particularly pain, edema, and fatigue, can also be significantly improved through targeted dietary strategies. Importantly, these improvements often occur independently of weight loss, suggesting that metabolic and inflammatory pathways may play a central role in symptom modulation. Among the most promising approaches are anti-inflammatory dietary patterns, including modified Mediterranean and ketogenic diets, which have consistently shown beneficial effects on pain, mobility, and QoL. In recognition of this emerging evidence, the newly published German S2k guidelines for lipedema now formally recommend specific dietary approaches – namely, anti-inflammatory, Mediterranean, and ketogenic diets – alongside more general nutritional guidance.[22, 23] These guidelines represent a significant step toward integrating nutrition as a core component of holistic lipedema management, highlighting the need for further research to refine and personalize dietary interventions for this complex disease.

Therapeutic priorities in nutritional intervention

Any nutritional intervention for lipedema must prioritize maintaining or restoring mobility and functional capacity, preventing disease progression, and achieving or preserving a healthy body composition. Equally critical is the reduction of pain and other distressing symptoms that impact QoL.

A substantial proportion of individuals with lipedema are also affected by overweight or obesity. While lipedema and obesity are distinct and co-occurring diseases, neither causing nor resulting from the other, their interaction is clinically significant. Emerging research suggests that weight gain may exacerbate limb volume in lipedema,[24] although this increase does not always correspond with symptom severity. Pain and discomfort are influenced by a variety of factors beyond volume, including hormonal changes, dietary habits, psychological health, and physical activity levels.

Coexisting obesity often contributes to reduced mobility and orthopedic issues, such as genu valgum (knock knees), and can be accompanied by metabolic complications, particularly when abdominal obesity is present. These may include insulin resistance, non-alcoholic fatty liver disease, hypertension, cardiovascular diseases, and in some cases, obesity-related lymphedema, all of which further compromise overall health and well-being.

For these reasons, effective weight management is a central pillar in the comprehensive treatment of lipedema. This should involve an integrative approach that combines individualized nutritional therapy, structured physical activity, and, when indicated, behavioral therapy. Interventions should address both the initial weight reduction phase and the long-term maintenance of healthy body composition to maximize and sustain therapeutic outcomes.[25, 26, 27]

To maintain a healthy body composition and to ensure that weight reduction occurs by reducing fat mass and not muscle mass, it is important to provide a sufficiently high quantity of protein. A healthy body composition is characterized by a balance between fat mass (FM) and fat-free mass (FFM), particularly body cell mass (BCM), which is appropriate for the patient's age and sex. Sarcopenic obesity is frequent and must be recognized and treated.[28, 29, 30, 31]

Given the high prevalence of eating disorders among individuals with lipedema, it is essential to monitor for signs of conditioned eating behaviors or distorted attitudes toward food. When such patterns are identified, timely psychological support should be offered to prevent further harm and promote healthier coping strategies.[22, 23, 32] Many patients with lipedema report a history of repeated, unsuccessful attempts at weight loss through restrictive or inappropriate dieting, often leading to the development of eating disorders or a sense of hopelessness and resignation regarding their bodies and weight.

Early education on the nature of lipedema and the importance of a healthy lifestyle is therefore crucial. Young girls and women, in particular, should be informed that while lipedema cannot be cured through diet alone, nutritional interventions can help slow disease progression, alleviate symptoms, and improve QoL. It is critical to emphasize that dietary management in lipedema is not merely about weight loss, but rather about reducing pain, enhancing physical function, and supporting overall well-being.

Patients should be encouraged to avoid unsustainable dietary patterns, such as 'crash diets' or cyclical 'yo-yo' dieting, which can be both physically and psychologically detrimental. Instead, a long-term, individualized nutrition plan that aligns with the patient's preferences, lifestyle, and medical needs should be promoted as a cornerstone of comprehensive lipedema care. In this context, healthcare professionals should strive to educate patients on the potential favorable or unfavorable effects of their eating habits on blood sugar and insulin levels, and consequently on lipogenesis and inflammatory processes.

Guidelines for healthy eating

Elevated insulin levels promote lipogenesis and contribute to sodium and water retention, both of which are particularly undesirable for individuals with lipedema. Moreover, insulin resistance is recognized as a highly pro-inflammatory state.[3, 33] As a result, dietary strategies for managing lipedema should aim to minimize fluctuations in blood glucose and insulin levels. This includes avoiding high-glycemic and high-carbohydrate diets that can trigger blood sugar and insulin spikes.

Reducing meal frequency may further help stabilize insulin and blood glucose levels by limiting the number of metabolic peaks throughout the day. This can be accomplished by eliminating snacks and ensuring adequate intervals between meals. Additionally, lowering the glycemic load of the diet may contribute to a decrease in systemic inflammation. For example, a low-glycemic, isocaloric diet led to a significant reduction of approximately 27% in high-sensitivity C-reactive protein (hs-CRP), a marker of inflammation, in obese individuals, while increasing levels of adiponectin, an anti-inflammatory adipokine that supports lymphatic health and insulin sensitivity.[34] Similarly, in a randomized 12-week study comparing a hypocaloric high-fat, low-carbohydrate (HFLC) diet with a low-fat, high-carbohydrate diet in obese participants, those following the HFLC diet experienced significant reductions in triglycerides and hs-CRP, along with increases in HDL cholesterol and adiponectin levels.[35]

Fat: good fats, bad fats

For decades, dietary fat was widely regarded as the primary culprit behind overweight and obesity. This belief was largely based on the fact that fat contains 9 kilocalories per gram, more than double the 4 kilocalories found in protein or carbohydrates. Influenced by the *Seven Countries Study* conducted by Ancel Keys,[36] nutrition societies and healthcare professionals promoted the misguided idea that dietary fat was a leading cause of hypercholesterolemia and cardiovascular disease. In contrast, the findings of British scientist John Yudkin, who warned of the dangers of sugar in his book, *Pure, White and Deadly*, were dismissed, and he was discredited.[37]

As a result of this prevailing anti-fat narrative, food manufacturers began reducing fat in their products and compensating with added sugar to maintain palatability. This shift in food processing was compounded by long-standing dietary recommendations that emphasized:

- counting calories
- eating low-fat, high-carbohydrate foods
- consuming multiple small meals throughout the day.

Although such strategies might reduce caloric intake in the short term, they often fail to support lasting satiety, making long-term adherence difficult and ineffective for sustainable weight management.

Rather than eliminating fat, the focus should shift toward consuming healthy fats. These include both unsaturated and saturated fatty acids. Of particular importance is the intake of anti-inflammatory omega-3 fatty acids, especially those from marine sources, and a reduction in pro-inflammatory omega-6 fatty acids, which are commonly found in vegetable oils such as grapeseed, sunflower, safflower, corn germ, and wheat germ oils. An optimal dietary omega-3 to omega-6 ratio is between 1:3 and 1:5. However, in the average western diet, this ratio is heavily skewed, often ranging from 1:15 to as high as 1:25, contributing to chronic inflammation and related health concerns.[38, 39]

Table 14.1 lists healthy fats and those to be avoided. Good sources of omega-3 fatty acids include fatty fish such as herring, mackerel, and wild salmon. However, tuna, although rich in omega-3 fatty acids, is no longer recommended due to its high heavy metal content. Flaxseed oil is not sufficient for an adequate intake of omega-3 fatty acids. The plant-based alpha-linolenic acid cannot replace marine omega-3 fatty acids, since it can only be converted into eicosapentaenoic acid (EPA) to a small extent and not at all into docosahexaenoic acid (DHA). However, it does reduce the pro-inflammatory arachidonic acid, which is an omega-6 fatty acid.[40]

Industrial trans fats, such as artificially hardened fats, are found in many baked goods, including croissants, cookies, donuts, French fries, pizza, crisps, and even granola bars, and should be avoided at all costs. In contrast, natural trans fats in dairy products have been shown to yield positive effects on HDL, inflammatory markers, and overall vascular health. Full-fat dairy products from pasture-raised animals are recommended due to their higher content of omega-3 fatty acids and conjugated linoleic acid.[41, 42]

Table 14.1: Examples of good (healthy) fats and bad (unhealthy fats).

Good fats	Bad fats
Omega-3 fatty acids in fatty fish, pasture-raised meat	Omega-6 rich oils (grape seed, sunflower, safflower, corn germ, and wheat germ oil).
Full-fat dairy products from pasture-raised animals with natural trans fats, omega-3 fatty acids, and conjugated linoleic acid	Industrial trans fats, i.e. artificially hardened fats
Olive oil, walnut oil, nuts, flaxseed oil (if cold pressed)	Hydrogenated vegetable oil (margarine, shortening)

Optimized protein intake

Dietary recommendations often express protein requirements as a percentage of total caloric intake, commonly around 15%. However, protein needs are more accurately determined by an individual's body weight and the amount of lean mass to be preserved, rather than by total energy intake. Recent studies[43] indicate that a daily intake of at least 1 to 1.2 grams of protein per kilogram of ideal body weight is necessary, particularly during periods of weight loss. This is because maintaining lean muscle mass is essential for preserving basal metabolic rate, which helps prevent one of the primary drivers of the 'yo-yo dieting' effect: reduction in basal metabolic rate.[43]

It is crucial to consume adequate amounts of all essential amino acids to support muscle preservation and ensure the body has the necessary components for vital functions such as hormone synthesis. Those that the body cannot produce on its own must be obtained through diet. One of the reasons for overeating can be the so-called 'protein dilution' typical of the often extremely palatable ultra-processed foods rich in carbohydrates and fats. This, in effect, lowers the percentage of protein, prompting the body to increase its appetite in an effort to obtain the necessary amount of protein. The less protein a meal contains, the more calories are eaten. This is referred to as protein leverage.[44] Proteins satiate earlier, better, and longer than carbohydrates or fats, leading to lower calorie intake at subsequent meals.[45, 46]

It is also important to allay doubts concerning protein and kidney health, and also regarding possible increased gluconeogenesis, which some fear could impede ketosis (see below). Damage to kidney function in healthy adults can be ruled out with an intake of 1.2–1.5 g/kg.[47] Only in advanced chronic kidney insufficiency should protein intake be limited to 0.8 to 1.0 g/kg.[48]

In cases of fatty liver disease, usually present in insulin resistance or prediabetes, the fat content of the liver can be reduced by increasing protein consumption, which can at the same time improve liver enzymes, inflammation parameters, and insulin resistance.[49]

Carbohydrates – necessary or risky?

Essential fatty acids and essential amino acids must be supplied by diet, but there are no essential carbohydrates. In principle, the body can supply the brain with the necessary glucose for 20–25% of its energy needs through gluconeogenesis. Additionally, in a low-carbohydrate or fasting context, the brain's remaining energy demands are met directly by the ketone body β-hydroxybutyrate (BHB), thereby decreasing the need for glucose when dietary intake is low.[50]

The amount and type of carbohydrates a person can tolerate without adverse effects may be influenced, in part, by genetic or epigenetic factors, and particularly by levels of physical activity.[51] Complex carbohydrates found in vegetables and leafy greens may be beneficial due to their fiber content, which can support a healthy gut microbiome. These intestinal bacteria can play a role in digestion, immune function, and overall well-being. A daily fiber intake of at least 30 grams is recommended.[52] However, when the body is chronically overloaded with carbohydrates, particularly refined or high-glycemic types, insulin resistance often develops as an inevitable consequence.

Satiation – what works best?

Satiety is regulated by a complex interplay between mechanical and chemical signals in the gastrointestinal tract, including the actions of chemoreceptors and hormones such as cholecystokinin (CCK), peptide YY (PYY), glucagon-like peptide-1 (GLP-1), and the hunger/satiety hormones ghrelin and leptin. Ghrelin and leptin act in opposition. Ghrelin, produced primarily by the parietal cells of the gastric mucosa and in the pancreas, is the only known peripheral hormone that signals hunger to the hypothalamus. In contrast, leptin, secreted by adipose tissue, signals the sensation of satiety. However, in individuals with obesity, leptin resistance often impairs this signaling, contributing to persistent overeating and further weight gain.

Satiety begins with the act of eating itself. The chewing process initiates satiety signals through orofacial muscle activity, which is why starting a meal with a large, fibrous salad can be beneficial, as it takes time to chew, satisfying the time-dependent component of satiety. Once food enters the stomach, ghrelin secretion decreases, but only if the stomach is sufficiently stretched. This effect is best achieved by consuming high-volume, low-energy-density foods, such as vegetables. In addition to volume, macronutrient composition matters: increasing protein intake while reducing carbohydrates has been shown to significantly suppress ghrelin levels.[53]

To effectively reduce ghrelin secretion and promote satiety, a food volume of approximately 500 mL, equivalent to about two large handfuls of vegetables, is needed. This may be one reason why many conventional calorie-restricted diets are unsustainable: the low food volume leads to insufficient gastric stretch, a rise in ghrelin, and persistent hunger. Alarmingly, ghrelin levels can remain elevated for more than a year after such diets, making long-term weight maintenance especially challenging.[54]

Among all macronutrients, protein has the most potent and lasting satiating effect. Research consistently shows that higher protein intake improves appetite regulation and reduces total calorie consumption. In several studies, replacing carbohydrates with protein resulted in a spontaneous reduction of up to 400 kcal per day during ad libitum eating, supporting the key role of protein in both short-term and long-term weight management.[53, 55, 56]

Time-restricted eating and intermittent fasting

Prolonged fasting over several days or weeks can result in undesirable losses of lean body mass. However, more moderate approaches, such as restricting the daily eating window to 8–10 hours or incorporating occasional fasting days, have been shown not only to support weight loss and improve insulin sensitivity, but also to exert anti-inflammatory effects,[57, 58, 59] provided that nutrient-dense, anti-inflammatory foods are consumed during the eating periods.

For most individuals, intermittent fasting, such as fasting for 10 to 14 hours, including overnight, is feasible and sustainable, especially when meals during the eating window are satisfying and nutritionally adequate. When combined with a low-carbohydrate, anti-inflammatory diet, intermittent fasting may be particularly beneficial for individuals with lipedema, supporting symptom management while preserving muscle mass and nutritional status.

Nutritional ketosis

Physiological ketosis is a natural metabolic state that occurs either during total fasting or when carbohydrate intake is restricted. Once blood glucose is depleted, the body then utilizes glycogen stores from the liver and muscles as an energy source. In the context of a high-carbohydrate diet, within one or two days, gluconeogenesis increases to support energy needs. Body fat stores are inaccessible in this state. Consequently, if sufficient dietary protein is not eaten, muscle protein is broken down and glucogenic amino acids, as well as glycerol, are converted into glucose. Thus, a gradual reduction of muscle mass leads to a decrease in the basal metabolic rate.

This strategy increased the survival chances for early humans. Precisely because energy consumption and metabolic rate are reduced, depletion of muscle tissue can be quickly replenished once food is available again. However, in the context of intended weight loss, muscle mass must be conserved by all means to avoid what is now known as yo-yo dieting. In a therapeutic ketogenic diet, providing sufficient amounts of protein is therefore mandatory to prevent endogenous protein breakdown.[60] This type of ketogenic diet is referred to as a protein-optimized ketogenic diet.[9]

In a state of therapeutic ketosis, the body converts its fat reserves into energy through beta-oxidation (see Figure 14.1). Free fatty acids, released from the breakdown of triglycerides, are converted into ketone bodies (acetoacetate, BHB, and acetone) and short-chain fatty acids. The ketosis threshold varies among individuals. However, most people can maintain ketosis by consuming fewer than 50 grams of carbohydrates per day.[61] Once in ketosis, large amounts of fatty acids are oxidized for energy in a process called ketogenesis, making fatty acids and ketone bodies the primary energy sources for most tissues. Many organs can efficiently utilize ketones, particularly BHB, as an energy substrate. Notably, the brain can derive 70–80% of its energy from ketones, with the remaining 20% provided by glucose produced through gluconeogenesis, on demand. Additionally, ketones have appetite-suppressing effects,[62] which may contribute significantly to the success and sustainability of long-term weight reduction.

Effects of ketosis

The anti-inflammatory effects of ketosis, including reduced inflammation markers and a decrease in cardiovascular risk factors, as well as favorable outcomes in neurodegenerative diseases, have been demonstrated in multiple studies.[60, 63, 64, 65, 66] Glucose and insulin are normalized at healthy levels. Pro-inflammatory enzymes (interleukins 6 and 8, TNFα) are reduced, diuresis and natriuresis increased, and the blood concentration of arachidonic acid, an

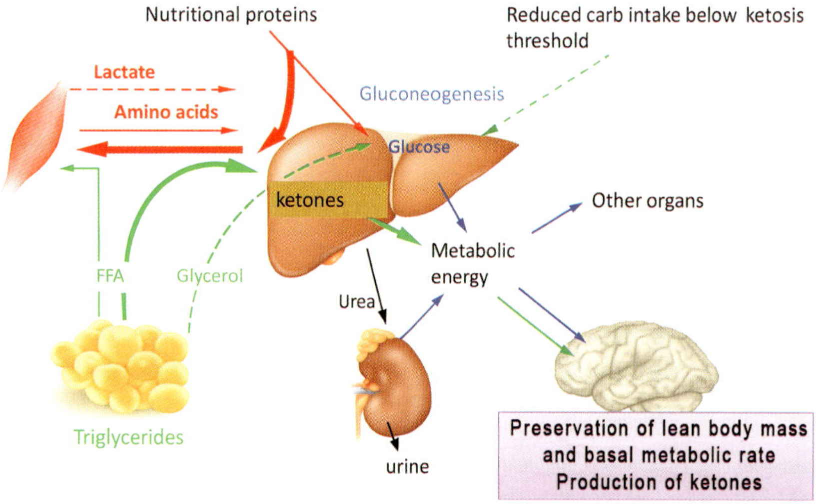

Figure 14.1: A state of ketosis due to a protein-optimized ketogenic diet. Courtesy of Dr. Faerber.

omega-6 fatty acid, decreases. Most importantly, BHB acts in a direct anti-inflammatory way by blocking the NLRP3 inflammasome, a part of the immune system involved in various inflammatory diseases.[64] These effects of nutritional ketosis are listed in Table 14.2.

Table 14.2: The effects of nutritional ketosis.

✓ Stable low levels of glucose and insulin
✓ Reduction of pro-inflammatory markers and enzymes (hsCRP, IL1, 6, 8, TNFα)
✓ Increased diuresis and natriuresis
✓ Reduced levels of arachidonic acid
✓ Reduced level of aromatase => reduction in estradiol production in adipose tissue
✓ Reduction of cortisol => increased pain threshold
✓ BHB blocks pro-inflammatory immune reaction (NLRP3 inflammasome–mediated inflammation)

Recent evidence confirms that a protein-optimized ketogenic diet not only supports effective weight reduction but also leads to a significant improvement in lipedema symptoms.[21, 67, 68] Notably, even normal-weight women with lipedema often report almost immediate relief from symptoms and pain after initiating a ketogenic diet. These improvements are clearly not solely attributable to weight loss but are likely the result of the anti-inflammatory and anti-edema effects associated with the metabolic shift induced by ketosis.[10, 11, 12, 13, 14, 15, 21] This makes the ketogenic diet a promising long-term strategy for managing pain in patients with lipedema. Importantly, in addition to reducing overall body weight and visceral fat, the ketogenic diet can lead to notable reductions in limb circumference and volume. This is due to the loss of alimentary fat, that is, subcutaneous fat in the extremities that is not exclusively related to lipedema, but influenced by diet[9, 22, 23] (Table 14.3).

Table 14.3: Reduction in body measurement circumference in patients with lipedema with protein-optimized ketogenic nutrition. Adapted from Faerber, 2017.[8]

Location of measurement (cm)	Baseline median (cm)	Baseline SD (cm)	Post- intervention median (cm)	Post-intervention SD (cm)	Amount of change (%)	p-value (t-test)	Effect size (d Cohen)
Distance between ankles	25.26	12.1	19.18	11.62	45.6	<0.001	-1.92
Proximal thigh	73.96	7.75	64.47	7.15	12.83	<0.001	-1.27
Mid-thigh	62.43	6.85	54.93	5.86	12.01	<0.001	-1.17
Knee	46.74	6.2	41.8	5.1	10.57	<0.001	-0.87
Calf	45.75	5.21	41.34	4.16	9.64	<0.001	-0.93

SD = standard deviation.

Balance between protein and fat

In cases where weight loss is not desired, such as in many neurological conditions, fat intake must be increased to meet caloric needs. Conversely, when weight loss is the goal, creating a moderate energy deficit may be necessary. These goals can be achieved by consuming appropriate amounts of healthy fats, including both unsaturated and saturated fats, as ketosis promotes lipolysis and supports the reduction of body fat.

To maximize the anti-inflammatory benefits of a ketogenic diet, protein sources should be selected based on their inflammatory potential. In addition to fatty cold-water fish, meat from pasture-raised animals, such as lamb, beef, or venison, contains higher levels of omega-3 fatty acids and significantly lower levels of arachidonic acid than pork, turkey, or meat from industrial livestock farming.

A daily intake of approximately 1.2 to 1.5 grams of protein per kilogram of ideal body weight is typically sufficient to preserve lean mass[43] and to support gluconeogenesis, which provides 20–25% of the glucose still required by the brain, despite its efficient use of ketones. However, excessive protein intake, generally more than 2 g/kg, may stimulate increased gluconeogenesis and insulin secretion, which could counteract some of the benefits of ketosis.

Problematic foods and ingredients

Artificial sweeteners are increasingly suspected of promoting, rather than preventing, obesity and diabetes and should therefore be avoided whenever possible. Despite containing no usable carbohydrates, their intense sweetness can trigger insulin secretion via the cephalic phase insulin response, which may ultimately be contributory to insulin resistance.[69, 70] Some sweeteners, such as sucralose, have also been shown to alter the gut microbiota.[71, 72] In contrast, polyols like erythritol and xylitol appear to have beneficial effects: erythritol has no impact on plasma glucose or insulin levels, and xylitol has only a minimal one. Both slow gastric emptying and stimulate the release of the satiety hormones CCK and GLP-1, contributing to greater feelings of fullness.[73]

Other chemical additives and preservatives can also negatively affect the gut microbiome, contributing to chronic inflammation and increased risk of obesity. These should be minimized or avoided whenever possible. One of the most effective strategies is to rely on whole, unprocessed foods rather than ready-made meals and industrial snacks, which are often loaded with sugar and additives that may trigger cravings and dysregulate appetite.

It has recently been hypothesized that lipedema may, at least in part, be linked to an accumulation of bacterial lipopolysaccharides (LPS), also known as endotoxins, in lipedema-prone fat deposits in the gluteal and femoral regions. This accumulation could lead to endotoxemia and chronic low-grade inflammation, potentially contributing to the abnormal expansion of fat tissue in lipedema.[74] Because LPS can enter the bloodstream when intestinal permeability is increased, a condition known as 'leaky gut', it is advisable to avoid food components that may compromise gut barrier integrity. These include lectins, trypsin inhibitors, and certain food additives. Anecdotal reports suggest that lipedema symptoms may improve on a lectin-free diet. Lectins and trypsin inhibitors serve as natural defense mechanisms in plants and are particularly abundant in grains, cereals, soybeans, and other legumes. As such, many ketogenic diets, which often exclude these foods, are inherently low in lectins.

To generally improve health, various habits can help achieve a healthy diet and lifestyle, such as reducing stress by getting enough sleep, increasing physical activity, eliminating snacks in between meals, avoiding unhealthy food choices, and increasing healthy ones. Additionally, inflammatory risk factors should be addressed, and micronutrients should be supplemented in cases of deficiency. See Table 14.4 for a list of lifestyle recommendations.

Table 14.4: Lifestyle and dietary recommendations for patients with lipedema.

Lifestyle recommendations	**Dietary recommendations**	**Supplements**
Reduce stress	**Avoid:**	Omega-3 oil
Improve sleep	Sugar, fructose, refined carbs, cereals, Transfats	Vitamin D, C
Exercise (aerobic, resistance)	Omega-6 oils	Possibly curcumin, ECGC, polyphenols
Reduce the number of meals per day	Ultra-processed food	According to lab values: vitamin B complex, zinc, magnesium, chromium, selenium
Try time-restricted eating	Additives, preservatives	Vitamin B complex, zinc, magnesium, chromium, selenium
Follow a protein-optimized ketogenic diet	Processed meats, meat from industrial farming	
	Artificial sweeteners	

Table 14.4: cont.

Lifestyle recommendations	Dietary recommendations	Supplements
	Prefer/increase:	
	Healthy fats	
	Wild-caught cold-water fish	
	Olive oil, nuts, seeds	
	Meat and (full-fat) dairy products (if tolerated) from pasture-raised animals	
	Fresh vegetables	
	Low glycemic berries	

Conclusion

Although a ketogenic diet as an intervention for lipedema is a new area of study, recent research with this population has highlighted its great potential for successfully managing symptoms. Because of the significant effect of nutritional ketosis on a plethora of diseases, including those commonly co-occurring with lipedema, a carbohydrate-reduced nutrition approach should be part of the holistic care of every patient with lipedema.

References

1. Cornely M. Lipedema of Arms and Legs. *Phlebologie*. 2017 Dec 30;40(3):146–51. DOI: https://doi.org/10.1055/s-0037-1621768
2. Stutz J. Liposuction in lipedema to prevent later joint complications. *Vasomed*. 2011 Jan;23. Available from: https://lipedema.net/wp-content/uploads/2024/12/liposuction20of20lipedema20to-20prevent20later20joint20complications.pdf
3. Blüher M, Fasshauer M, Tönjes A, Kratzsch J, Schön MR, Paschke R. Association of interleukin-6, C-reactive protein, interleukin-10 and adiponectin plasma concentrations with measures of obesity, insulin sensitivity and glucose metabolism. *Exp Clin Endocrinol Diabetes*. 2005 Oct 19;113:534–7. DOI: https://doi.org/10.1055/s-2005-872851
4. Al-Ghadban S, Cromer W, Allen M, Ussery C, Badowski M, Harris D, et al. Dilated blood and lymphatic microvessels, angiogenesis, increased macrophages, and adipocyte hypertrophy in lipedema thigh skin and fat tissue. *J Obes*. 2019 Mar 3;2019:1–10. DOI: https://doi.org/10.1155/2019/8747461
5. Felmerer G, Stylianaki A, Hägerling R, Wang A, Ströbel P, Hollmén M, et al. Adipose tissue hypertrophy, an aberrant biochemical profile and distinct gene expression in lipedema. *J Surg Res*. 2020 Sep 1;253:294–303. DOI: https://doi.org/10.1016/j.jss.2020.03.055
6. Felmerer G, Stylianaki A, Hollmén M, Ströbel P, Stepniewski A, Wang A, et al. Increased levels of VEGF-C and macrophage infiltration in lipedema patients without changes in lymphatic vascular morphology. *Sci Rep*. 2020 Jul 2;10(1):10947. DOI: https://doi.org/10.1038/s41598-020-67987-3
7. Nankam PAN, Cornely M, Klöting N, Blüher M. Is

subcutaneous adipose tissue expansion in people living with lipedema healthier and reflected by circulating parameters? *Front Endocrinol*. 2022 Oct 31;13. Available from: https://www.frontiersin.orghttps://www.frontiersin.org/journals/endocrinology/articles/10.3389/fendo.2022.1000094/full

8. Faerber G. Anti-inflammatory diet, what is it and what benefits does it have for lipedema? *Vasomed*. 2017;29:228. Available from: https://library.lipedema.org/bibliography/RNDGIIKX
9. Faerber G. [Nutritional therapy for lipedema and obesity – results of a guideline-based treatment concept]. *Vasomed*. 2017;29(4):176–7. Available from: https://library.lipedema.org/bibliography/YR8I2DME
10. Cannataro R, Cione E. Lipedema and nutrition: what's the link? *ACTA Sci Nutr Health*. 2020;4(11):86–9. DOI: https://doi.org/10.31080/ASNH.2020.04.0781
11. Di Renzo L, Cinelli G, Romano L, Zomparelli S, Lou De Santis G, Nocerino P, et al. Potential effects of a modified mediterranean diet on body composition in lipoedema. *Nutrients*. 2021 Feb;13(2):358. DOI: https://doi.org/10.3390/nu13020358
12. Keith L, Seo CA, Rowsemitt C, Pfeffer M, Wahi M, Staggs M, et al. Ketogenic diet as a potential intervention for lipedema. *Med Hypotheses*. 2021 Jan 1;146:110435. DOI: https://doi.org/10.1016/j.mehy.2020.110435
13. Amato ACM, Benitti DA. Lipedema can be treated non-surgically: a report of 5 cases. *Am J Case Rep*. 2021 Dec 6;22:e934406-1-e934406-8. DOI: https://doi.org/10.12659/AJCR.934406
14. Cannataro R, Michelini S, Ricolfi L, Caroleo MC, Gallelli L, De Sarro G, et al. Management of lipedema with ketogenic diet: 22-month follow-up. *Life*. 2021 Dec;11(12):1402. DOI: https://doi.org/10.3390/life11121402
15. Sørlie V, De Soysa AK, Hyldmo ÅA, Retterstøl K, Martins C, Nymo S. Effect of a ketogenic diet on pain and quality of life in patients with lipedema: the LIPODIET pilot study. *Obes Sci Pract*. 2022;8(4):483–93. DOI: https://doi.org/10.1002/osp4.580
16. Lundanes J, Gårseth M, Taylor S, Crescenzi R, Pridmore M, Wagnild R, et al. The effect of a low-carbohydrate diet on subcutaneous adipose tissue in females with lipedema. *Front Nutr*. 2024 Nov 7;11. Available from: https://www.frontiersin.org/journals/nutrition/articles/10.3389/fnut.2024.1484612/full
17. Lundanes J, Nes VF, Aakervik O, Ryan L, Hansson P, Rokstad AM, et al. Changes in cytokines and fibrotic growth factors after low-carbohydrate or low-fat low-energy diets in females with lipedema. *Curr Dev Nutr*. 2025 Mar 1;9(3):104571. DOI: https://doi.org/10.1016/j.cdnut.2025.104571
18. Lundanes J, Storliløkken GE, Solem MS, Dankel SN, Tangvik RJ, Ødegård R, et al. Gastrointestinal hormones and subjective ratings of appetite after low-carbohydrate vs. low-fat low-energy diets in females with lipedema – a randomized controlled trial. *Clin Nutr ESPEN*. 2025 Feb 1;65:16–24. DOI: https://doi.org/10.1016/j.clnesp.2024.11.018
19. Jeziorek M, Szuba ,Andrzej, Kujawa ,Krzysztof, and Regulska-Ilow B. The effect of a low-carbohydrate, high-fat diet versus moderate-carbohydrate and fat diet on body composition in patients with lipedema. *Diabetes Metab Syndr Obes*. 2022 Jan 1;15:2545–61. DOI: https://doi.org/10.2147/DMSO.S377720
20. Jeziorek M, Szuba A, Sowicz M, Adaszyńska A, Kujawa K, Chachaj A. The effect of a low-carbohydrate high-fat diet on laboratory parameters in women with lipedema in comparison to overweight/obese women. *Nutrients*. 2023 Jan;15(11):2619. DOI: https://doi.org/10.3390/nu15112619
21. Jeziorek M, Chachaj A, Sowicz M, Adaszyńska A, Truszyński A, Putek J, et al. The benefits of low-carbohydrate, high-fat (LCHF) diet on body composition, leg volume, and pain in women with lipedema. *J Obes*. 2023;2023(1):5826630. DOI: https://doi.org/10.1155/2023/5826630
22. AWMF. *S2k Guideline lipoedema of the German Society of Phlebology and Lymphology*. Association of the Scientific Medical Societies in Germany; 2024. Available from: https://register.awmf.org/assets/guidelines/037_D_Ges_fuer_Phlebologie/037-012le_S2k_Lipoedema__2024-08.pdf
23. Faerber G, Cornely M, Daubert C, Erbacher G, Fink J, Hirsch T, et al. S2k guideline lipedema. *JDDG J Dtsch Dermatol Ges*. 2024;22(9):1303–15. DOI: https://doi.org/10.1111/ddg.15513
24. Forner-Cordero I, Perez-Pomares MV, Forner A,

Ponce-Garrido AB, Munoz-Langa J. Prevalence of clinical manifestations and orthopedic alterations in patients with lipedema: a prospective cohort study. *Lymphology*. 2021;54(4):170–81. DOI: https://doi.org/10.2458/lymph.4838
25. Centre for Public Health Excellence at NICE (UK), National Collaborating Centre for Primary Care (UK). *Obesity: the prevention, identification, assessment and management of overweight and obesity in adults and children*. London: National Institute for Health and Clinical Excellence (UK); 2006. (National Institute for Health and Clinical Excellence: Guidance). Available from: http://www.ncbi.nlm.nih.gov/books/NBK63696/
26. Ditschuneit HH, Flechtner-Mors M, Johnson TD, Adler G. Metabolic and weight-loss effects of a long-term dietary intervention in obese patients. *Am J Clin Nutr*. 1999 Feb 1;69(2):198–204. DOI: https://doi.org/10.1093/ajcn/69.2.198
27. Ross Middleton KM, Patidar SM, Perri MG. The impact of extended care on the long-term maintenance of weight loss: a systematic review and meta-analysis. *Obes Rev*. 2012;13(6):509–17. DOI: https://doi.org/10.1111/j.1467-789X.2011.00972.x
28. Claussen M, Friese G, Theis S. Outpatient weight reduction through meal replacement therapy in medical practice: 2-year results of a non-controlled observational study. *Aktuelle Ernährungsmedizin*. 2022 Apr 12;47:122–34. DOI: https://doi.org/10.1055/a-1740-3572
29. Ebbeling CB, Feldman HA, Klein GL, Wong JMW, Bielak L, Steltz SK, et al. Effects of a low carbohydrate diet on energy expenditure during weight loss maintenance: randomized trial. *BMJ*. 2018 Nov 14;k4583. DOI: https://doi.org/10.1136/bmj.k4583
30. Faerber G. The overweight patient with chronic vein insufficiency or lymphedema: Risk factor or cause? *Vasomed*. 2014;26(1):19. Available from: https://www.researchgate.net/publication/293147822_The_overweight_patient_with_chronic_vein_insufficiency_or_lymphedema_Risk_factor_or_cause
31. Larsen TM, Dalskov SM, Baak M van, Jebb SA, Papadaki A, Pfeiffer AFH, et al. Diets with high or low protein content and glycemic index for weight-loss maintenance. *N Engl J Med*. 2010 Nov 25;363(22):2102–13. DOI: https://doi.org/10.1056/NEJMoa1007137
32. Stutz J. [Lipoedema: cause of serious eating disorders]. *Phlebologie*. 2013;5:A10–11.
33. Feinman RD, Pogozelski WK, Astrup A, Bernstein RK, Fine EJ, Westman EC, et al. Dietary carbohydrate restriction as the first approach in diabetes management: critical review and evidence base. *Nutrition*. 2015 Jan 1;31(1):1–13. DOI: https://doi.org/10.1016/j.nut.2014.06.011
34. Neuhouser ML, Schwarz Y, Wang C, Breymeyer K, Coronado G, Wang CY, et al. A low-glycemic load diet reduces serum c-reactive protein and modestly increases adiponectin in overweight and obese adults. *J Nutr*. 2012 Feb 1;142(2):369–74. DOI: https://doi.org/10.3945/jn.111.149807
35. Ruth MR, Port AM, Shah M, Bourland AC, Istfan NW, Nelson KP, et al. Consuming a hypocaloric high fat low carbohydrate diet for 12 weeks lowers C-reactive protein, and raises serum adiponectin and high density lipoprotein-cholesterol in obese subjects. *Metabolism*. 2013 Dec 1;62(12):1779–87. DOI: https://doi.org/10.1016/j.metabol.2013.07.006
36. Keys A, Menotti A, Aravanis C, Blackburn H, Djordevič BS, Buzina R, et al. The seven countries study: 2,289 deaths in 15 years. *Prev Med*. 1984 Mar 1;13(2):141–54. DOI: https://doi.org/10.1016/0091-7435(84)90047-1
37. Yudkin J. *Pure, White, and Deadly: How Sugar Is Killing Us and What We Can Do to Stop It*. Penguin; 2012. 149 p. Available from: https://www.amazon.com/Pure-White-Deadly-Sugar-Killing/dp/0143125184
38. Schulze MB, Minihane AM, Saleh RNM, Risérus U. Intake and metabolism of omega-3 and omega-6 polyunsaturated fatty acids: nutritional implications for cardiometabolic diseases. *Lancet Diabetes Endocrinol*. 2020 Nov 1;8(11):915–30. DOI: https://doi.org/10.1016/S2213-8587(20)30148-0
39. DiNicolantonio JJ, O'Keefe J. The importance of maintaining a low omega-6/omega-3 ratio for reducing the risk of autoimmune diseases, asthma, and allergies. *Mo Med*. 2021;118(5):453–9. Available from: https://www.ncbi.nlm.nih.gov/pmc/articles/PMC8504498/
40. Stossier H, Bayer W. [Study on the influence of linseed oil and fish oil as sources of omega-3 fatty acids on fatty acid status]. *Z Für Orthomolekulare*

Med. 2009 Dec 3;7:11–5.
DOI: https://doi.org/10.1055/s-0029-1186170

41. Hoenselaar R. Saturated fat and cardiovascular disease: the discrepancy between the scientific literature and dietary advice. *Nutrition*. 2012 Feb 1;28(2):118–23.
DOI: https://doi.org/10.1016/j.nut.2011.08.017
42. Sofi F, Buccioni A, Cesari F, Gori AM, Minieri S, Mannini L, et al. Effects of a dairy product (pecorino cheese) naturally rich in cis-9, trans-11 conjugated linoleic acid on lipid, inflammatory and haemorheological variables: a dietary intervention study. *Nutr Metab Cardiovasc Dis*. 2010 Feb 1;20(2):117–24. DOI: https://doi.org/10.1016/j.numecd.2009.03.004
43. Westerterp-Plantenga MS, Lemmens SG, Westerterp KR. Dietary protein – its role in satiety, energetics, weight loss and health. *Br J Nutr*. 2012 Aug;108(S2):S105–12.
DOI: https://doi.org/10.1017/S0007114512002589
44. Raubenheimer D, Simpson SJ. Protein leverage: theoretical foundations and ten points of clarification. *Obesity*. 2019;27(8):1225–38.
DOI: https://doi.org/10.1002/oby.22531
45. Anderson GH, Moore SE. Dietary proteins in the regulation of food intake and body weight in humans. *J Nutr*. 2004 Apr 1;134(4):974S–979S.
DOI: https://doi.org/10.1093/jn/134.4.974S
46. Leidy HJ, Hoertel HA, Douglas SM, Higgins KA, Shafer RS. A high-protein breakfast prevents body fat gain, through reductions in daily intake and hunger, in 'Breakfast skipping' adolescents. *Obesity*. 2015;23(9):1761–4.
DOI: https://doi.org/10.1002/oby.21185
47. Devries MC, Sithamparapillai A, Brimble KS, Banfield L, Morton RW, Phillips SM. 'Changes in kidney function do not differ between healthy adults consuming higher- compared with lower- or normal-protein diets: a systematic review and meta-analysis. *J Nutr*. 2018 Nov 1;148(11):1760–75. DOI: https://doi.org/10.1093/jn/nxy197
48. Hamdy O, Carver C. The why WAIT program: Improving clinical outcomes through weight management in type 2 diabetes. *Curr Diab Rep*. 2008 Oct 1;8(5):413–20.
DOI: https://doi.org/10.1007/s11892-008-0071-5
49. Markova M, Pivovarova O, Hornemann S, Sucher S, Frahnow T, Wegner K, et al. Isocaloric diets high in animal or plant protein reduce liver fat and inflammation in individuals with type 2 diabetes. *Gastroenterology*. 2017 Feb 1;152(3):571–585.e8.
DOI: https://doi.org/10.1053/j.gastro.2016.10.007
50. LaManna JC, Salem N, Puchowicz M, Erokwu B, Koppaka S, Flask C, et al. Ketones suppress brain glucose consumption. *Adv Exp Med Biol*. 2009;645:301–6. DOI: https://doi.org/10.1007/978-0-387-85998-9_45
51. Barrès R, Zierath JR. The role of diet and exercise in the transgenerational epigenetic landscape of T2DM. *Nat Rev Endocrinol*. 2016 Aug;12(8):441–51. DOI: https://doi.org/10.1038/nrendo.2016.87
52. Duncan SH, Belenguer A, Holtrop G, Johnstone AM, Flint HJ, Lobley GE. Reduced dietary intake of carbohydrates by obese subjects results in decreased concentrations of butyrate and butyrate-producing bacteria in feces. *Appl Environ Microbiol*. 2007;73:1073–8.
DOI: https://doi.org/10.1128/AEM.02340-06
53. Weigle DS, Breen PA, Matthys CC, Callahan HS, Meeuws KE, Burden VR, et al. A high-protein diet induces sustained reductions in appetite, ad libitum caloric intake, and body weight despite compensatory changes in diurnal plasma leptin and ghrelin concentrations. *Am J Clin Nutr*. 2005 Jul 1;82(1):41–8.
DOI: https://doi.org/10.1093/ajcn/82.1.41
54. Cummings DE, Weigle DS, Frayo RS, Breen PA, Ma MK, Dellinger EP, et al. Plasma ghrelin levels after diet-induced weight loss or gastric bypass surgery. *N Engl J Med*. 2002 May 23;346(21):1623–30.
DOI: https://doi.org/10.1056/NEJMoa012908
55. Rolls BJ, Hetherington M, Burley VJ. The specificity of satiety: the influence of foods of different macronutrient content on the development of satiety. *Physiol Behav*. 1988 Jan 1;43(2):145–53. DOI: https://doi.org/10.1016/0031-9384(88)90230-2
56. Schoeller DA, Buchholz AC. Energetics of obesity and weight control: does diet composition matter? *J Am Diet Assoc*. 2005 May 1;105(5, Supplement):24–8.
DOI: https://doi.org/10.1016/j.jada.2005.02.025
57. Harvie M, Wright C, Pegington M, McMullan D, Mitchell E, Martin B, et al. The effect of intermittent energy and carbohydrate restriction v. daily energy restriction on weight loss and metabolic disease risk markers in overweight women. *Br J*

Nutr. 2013 Oct;110(8):1534–47.
DOI: https://doi.org/10.1017/S0007114513000792
58. Klempel MC, Kroeger CM, Bhutani S, Trepanowski JF, Varady KA. Intermittent fasting combined with calorie restriction is effective for weight loss and cardio-protection in obese women. *Nutr J*. 2012 Nov 21;11(1):98.
DOI: https://doi.org/10.1186/1475-2891-11-98
59. Mizushima N, Noda T, Yoshimori T, Tanaka Y, Ishii T, George MD, et al. A protein conjugation system essential for autophagy. *Nature*. 1998 Sep;395(6700):395–8.
DOI: https://doi.org/10.1038/26506
60. Westman EC, Feinman RD, Mavropoulos JC, Vernon MC, Volek JS, Wortman JA, et al. Low-carbohydrate nutrition and metabolism. *Am J Clin Nutr*. 2007 Aug 1;86(2):276–84.
DOI: https://doi.org/10.1093/ajcn/86.2.276
61. Westman EC, Mavropoulos J, Yancy WS, Volek JS. A review of low-carbohydrate ketogenic diets. *Curr Atheroscler Rep*. 2003 Nov;5(6):476–83. DOI: https://doi.org/10.1007/s11883-003-0038-6
62. Volek JS, Sharman MJ, Love DM, Avery NG, Gómez AL, Scheett TP, et al. Body composition and hormonal responses to a carbohydrate-restricted diet. *Metabolism*. 2002 Jul;51(7):864–70.
DOI: https://doi.org/10.1053/meta.2002.32037
63. Noakes TD. Low-carbohydrate and high-fat intake can manage obesity and associated conditions: occasional survey. *South Afr Med J Suid-Afr Tydskr Vir Geneeskd*. 2013 Sep 30;103(11):826–30. DOI: https://doi.org/10.7196/samj.7302
64. Yancy WS, Olsen MK, Guyton JR, Bakst RP, Westman EC. A low-carbohydrate, ketogenic diet versus a low-fat diet to treat obesity and hyperlipidemia: a randomized, controlled trial. *Ann Intern Med*. 2004 May 1;140(10):769–77. DOI: https://doi.org/10.7326/0003-4819-140-10-200405180-00006
65. Maalouf M, Rho JM, Mattson MP. The neuroprotective properties of calorie restriction, the ketogenic diet, and ketone bodies. *Brain Res Rev*. 2009 Mar 1;59(2):293–315. DOI: https://doi.org/10.1016/j.brainresrev.2008.09.002
66. Stafstrom CE, Rho CE. The ketogenic diet as a treatment paradigm for diverse neurological diseases. *Front Pharmacol*. 2012 Apr 9;3. Available from: https://www.frontiersin.org/journals/pharmacology/articles/10.3389/fphar.2012.00059/full
67. Faerber G. Obesity and chronic inflammation in phlebological and lymphatic diseases. *Phlebologie*. 2018 Feb;47(02):55–65.
DOI: https://doi.org/10.12687/phleb2413-2-2018
68. Lundanes J, Sandnes F, Gjeilo KH, Hansson P, Salater S, Martins C, et al. Effect of a low-carbohydrate diet on pain and quality of life in female patients with lipedema: a randomized controlled trial. *Obesity*. 2024;32(6):1071–82.
DOI: https://doi.org/10.1002/oby.24026
69. Just T, Pau HW, Engel U, Hummel T. Cephalic phase insulin release in healthy humans after taste stimulation? *Appetite*. 2008 Nov 1;51(3):622–7.
DOI: https://doi.org/10.1016/j.appet.2008.04.271
70. Pepino MY, Tiemann CD, Patterson B, Wice BM, Klein S. Sucralose affects glycemic and hormonal responses to an oral glucose load. *Diabetes Care*. 2013;36(9):2529–30. Available from: https://dialnet.unirioja.es/servlet/articulo?codigo=5429799
71. Abou-Donia MB, El-Masry ,Eman M., Abdel-Rahman ,Ali A., McLendon ,Roger E., and Schiffman SS. Splenda alters gut microflora and increases intestinal P-glycoprotein and cytochrome P-450 in male rats. *J Toxicol Environ Health A*. 2008 Sep 22;71(21):1415–29.
DOI: https://doi.org/10.1080/15287390802328630
72. Suez J, Korem T, Zeevi D, Zilberman-Schapira G, Thaiss CA, Maza O, et al. Artificial sweeteners induce glucose intolerance by altering the gut microbiota. *Nature*. 2014 Oct;514(7521):181–6. DOI: https://doi.org/10.1038/nature13793
73. Wölnerhanssen BK, Cajacob L, Keller N, Doody A, Rehfeld JF, Drewe J, et al. Gut hormone secretion, gastric emptying, and glycemic responses to erythritol and xylitol in lean and obese subjects. *Am J Physiol Endocrinol Metab*. 2016 Jun 1;310(11):E1053–1061.
DOI: https://doi.org/10.1152/ajpendo.00037.2016
74. Kruglikov IL, Scherer PE. Is the endotoxin–complement cascade the major driver in lipedema? *Trends Endocrinol Metab*. 2024 Sep 1;35(9):769–80.
DOI: https://doi.org/10.1016/j.tem.2024.04.004

Chapter Fifteen
A holistic approach to diagnosis, care, and treatment

Matthew Carmody and Siobhan Huggins

Introduction

Holistic medical care refers to a comprehensive, integrative approach that considers the whole person – body, mind, emotions, social context, and spirit – in the prevention, diagnosis, and treatment of illness. Rather than focusing solely on disease symptoms, holistic care seeks to promote overall well-being and functional capacity. A growing body of research supports the value of this approach, particularly for individuals with multiple chronic diseases. Studies have shown that multidisciplinary, holistic care is associated with improved health outcomes, enhanced self-management, and reduced hospitalizations.[1]

This chapter presents a holistic, patient-centered model for managing lipedema, grounded in five interrelated domains of health: physical, mental/psychological, emotional, social, and spiritual,[2] as depicted in Figure 15.1.

Each domain is explored in terms of the relevant symptoms, diagnoses, and challenges – referred to here as 'topics' – such as pain, swelling, or excess adiposity within the physical domain. Suggested interventions, referral strategies, and supportive measures are provided to help clinicians tailor care to the individual needs of each patient. Table 15.1 lists the five domains along with their areas of focus.

Table 15.1: Five domains of holistic lipedema care and their focus areas.

Holistic approach domain	Focus areas
Physical	Swelling, pain, excess adipose tissue, weight management
Emotional	Emotional regulation, body image, managing emotions
Mental/ psychological	Depression, anxiety, disordered eating
Social	Social support, isolation, peer groups
Spiritual	Purpose, sense of self, life meaning, aliveness

While this chapter offers an overview, these domains are examined in greater detail elsewhere in this book, which includes clinical evidence, estimated prevalence rates where available, and practical considerations for implementation. As each domain is explored, readers are invited to consider how lipedema care can be broadened to support patients in realizing a fuller sense of well-being. By identifying and nurturing strengths – even those that may lie dormant – clinicians can play a vital role in helping patients reclaim

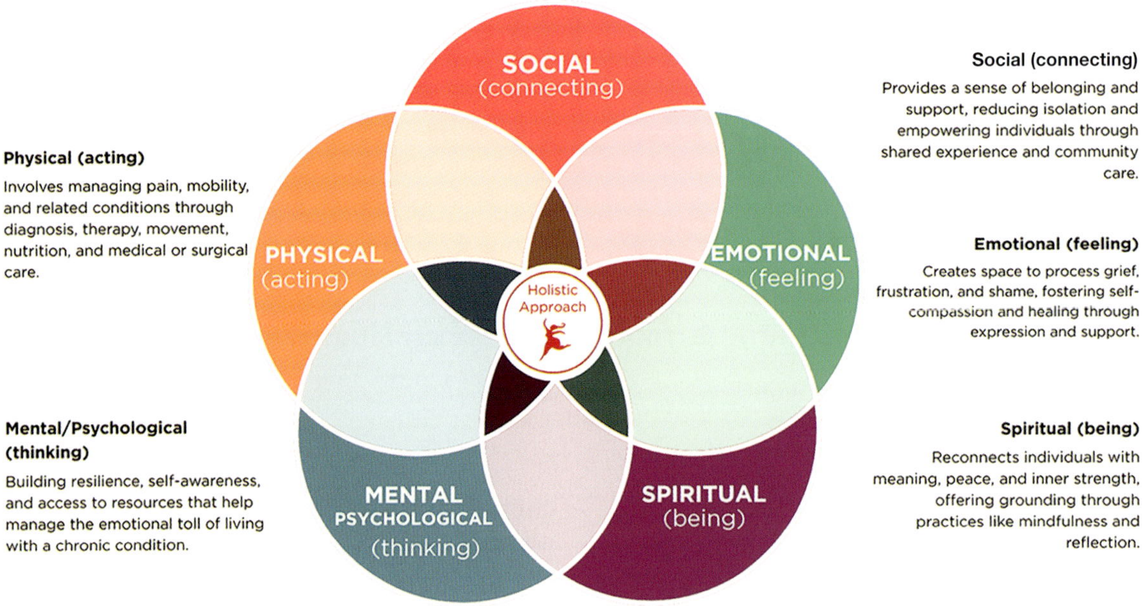

Figure 15.1: Holistic approach. Used with permission from Lipedema Simplified LLC.

function, confidence, and purpose. This chapter offers a summary of that comprehensive, multidimensional approach.

The physical domain

The physical domain primarily focuses on addressing the physical symptoms of lipedema, including swelling, pain, and excess adipose tissue, and may also include physical difficulties that are a consequence of lipedema symptoms, such as gait abnormalities and mobility impairments. Other topics discussed are treatment strategies and long-term weight management (see Table 15.2).

Table 15.2: Common physical symptoms and suggested interventions.

Physical symptom	Suggested interventions
Swelling	Compression, movement, non-inflammatory diet
Pain	Compression garments, manual lymph drainage (MLD), ketogenic diet, low-carb diet, topical treatments
Excessive adipose tissue	Weight management, decongestive therapy, surgery
Mobility impairment	Joint care, physical therapy

Swelling

Patients with lipedema commonly report sensations of swelling in areas where they have excess adipose tissue resulting from lipedema (e.g. lower body, arms).[3, 4, 5] This swelling may interfere with daily activities and result in significant discomfort.[6] For instance, a patient may describe their legs as feeling heavy, or 'like concrete,' 'puffy,' or report experiencing swollen ankles or legs. Impacts on daily activities may include difficulty with prolonged standing or walking for extended periods, climbing stairs, or getting in and out of a car. Similarly, if the patient experiences swelling in their arms, they may notice difficulty with tasks that involve lifting objects or reaching high shelves. The sensation of swelling may vary day-to-day, often worsening in heat and humidity, with increased activity, or as the day progresses.[7]

Initially, the main strategy will be to discuss with the patient what interventions have provided relief in the past. Understanding the patient experience can help guide the use of practical symptom relief measures that the patient may want to integrate into their daily routine. Additionally, this can help highlight factors the patient may want to avoid or minimize if they exacerbate swelling. Other management strategies may include elevation, movement/exercise, compression garments, pneumatic compression, reduced intake of inflammatory foods, and referral to a certified lymphedema therapist.

Pain

Exact causes of pain in lipedema are not currently well understood.[8] Current evidence indicates that pain is experienced by the majority of patients with lipedema[9, 10] and may also significantly impact many aspects of the patient's life, including mental and physical health[11] and overall quality of life,[12] making pain management an important focus of holistic lipedema care.

Despite the significant impact pain can have, some patients may not always spontaneously divulge the presence of pain. This may be because the patient is unaware that the pain is due to an underlying disease, or because they may assume that the pain is a common experience. Therefore, a thorough clinical examination, including physical palpation and targeted questions, can help establish the severity of pain that a patient is experiencing.

While pain is inherently subjective, some commonalities can be found in lipedema-related pain. Patients typically report pain in areas impacted by lipedema, such as the lower body and arms. Patients may also describe the pain as being right below the surface, in fatty regions, or that their fat is tender or painful. Additionally, while this pain may be spontaneous or constant, pain may also intensify with even light touch or pressure.

Because lipedema is a chronic disease, and pain may be a chronic symptom, the authors currently believe that options used should ideally be safe for long-term use, non-habit-forming, and not contraindicated for co-morbidities or other medications the patient is presently taking. There are currently no specific recommendations for the use of medications aimed primarily at pain reduction for patients with lipedema.[13] Patients should be encouraged to share any pain relief methods they are using, including oral or topical pain relievers.

Several other approaches may help manage lipedema-related pain. Dietary strategies, such as carbohydrate-restricted diets, have been shown to reduce pain in some patients.[14, 15] This approach is discussed further in Chapter 14. For personalized guidance, consider referring patients to a nutritionist, ideally one experienced with these diets.

Therapies such as manual lymph drainage, intermittent pneumatic compression, and short-stretch compression wrapping may help relieve pain. Compression garments, commonly used to reduce swelling, are also reported by many patients to alleviate discomfort (further discussed in Chapters 12 and 18). Referral to a certified lymphatic therapist can also assist the patient with accessing appropriate compression tools and therapies.

Excess adipose tissue

Excess adipose tissue in lipedema has distinct clinical implications, with effects largely influenced by the volume and anatomical distribution of the tissue. For example, adipose accumulation around the hips and legs can increase mechanical load on weight-bearing joints, leading to pain in the knees or ankles. Current literature on these effects in lipedema is limited. However, Forner-Cordero et al.[16] observed a positive correlation between the stage of lipedema and the severity of knee osteoarthritis. Additionally, fat deposition around the inner knees and thighs may alter gait mechanics, increasing joint stress and contributing to abnormal movement patterns. Chachaj et al.[17] reported that a greater leg volume in individuals with lipedema was associated with impaired physical functioning, difficulties with self-care, and reduced ability to perform work and household activities. These functional impairments, resulting from joint strain, gait abnormalities, and compromised balance, may necessitate the use of mobility aids, such as walkers or wheelchairs, and, in severe cases, may lead to immobility or confinement to bed.

Management strategies for patients with excess adipose tissue in lipedema should be tailored to both the underlying disease and any co-morbid conditions. In cases where obesity coexists with lipedema, weight management may help reduce overall adipose burden and improve joint function. Nutritional interventions, such as ketogenic diets, and conservative measures like complete decongestive therapy, may assist in reducing limb volume and alleviating pressure on joints.

In more advanced cases, where conservative approaches are insufficient, surgical interventions may be warranted. Total knee arthroplasty, although not extensively studied in lipedema, has shown promising results in a small cohort.[18] A follow-up study involving five patients with lipedema undergoing knee replacement surgery reported low complication rates and improvements in pain and mobility.[18] Given the lack of robust, large-scale data, referral to an orthopedic surgeon with experience in managing lipedema is advised. Such specialists can offer individualized pre- and post-operative guidance to accommodate the unique anatomical and physiological considerations of lipedema.

Together, a multidisciplinary approach that integrates weight management, conservative therapies, and, when appropriate, surgical interventions, offers the most comprehensive strategy to address the musculoskeletal and functional challenges associated with excess adipose tissue in lipedema.

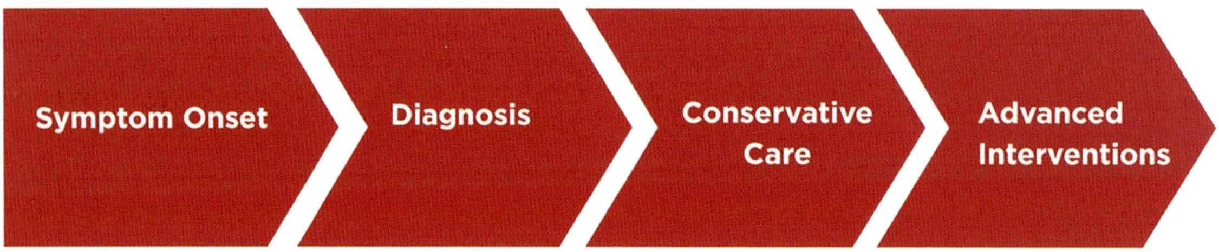

Figure 15.2: The journey of a patient with lipedema, from the onset of symptoms to diagnosis and care.

Beyond conservative care

Conservative measures, while foundational in lipedema management, may not be sufficient to fully address all physical symptoms. In such cases, lipedema reduction surgery can serve as an additional therapeutic option. It is important to emphasize, however, that surgical options should not generally be the first-line intervention. As depicted in Figure 15.2, the journey of managing lipedema starts with the onset of symptoms and diagnosis and continues with exploring and experimenting with conservative treatment measures before moving toward advanced interventions like surgery.

Surgical interventions are explored in greater detail in Chapters 16 and 17. Lipedema surgeries aim to remove excess adipose tissue and may help alleviate issues related to mobility, balance, and joint strain. Some reports also suggest a reduction in pain following surgery, contributing to improved quality of life.[13, 19]

When surgery is being considered, application of the holistic care model remains essential. The patient's physical readiness, psychological state, emotional well-being, and expectations should all be assessed. A referral to a surgeon may be appropriate if the patient expresses interest in surgical intervention. Due to the unique nature of lipedema tissue and the complexity of the disease, referral to a surgeon who specializes in lipedema is strongly recommended. The specialist can evaluate the patient to determine surgical candidacy and begin planning appropriate pre- and post-operative care.

Even when surgery is pursued, conservative therapies are typically maintained as part of a comprehensive treatment plan rather than used in isolation. Conservative measures may serve as pre-operative preparation, improving surgical outcomes, or as part of the post-operative recovery process to support healing and long-term management.

During the decision-making process, it is important to explore the patient's goals and expectations to ensure they are realistic. For instance, if a patient believes surgery will eliminate the need for ongoing conservative therapy, this should be addressed, as it may not reflect clinical reality. Establishing a realistic and healthy mindset before surgery can positively influence both the surgical experience and long-term satisfaction.

Finally, psychological and emotional factors – discussed further in a later section of this chapter – may significantly impact post-operative outcomes and patient satisfaction. Integrating these considerations into pre-surgical counseling reinforces the value of a holistic, patient-centered approach to care.

Long-term weight management

Long-term weight stabilization may be beneficial for individuals with lipedema, as weight gain, regardless of its cause, can exacerbate symptoms and potentially contribute to disease progression.[4] When discussing weight management with patients, it is helpful to begin by exploring their previous experiences. For instance, patients may recall periods of weight stability or gain and identify contributing factors, such as dietary patterns or stress. These insights can inform the development of a sustainable, individualized weight management plan.

Specialized nutritional approaches that address troubling lipedema symptoms and promote weight management may be appropriate, such as carbohydrate-restricted diets (discussed in Chapter 14). Ongoing monitoring is recommended for patients following specialized diets, both to assess clinical effectiveness and ensure nutritional adequacy. Referral to a dietitian or nutritionist with expertise in the chosen dietary approach can support this process, offering tailored guidance and monitoring of nutrient status.

Support systems are also important for long-term adherence. Connecting patients with support groups, whether general weight loss communities or those focused specifically on lipedema, can provide practical advice, motivation, and social reinforcement. Meta-analyses of successful long-term weight loss maintenance consistently identify support groups as a key factor in sustaining results.[20] Lipedema-focused groups, in particular, may offer shared experiences and strategies uniquely relevant to the challenges faced by this patient population.

The emotional domain

The emotional domain primarily focuses on addressing the emotional impacts of lipedema. These include the emotional toll of managing a chronic disease as well as the impacts on physical appearance and self-esteem. Emotional challenges are common among patients with lipedema and may stem from both the diagnosis itself and the demands of managing a chronic illness. Difficulty recognizing and regulating emotions can negatively affect symptom management, overall well-being, and quality of life. Table 15.3 lists the emotional challenges and psychological issues (discussed in the next section).

Emotional regulation

Emerging research suggests that emotional dysregulation may not be uncommon in this population. For instance, 28% of 1,362 individuals with self-identified lipedema reported emotional lability, and 75% noted increased sensitivity and irritability, potential indicators of impaired emotional regulation.[21] A 2022 case-control study also found that patients with lipedema experienced greater difficulty with emotional regulation, impulse control, and goal-directed behavior compared to the control group.[22] While the origins of emotional dysregulation in lipedema are unclear, it is plausible that it may stem from the chronic nature of the disease, given the potential interplay between chronic disease and emotional dysregulation more generally, as discussed by Conversano.[23] However, studies comparing rates of emotional dysregulation in lipedema compared to rates in other chronic diseases are not currently available to elucidate this possibility.

Table 15.3: Emotional and psychological challenges experienced by patients with lipedema.

Challenge	Possible indicators	Suggested support
Emotional dysregulation	Irritability, mood swings	Mindfulness therapy, yoga
Body image issues	Avoiding mirrors, shame	Body-positive counseling, acceptance and commitment therapy (ACT)
Depression	Fatigue, hopelessness	Cognitive behavior therapy (CBT), medication support
Anxiety	Worry, sleep issues	Meditation, relaxation techniques
Disordered eating	Yo-yo dieting, bingeing	Specialist therapy, nutritional monitoring

Impaired body image

The disfiguring nature of lipedema often contributes to body image issues, which can cause significant emotional distress and impact daily life. Patients may express this through self-critical language, shame about their appearance, or avoidance of activities that expose the body, such as going to the beach or engaging in physical intimacy.

A report from the UK advocacy group Lipoedema UK presented insights generated from patient focus groups and highlighted common themes of low self-esteem, self-consciousness, and social withdrawal due to body image concerns.[24] Some participants avoided activities like swimming to prevent others from seeing their bodies. These findings suggest that body image issues in lipedema can interfere not only with emotional well-being but also with symptom management and social participation. Qualitative research further supports these experiences, with patients describing feelings of being trapped in their bodies, self-judgment, and fear of external judgment related to their size and shape.[25]

Managing emotions around lipedema

Given the potential impact on mental and physical health, referral to a mental health professional, particularly one experienced in mindfulness-based therapies, may be beneficial. Mindfulness practices, such as meditation or yoga, can also support emotional regulation. For patients with mobility limitations, virtual classes and resources may provide accessible alternatives.

The mental/psychological domain

The mental/psychological domain focuses on recognizing patients' psychological needs and providing support for challenges and difficulties that may interfere with lipedema care. Psychological factors may result from experiences related to lipedema, or they may be the result of a co-morbid psychiatric diagnosis. Both can profoundly impact lipedema management. Refer to Table 15.3 for a listing of the common challenges faced by patients with lipedema in the mental/psychological domains.

Depression

The relationship between lipedema and depression is not yet fully understood. It remains unclear whether depression arises directly from lipedema's physiological mechanisms or as a psychological response to living with a chronic disease. In other chronic illnesses, such as diabetes and coronary artery disease, a bi-directional link with depression has been proposed, though this has not been thoroughly explored in lipedema.[26]

Plausible biological pathways may exist. Lipedema involves chronic pain, inflammation, and possible lymphatic dysfunction, factors that have also been associated with major depressive disorder (MDD).[27, 28] Depression may also stem from the emotional toll of managing a chronic, painful disease, as pain levels correlate with depression symptoms in lipedema.[29]

Studies suggest that depression is more prevalent among individuals with lipedema than in the general population. A German retrospective study reported a 25.5% depression rate in patients with lipedema, while a Polish survey found signs of depression in nearly 60% of respondents, with 11% potentially experiencing severe symptoms.[30, 31]

Depression can significantly impair quality of life and interfere with lipedema management.[31] Symptoms such as hopelessness, fatigue, low motivation, and difficulty initiating tasks may prevent patients from engaging in necessary self-care. Emotional withdrawal, persistent sadness, or loss of interest in daily activities are also common. In severe cases, depression may lead to self-harm or suicidal thoughts.

When signs of depression are present, it is important to explore coping strategies that the patient has used in the past, if any. Some patients may have found relief through physical activity, therapy, or medication during previous episodes of their condition. On the other hand, some patients may have never sought support before, in which case a referral to a therapist or psychologist may be beneficial to help them identify possible interventions to try. Identifying these resources can guide appropriate referrals and support holistic care.

Anxiety

Anxiety is commonly reported among individuals with lipedema. For instance, a Brazilian study found that 60% of women who met diagnostic criteria for lipedema reported experiencing anxiety symptoms.[32] Similarly, other studies have shown that women with lipedema often exhibit significantly higher levels of anxiety compared to non-lipedema controls.[22] This heightened vulnerability may stem from the chronic pain, progressive changes in body shape, and potential mobility limitations associated with the disease, as factors like disability and symptom severity predict health anxiety in individuals with chronic disease.[33] Together, these challenges can contribute to health-related anxiety, which has been connected to diminished quality of life in those with chronic diseases.[34]

Anxiety in this population may manifest in a range of ways. Some patients may appear reluctant to try new treatments, express persistent worries such as 'What if this doesn't work?' or exhibit fear about worsening symptoms. Others may report physical symptoms, such as shortness of breath, rapid heartbeat, difficulty sleeping, or gastrointestinal disturbances, that are often linked to their anxiety. When unaddressed, these concerns can lead to feelings of hopelessness and reduce adherence to treatment plans.

Although research into specific modalities for health anxiety in patients with lipedema is not currently available, patients may find that mindfulness therapies, such as meditation classes or groups, may be an approachable way to address health anxiety as a starting point. If additional support is needed or desired, cognitive behavior therapy (CBT) and mindfulness therapies have shown benefit in individuals with health anxiety more generally.[35, 36] A referral to a specialist, such as a therapist or psychologist familiar with these techniques, may be appropriate.

Disturbed relationship with food

Multiple surveys have documented a notable prevalence of eating disorders among individuals with lipedema, though reported rates vary widely. For example, a survey of 250 women diagnosed with lipedema by a healthcare professional found that 45% reported having an eating disorder.[37] In contrast, a larger study involving 1,298 participants reported a significantly lower rate of 16%.[21]

The origins of eating disorders in the context of lipedema are not yet fully understood. However, persistent challenges with weight management and body image, especially given lipedema's resistance to traditional weight loss methods, are likely contributing factors. Some patients also report that their disclosures about conditioned eating are dismissed or not taken seriously, which may reflect anti-fat bias and the misconception that individuals with lipedema are simply obese.[38] Without appropriate recognition and support, repeated, unsuccessful weight loss attempts can foster frustration and promote an unhealthy relationship with food.

Eating disorders carry serious health risks. Anorexia nervosa (AN) can impair bone density and muscle health, while binge eating disorder (BED) is associated with obesity, metabolic syndrome, and related complications. [39, 40, 41, 42] Early identification and compassionate, individualized treatment are essential to improving outcomes for those affected.

Certain therapy avenues for eating disorders, such as AN, bulimia nervosa (BN), and BED, have been researched more generally. For example, CBT, alone or as part of an integrated approach, is a potentially useful tool in both AN and BED.[35, 43] Currently, it is unknown whether specific interventions are more effective in patients with lipedema who exhibit patterns of conditioned eating. As such, if conditioned eating is suspected, a referral to a psychologist or therapist specializing in conditioned eating can be made. A specialist who offers interventions like CBT or guided self-help may be especially beneficial. Additionally, possible nutritional intervention strategies are suggested below.

Nutritional therapies in patients at risk of disordered eating

Given the high prevalence of disordered eating in patients with lipedema, the best way to integrate nutrition plans for symptom management remains unclear. Carbohydrate-restricted diets, such as Mediterranean, low-carb, and ketogenic diets, are often recommended for lipedema (see Chapter 14), but their appropriateness in patients with disordered eating requires further exploration.

Preliminary studies have examined ketogenic diets in diseases like AN and BED. [44, 45, 46] In AN, ketogenic diets are proposed to target both metabolic and psychiatric drivers, including anxiety.[47] In BED, some early reports suggest reduced cravings.[48] While these findings are promising, they come primarily from case series and pilot trials. Robust evidence from randomized controlled trials is lacking, making it premature to recommend ketogenic diets for patients with lipedema and co-occurring disordered eating.

Given the limited research, general recommendations are more appropriate at this stage. For example, if a patient finds symptom relief from a certain dietary approach but also experiences reemerging disordered eating patterns, additional support is crucial. Therefore, a personalized, patient-centered approach is recommended. Patients may benefit from working with a multidisciplinary team, including a psychologist, therapist, and/or dietitian, to tailor a dietary plan that supports both physical and mental health. This includes identifying and modifying potentially triggering aspects of a diet while preserving its symptom-relieving benefits. Ultimately, this approach ensures that dietary interventions for lipedema are balanced with appropriate mental health support, especially in the presence of comorbid eating disorders.

Special note on psychiatric medications

Recent research has explored the use of metabolic therapies, including ketogenic diets, in mental health conditions such as depression and anxiety. While the links between metabolic dysfunction, insulin resistance, and mental illness are beyond the scope of this chapter, reviews by Watson et al.[49] and Laurent et al.[50] provide further insight.

It remains unclear whether ketogenic diets can effectively treat depression or anxiety in patients with lipedema. Although promising, the field of metabolic psychiatry is still emerging, and ketogenic diets cannot yet be recommended as standard treatment for mental illness. However, ketogenic diets are commonly suggested for lipedema management. Therefore, a patient with both lipedema and a co-occurring mental health condition may consider this approach for its potential physical benefits.

In such cases, additional monitoring may be necessary. For example, in a study of 31 patients with treatment-resistant mental illness, 64% required psychiatric medication adjustments after starting a ketogenic diet, including 5 of 6 patients with major depressive disease.[51] Because ketogenic diets can impact medication needs, patients on psychiatric medications should be supervised by a qualified healthcare provider, ideally their psychiatrist.

If the treating psychiatrist is unfamiliar with ketogenic diets or metabolic psychiatry, referral to a specialist with relevant experience is advised. This ensures proper monitoring of mental health, medication adjustments if needed, and overall support during dietary changes. The goal of this approach is to safeguard psychological well-being while supporting symptom management of lipedema through nutritional therapy.

The social domain

The social domain focuses on addressing the impact of lipedema on the patient's relationships with others. These could include relationships with family, friends, and peers. The social domain also focuses on social isolation that can occur in patients with lipedema.

The role of social support in lipedema management

Support from loved ones, including validation, emotional encouragement, and help accommodating limitations, can play a key role in lipedema management. Although the impact of inadequate support remains underexplored, Christoffersen et al.[38] found that patients view strong social support as critical to their success. Grey et al.[52] suggest that family involvement becomes particularly valuable when the perceived burden of the diagnosis is high, or the patient is dealing with depression. More broadly, studies across chronic illnesses have linked family support to better outcomes, especially when it includes encouragement and open communication.[53] In contrast, criticism or anger toward symptoms correlates with worse long-term outcomes. While specific research on family support in lipedema is limited, these findings highlight its potential importance.

However, many patients report a lack of understanding from family or friends, some even stating their disease is dismissed or not believed to be a true malady.[25] This lack of awareness can undermine care, as loved ones may not recognize how their support influences treatment adherence. Feeling unsupported may leave patients feeling overwhelmed, isolated, or even sabotaged in their efforts to manage their disease.

In such cases, peer support can be invaluable. Support groups offer connection, validation, and emotional relief from those who truly understand the challenges of lipedema. These communities can empower patients, even if family support is lacking. If appropriate, patients can be referred to local or online support groups for lipedema. A list of resources is provided in Chapter 19.

Social isolation and lipedema

The full health impact of social isolation in lipedema is not yet known. However, survey data show that nearly 40% of women with self-reported lipedema feel lonelier due to their disease, and over half report staying home more often,[21] both indicators of reduced social functioning. Social isolation in lipedema can stem from psychological factors like depression, anxiety, or poor body image. It may also result from physical barriers such as pain, reduced mobility, or fatigue, which limit participation in previously enjoyed activities.

In one study comparing women with lipedema to overweight/obese peers, those with lipedema were less likely to engage in work, school, and community activities, likely due to mobility challenges.[17] When these activities serve as a primary source of social interaction, withdrawal can lead to loneliness and isolation. More broadly, research has linked social isolation to negative health outcomes, including cognitive decline and changes in brain function.[54, 55] Notably, isolation may heighten pain perception due to the reduced 'pain-buffering' effects of social connection.[56]

Patients may not always identify themselves as socially isolated, but they may describe feeling lonely, 'stuck at home,' or having no one to talk to. They may also mention difficulty participating in hobbies or social events. These cues can help identify patients who may benefit from additional social or psychological support.

If patients feel socially isolated or are hesitant to engage in public settings, exploring alternative forms of connection can be helpful. Online communities, such as hobby groups, book clubs, or wellness classes like yoga and meditation, can provide enjoyable social interaction from the comfort of your own home. Many of these also offer time for informal conversation, which can foster connection. Joining or starting a lipedema-specific support group, either virtually or locally, may be especially valuable. These spaces can help alleviate feelings of judgment and foster understanding among those who share similar experiences. Refer to Chapter 19 for additional suggestions on resources.

For patients facing mental health challenges contributing to isolation, group therapy, whether for lipedema or chronic illness more broadly, can offer a safe and supportive environment. If underlying physical or psychological barriers to socialization exist, these should be addressed directly. However, seeking connection through alternative means may still offer meaningful support while those issues are being managed.

The spiritual domain

The spiritual domain may include connection to religious or spiritual practices but may also include a more general sense of overall well-being. This could include factors like a sense of greater purpose and meaning, and the patient living beyond their disease. The role of these factors in holistic care will be discussed in this section.

Loss of life enjoyment

Lipedema care can be time- and energy-intensive, often requiring daily or weekly interventions. As a result, other aspects of life, such as family time, careers, or hobbies, may be neglected. When symptom management becomes the sole focus, it can be challenging to maintain during periods of stress and may ultimately lead to reduced overall well-being and life satisfaction.

Patients may report giving up hobbies they once enjoyed, not due to a loss of interest, but because they feel that management takes priority. Others may struggle to engage in leisure activities due to symptoms like pain or reduced mobility. In chronic illness more broadly, these factors are commonly cited as barriers to maintaining enjoyable activities.[57]

Referral to a psychologist or counselor trained in narrative therapy can help patients make sense of their experiences along with encouraging re-engagement in leisure activities, if possible for the patient. This approach enables them to reframe their personal story, emphasizing the strengths they've demonstrated during past challenges and identifying hopeful or positive aspects of their situation. By reshaping their narrative, patients may regain a sense of agency and control, which can be especially valuable in addressing feelings of lost enjoyment or purpose in life.[58]

Existential suffering in lipedema

Existential suffering involves distress related to questions of meaning, identity, and purpose. While not widely studied in lipedema, it has been observed in similar contexts, such as chronic pain[59, 60] where patients often grieve the loss of their envisioned future or struggle with self-identity after diagnosis. Lipedema, like many chronic illnesses, brings uncertainty about symptoms and progression, which can undermine a patient's confidence in their future or previously held goals.

Patients may also experience a disrupted sense of self. For example, someone who identifies as energetic and career-driven may feel their identity is challenged if lipedema symptoms or daily care demands limit their ability to work or stay active. Some may experience deeper distress, questioning the meaning of life while coping with a chronic disease. In these cases, patients may express that their life feels defined by managing lipedema rather than by a broader sense of purpose.

If a patient is grappling with existential concerns and belongs to a spiritual or religious community, they may benefit from discussing these topics with a trusted spiritual leader, provided they feel comfortable doing so. If the patient is not part of a spiritual or religious community, referral to a therapist can be given instead to discuss sense of purpose and meaning from a practical or personal view. Spiritual leaders can offer guidance that aligns with the patient's beliefs and values, helping them find meaning and direction within their faith. Spiritual counseling may also provide a broader perspective and foster a sense of connection to something larger than themselves.

Support and purpose through community

Patients who wish to discuss their experiences with others may benefit from joining a support group, especially one focused on lipedema. Connecting with others who share the same condition in a supportive community, whether online or in person, can encourage practical insights and examples of individuals who have found ways to thrive while managing the disease. Resources for support groups are listed in Chapter 19.

Many lipedema support communities also focus on raising awareness and advocating for change. While participation varies, these activities may be especially meaningful for patients seeking a sense of purpose. By identifying advocacy goals that resonate with them, patients can regain a sense of agency and connection. Engaging in these efforts may help them find renewed purpose and empowerment as they contribute to broader change.

Additional considerations in the holistic approach

As you can see, the holistic approach focuses on a whole person in a multi-faceted manner. This chapter introduces core concepts to this process, but the holistic approach can cover areas beyond what was discussed here. Some examples, in brief, are presented here.

The role of co-morbidities in lipedema care

Addressing co-morbidities is an important part of holistic lipedema management, as they can affect both symptoms and overall well-being. For example, hypothyroidism, present in up to a third of patients with lipedema, may hinder weight loss efforts. Treating it can also improve overall health and energy levels. Another common comorbidity is lymphedema. While it shares treatment approaches with lipedema, its presence increases the risk of skin infections and requires added attention to skincare. In such cases, co-morbidities may guide treatment priorities, even if they don't directly alter lipedema goals. These examples illustrate how managing co-morbidities can support wellness, influence symptom management, and help shape individualized care strategies.

Addressing co-morbidities can be considered part of a holistic approach to lipedema management, as some co-morbidities can impact lipedema symptoms or interfere with the patient's overall well-being and health. The reader is referred to Chapter 9 for a more in-depth discussion of common co-morbidities seen with lipedema.

The role of monitoring in lipedema holistic care

In certain situations, additional monitoring may be beneficial to track the impact of specific interventions or life events on lipedema symptoms. This proactive approach enables timely adjustments to care if symptoms worsen and helps identify when more conservative treatments might be beneficial. Monitoring is especially useful when a potential exacerbation is suspected, but its exact effect is unclear. A typical example involves hormonal changes, which some patients report as triggering or worsening symptoms, such as during puberty, pregnancy, perimenopause, or while using hormonal contraception.[4,30] This raises the possibility of other hormonal interventions being a possible trigger for lipedema symptoms, such as when undergoing infertility treatments or hormone replacement therapy. However, this has yet to be studied.

Since the relationship between hormones and lipedema is still not fully understood, close observation during these interventions can provide valuable insight. For example, if symptoms worsen during hormonal therapy, adjustments can be considered. Discussing potential effects in advance also helps patients feel more prepared and less stressed by unexpected changes.

Without awareness of these possible connections, patients may view symptom changes as random and uncontrollable. Monitoring helps bring clarity and empowers patients to understand, manage, and potentially prevent future flare-ups.

Monitoring can be done by the clinician or independently by the patient. This may include brief symptom check-ins, pain or mobility surveys, symptom journals, or verbal updates during appointments. Regular tracking helps validate the patient's experience and supports a more informed, responsive approach to care. Monitoring for significant events or changes is suggested in Table 15.4.

Table 15.4: Suggested monitoring for significant events or changes for a patient with lipedema.

Event or change	Potential impact	Monitoring strategy
Hormonal changes (e.g. menopause)	Symptom flare-ups	Symptom journal, regular check- ins
Dietary shift (e.g. ketogenic diet)	Improved symptoms or risks	Diet log, weight/ pain tracking
Starting therapy or medication	Mood or symptoms shifts	Mental health surveys, verbal updates
Surgery	Improved function, Healing challenges	Follow-up appointments, patient-reported outcomes
Increased isolation	Mental health decline	Social engagement checklists, support group referrals

Conclusion

Lipedema affects multiple aspects of a patient's life, often encompassing all five domains discussed in this chapter. A holistic, patient-centered approach allows clinicians to identify and address these challenges more effectively, supporting the patient as a whole rather than focusing solely on the disease. (The reader is reminded to see elsewhere in this book, for a more detailed look at each domain.) As we have demonstrated, progress in one domain can alleviate challenges in another. Patients may also benefit from shifting focus between domains over time, such as first addressing their relationship with food before implementing a structured nutrition plan. This flexibility is central to holistic care. Empowering patients to lead their care decisions fosters agency and supports long-term engagement. It also helps rebuild trust, especially important for those who have experienced dismissive or invalidating encounters with healthcare providers in the past. Ultimately, holistic care aims to support each patient's unique journey toward wellness. By respecting their pace, priorities, and evolving needs, clinicians can help patients with lipedema find the path that works best for them.

References

1. Kuipers SJ, Cramm JM, Nieboer AP. The importance of patient-centered care and co-creation of care for satisfaction with care and physical and social well-being of patients with multi-morbidity in the primary care setting. *BMC Health Serv Res.* 2019 Jan 8;19(1):13. DOI: https://doi.org/10.1186/s12913-018-3818-y
2. Zamanzadeh V, Jasemi M, Valizadeh L, Keogh B, Taleghani F. Effective factors in providing holistic care: a qualitative study. *Indian J Palliat Care.* 2015;21(2):214–24. DOI: https://doi.org/10.4103/0973-1075.156506
3. Alosaimi K, Mortada H, Alshomer F. Characteristics and clinical features of patients with lipedema in saudi arabia: a cross-sectional comprehensive assessment. *Plast Reconstr Surg – Glob Open.* 2024 Sep;12(9):e6173. DOI: https://doi.org/10.1097/GOX.0000000000006173
4. Patton L, Ricolfi L, Bortolon M, Gabriele G, Zolesio P, Cione E, et al. Observational study on a large Italian population with lipedema: biochemical and hormonal profile, anatomical and clinical evaluation, self-reported history. *Int J Mol Sci.* 2024 Jan;25(3):1599. DOI: https://doi.org/10.3390/ijms25031599
5. Aday AW, Donahue PM, Garza M, Crain VN, Patel NJ, Beasley JA, et al. National survey of patient symptoms and therapies among 707 women with a lipedema phenotype in the United States. *Vasc Med.* 2024 Feb 1;29(1):36–41. DOI: https://doi.org/10.1177/1358863X231202769
6. Melander C, Juuso, Päivi, and Olsson M. Women's experiences of living with lipedema. *Health Care Women Int.* 2022 Mar 4;43(1–3):54–69. DOI: https://doi.org/10.1080/07399332.2021.1932894
7. Forner-Cordero I, Szolnoky G, Forner-Cordero A, Kemény L. Lipedema: an overview of its clinical manifestations, diagnosis and treatment of the disproportional fatty deposition syndrome – systematic review. *Clin Obes.* 2012;2(3–4):86–95. DOI: https://doi.org/10.1111/j.1758-8111.2012.00045.x
8. Aksoy H, Karadag AS, Wollina U. Cause and management of lipedema-associated pain. *Dermatol Ther.* 2021 Jan;34(1):e14364. DOI: https://doi.org/10.1111/dth.14364
9. Bauer AT, von Lukowicz D, Lossagk K, Aitzetmueller M, Moog P, Cerny M, et al. New insights on lipedema: the enigmatic disease of the peripheral fat. *Plast Reconstr Surg.* 2019 Dec;144(6):1475–84. DOI: https://doi.org/10.1097/PRS.0000000000006280
10. Chakraborty A, Crescenzi R, Usman TA, Reyna AJ, Garza ME, Al-Ghadban S, et al. Indications of peripheral pain, dermal hypersensitivity, and neurogenic inflammation in patients with lipedema. *Int J Mol Sci.* 2022 Jan;23(18):10313. DOI: https://doi.org/10.3390/ijms231810313
11. Aitzetmüller-Klietz ML, Busch L, Hamatschek M, Paul M, Schriek C, Wiebringhaus P, et al. Understanding the vicious circle of pain, physical activity, and mental health in lipedema patients – a response surface analysis. *J Clin Med.* 2023 Jan;12(16):5319. DOI: https://doi.org/10.3390/jcm12165319
12. Alwardat N, Di Renzo L, Alwardat M, Romano L, De Santis GL, Gualtieri P, et al. The effect of lipedema on health-related quality of life and psychological status: a narrative review of the literature. *Eat Weight Disord EWD.* 2020 Aug;25(4):851–6. DOI: https://doi.org/10.1007/s40519-019-00703-x
13. Herbst KL, Kahn LA, Iker E, Ehrlich C, Wright T, McHutchison L, et al. Standard of care for lipedema in the United States. *Phlebology.* 2021 Dec 1;36(10):779–96. DOI: https://doi.org/10.1177/02683555211015887
14. Cannataro R, Michelini S, Ricolfi L, Caroleo MC, Gallelli L, De Sarro G, et al. Management of lipedema with ketogenic diet: 22-month follow-up. *Life.* 2021 Dec;11(12):1402. DOI: https://doi.org/10.3390/life11121402
15. Lundanes J, Sandnes F, Gjeilo KH, Hansson P, Salater S, Martins C, et al. Effect of a low-carbohydrate diet on pain and quality of life in female patients with lipedema: a randomized controlled trial. *Obesity.* 2024;32(6):1071–82. DOI: https://doi.org/10.1002/oby.24026
16. Forner-Cordero I, Perez-Pomares MV, Forner A, Ponce-Garrido AB, Munoz-Langa J. Prevalence of clinical manifestations and orthopedic alterations in patients with lipedema: a prospective cohort study. *Lymphology.* 2021;54(4):170–81.

DOI: https://doi.org/https://doi.org/10.2458/lymph.4838

17. Chachaj A, Jeziorek M, Dudka I, Sowicz M, Adaszyńska A, Truszyński A, et al. Disability and emotional symptoms in women with lipedema: a comparison with overweight/obese women. *Adv Clin Exp Med*. 2024;33(12):1367–77. DOI: https://doi.org/10.17219/acem/181146
18. Granger L, Bolam SM, Sur A, Mitchell P, Hutt J, Sandiford NA. Five-year results after total knee arthroplasty in lymphoedema and lipoedema: encouraging functional and clinical outcomes and low rates of infection. *Int Orthop*. 2022 Dec;46(12):2815–20. DOI: https://doi.org/10.1007/s00264-022-05575-y
19. Wright T, Babula M, Schwartz J, Wright C, Danesh N, Herbst K. Lipedema reduction surgery improves pain, mobility, physical function, and quality of life: case series report. *Plast Reconstr Surg – Glob Open*. 2023 Nov;11(11):e5436. DOI: https://doi.org/10.1097/GOX.0000000000005436
20. Spreckley M, Seidell J, Halberstadt J. Perspectives into the experience of successful, substantial long-term weight-loss maintenance: a systematic review. *Int J Qual Stud Health Well-Being*. 16(1):1862481. DOI: https://doi.org/10.1080/17482631.2020.1862481
21. Clarke C, Kirby JN, Smidt T, Best T. Stages of lipoedema: experiences of physical and mental health and health care. *Qual Life Res*. 2023 Jan 1;32(1):127–37. DOI: https://doi.org/10.1007/s11136-022-03216-w
22. Al-Wardat M, Clarke C, Alwardat N, Kassab M, Salimei C, Gualtieri P, et al. The difficulties in emotional regulation among a cohort of females with lipedema. *Int J Environ Res Public Health*. 2022 Oct 21;19(20):13679. DOI: https://doi.org/10.3390/ijerph192013679
23. Conversano C. Common psychological factors in chronic diseases. *Front Psychol* . 2019 Dec 6;10. Available from: https://www.frontiersin.org/journals/psychology/articles/10.3389/fpsyg.2019.02727/full
24. Fetzer A. Women in dire need: the far-reaching impact of lipoedema on women's lives. *Br J Community Nurs*. 2020 Apr 1;25(Sup4):S6–9. DOI: https://doi.org/10.12968/bjcn.2020.25.Sup4.S6
25. Dahlberg J, Nylander ,Elisabet, Persson ,Margareta, and Shayesteh A. An uncertain uphill battle – experiences and consequences of living with lipedema. *Int J Qual Stud Health Well-Being*. 2024 Dec 31;19(1):2300152. DOI: https://doi.org/10.1080/17482631.2023.2300152
26. J. Katon Wayne. Epidemiology and treatment of depression in patients with chronic medical illness. *Dialogues Clin Neurosci*. 2011 Mar 31;13(1):7–23. DOI: https://doi.org/10.31887/DCNS.2011.13.1/wkaton
27. Barlattani T, Grandinetti P, Cintio AD, Montemagno A, Testa R, D'Amelio C, et al. Glymphatic system and psychiatric disorders: a rapid comprehensive scoping review. *Curr Neuropharmacol*. 2024 Oct 1;22(12):2016–33. DOI: https://doi.org/10.2174/1570159X22666240130091235
28. Gu S, Li Y, Jiang Y, Huang JH, Wang F. Glymphatic dysfunction induced oxidative stress and neuro-inflammation in major depression disorders. *Antioxidants*. 2022 Nov;11(11):2296. DOI: https://doi.org/10.3390/antiox11112296
29. Kempa S, Gross M, Oliinyk D, Siegmund A, Müller M, Prantl L, et al. Health implications of lipedema: analysis of patient questionnaires and population-based matched controls. *Life*. 2024 Mar;14(3):295. DOI: https://doi.org/10.3390/life14030295
30. Ghods M, Georgiou I, Schmidt J, Kruppa P. Disease progression and comorbidities in lipedema patients: a 10-year retrospective analysis. *Dermatol Ther*. 2020;33(6):e14534. DOI: https://doi.org/10.1111/dth.14534
31. Dudek JE, Białaszek W, Ostaszewski P, Smidt T. Depression and appearance-related distress in functioning with lipedema. *Psychol Health Med*. 2018 Aug 9;23(7):846–53. DOI: https://doi.org/10.1080/13548506.2018.1459750
32. Amato ACM, Amato FCM, Amato JLS, Benitti DA. Lipedema prevalence and risk factors in Brazil. *J Vasc Bras*. 2022 May 23;21:e20210198. DOI: https://doi.org/https://doi.org/10.1590/1677-5449.202101982
33. Lebel S, Mutsaers B, Tomei C, Leclair CS, Jones G, Petricone-Westwood D, et al. Health anxiety and illness-related fears across diverse chronic illnesses: a systematic review on conceptualization, measurement, prevalence, course, and correlates.

PloS ONE. 2020 Jul 27;15(7):e0234124. DOI: https://doi.org/10.1371/journal.pone.0234124

34. Sherbourne CD, Wells KB, Meredith LS, Jackson CA, Camp P. Comorbid anxiety disorder and the functioning and well-being of chronically ill patients of general medical providers. *Arch Gen Psychiatry*. 1996 Oct 1;53(10):889–95. DOI: https://doi.org/10.1001/archpsyc.1996.01830100035005
35. Petricone-Westwood D, Jones G, Mutsaers B, Leclair CS, Tomei C, Trudel G, et al. A systematic review of interventions for health anxiety presentations across diverse chronic illnesses. *Int J Behav Med*. 2019 Feb 1;26(1):3–16. DOI: https://doi.org/10.1007/s12529-018-9748-6
36. Cooper K, Gregory JD, Walker I, Lambe S, Salkovskis PM. Cognitive behaviour therapy for health anxiety: a systematic review and meta-analysis. *Behav Cogn Psychother*. 2017 Mar;45(2):110–23. DOI: https://doi.org/10.1017/S1352465816000527
37. Fetzer A, Fetzer, Sharie. *Lipoedema UK Big Survey 2014 Research Report*. Lipoedema UK; 2016 Jul p. 1–8. Available from: https://lipoedema.co.uk/wp-content/uploads/2024/05/LATEST-LUK000-UK-Big-Survey16-Mar24-web.pdf
38. Christoffersen V, Tennfjord MK. Younger women with lipedema, their experiences with healthcare providers, and the importance of social support and belonging: a qualitative study. *Int J Environ Res Public Health*. 2023 Jan;20(3):1925. DOI: https://doi.org/10.3390/ijerph20031925
39. McLoughlin DM, Spargo E, Wassif WS, Newham DJ, Peters TJ, Lantos PL, et al. Structural and functional changes in skeletal muscle in anorexia nervosa. *Acta Neuropathol (Berl)*. 1998 May 1;95(6):632–540. DOI: https://doi.org/10.1007/s004010050850
40. McLoughlin DM, Wassif WS, Morton J, Spargo E, Peters TJ, Russell GFM. Metabolic abnormalities associated with skeletal myopathy in severe anorexia nervosa. *Nutrition*. 2000 Mar 1;16(3):192–6. DOI: https://doi.org/10.1016/S0899-9007(99)00286-5
41. Mehler PS, Brown C. Anorexia nervosa – medical complications. *J Eat Disord*. 2015 Mar 31;3(1):11. DOI: https://doi.org/10.1186/s40337-015-0040-8
42. Wassenaar E, Friedman J, Mehler PS. Medical complications of binge eating disorder. *Psychiatr Clin North Am*. 2019 Jun;42(2):275–86. DOI: https://doi.org/10.1016/j.psc.2019.01.010
43. Russell H, Aouad P, Le A, Marks P, Maloney D, Aouad P, et al. Psychotherapies for eating disorders: findings from a rapid review. *J Eat Disord*. 2023 Oct 4;11(1):175. DOI: https://doi.org/10.1186/s40337-023-00886-w
44. Rostanzo E, Marchetti M, Casini I, Aloisi AM. Very-low-calorie ketogenic diet: a potential treatment for binge eating and food addiction symptoms in women. a pilot study. *Int J Environ Res Public Health*. 2021 Jan;18(23):12802. DOI: https://doi.org/10.3390/ijerph182312802
45. Calabrese L, Scolnick B, Zupec-Kania B, Beckwith C, Costello K, Frank GKW. Ketogenic diet and ketamine infusion treatment to target chronic persistent eating disorder psychopathology in anorexia nervosa: a pilot study. *Eat Weight Disord – Stud Anorex Bulim Obes*. 2022 Dec 1;27(8):3751–7. DOI: https://doi.org/10.1007/s40519-022-01455-x
46. Norwitz NG, Hurn M, Forcen FE. Animal-based ketogenic diet puts severe anorexia nervosa into multi-year remission: a case series. J Metab Health. 2023 Jun 14;6(1):8. DOI: https://doi.org/10.4102/jir.v6i1.84
47. Frank GKW, Scolnick B. Therapeutic ketogenic diet as treatment for anorexia nervosa. *Front Nutr* . 2024 Sep 4;11. Available from: https://www.frontiersin.org/journals/nutrition/articles/10.3389/fnut.2024.1392135/full
48. Carmen M, Safer DL, Saslow LR, Kalayjian T, Mason AE, Westman EC, et al. Treating binge eating and food addiction symptoms with low-carbohydrate ketogenic diets: a case series. *J Eat Disord*. 2020 Jan 29;8(1):2. DOI: https://doi.org/10.1186/s40337-020-0278-7
49. Watson K, Nasca C, Aasly L, McEwen B, Rasgon N. Insulin resistance, an unmasked culprit in depressive disorders: Promises for interventions. *Neuropharmacology*. 2018 Jul 1;136:327–34. DOI: https://doi.org/10.1016/j.neuropharm.2017.11.038
50. Laurent N, Bellamy EL, Hristova D, Houston A. Ketogenic diets in clinical psychology: examining the evidence and implications for practice. *Front Psychol* . 2024 Sep 26;15. Available from:

https://www.frontiersin.org/journals/psychology/articles/10.3389/fpsyg.2024.1468894/full
51. Danan A, Westman EC, Saslow LR, Ede G. The ketogenic diet for refractory mental illness: a retrospective analysis of 31 inpatients. *Front Psychiatry* . 2022 Jul 6;13. Available from: https://www.frontiersin.org/journals/psychiatry/articles/10.3389/fpsyt.2022.951376/full
52. Grey M, Knafl K, McCorkle R. A framework for the study of self- and family management of chronic conditions. *Nurs Outlook*. 2006 Sep 1;54(5):278–86. DOI: https://doi.org/10.1016/j.outlook.2006.06.004
53. Rosland AM, Piette JD. Emerging models for mobilizing family support for chronic disease management: a structured review. *Chronic Illn*. 2010 Mar 1;6(1):7–21. DOI: https://doi.org/10.1177/1742395309352254
54. Holt-Lunstad J, Steptoe A. Social isolation: An underappreciated determinant of physical health. *Curr Opin Psychol*. 2022 Feb 1;43:232–7. DOI: https://doi.org/10.1016/j.copsyc.2021.07.012
55. Lammer L, Beyer F, Luppa M, Sanders C, Baber R, Engel C, et al. Impact of social isolation on grey matter structure and cognitive functions: a population-based longitudinal neuroimaging study. Zhou H, Roiser J, editors. *eLife*. 2023 Jun 20;12:e83660. DOI: https://doi.org/10.7554/eLife.83660
56. Karayannis NV, Baumann I, Sturgeon JA, Melloh M, Mackey SC. The impact of social isolation on pain interference: a longitudinal study. *Ann Behav Med*. 2019 Jan 1;53(1):65–74. DOI: https://doi.org/10.1093/abm/kay017
57. Snelgrove R, Wood, Laura, and Carr K. Emerging adults with chronic illness pursuing and enhancing leisure. *Leis Sci*. 2016 Jan 1;38(1):34–49. DOI: https://doi.org/10.1080/01490400.2015.1057660
58. Etchison M, Kleist DM. Review of narrative therapy: research and utility. *Fam J*. 2000 Jan 1;8(1):61–6. DOI: https://doi.org/10.1177/1066480700081009
59. Lundberg M, Styf J. Experiences of moving with persistent pain –a qualitative study from a patient perspective. *Physiother Theory Pract*. 2007 Jan 1;23(4):199–209. DOI: https://doi.org/10.1080/09593980701209311
60. Kieselbach K, Koesling D, Wabel T, Frede U, Bozzaro C. [Chronic pain as an existential challenge]. *Schmerz Berl Ger*. 2023 Apr;37(2):116–22. DOI: https://doi.org/10.1007/s00482-022-00632-2

VI
Surgical options for lipedema

Chapter Sixteen
Surgical treatment pathways for lipedema

Ramin Shayan and Tara Karnezis

Introduction

Lipedema is a chronic disease characterized by the abnormal and disproportionate accumulation of adipose tissue primarily in the lower extremities, but also in the arms and potentially the truncal areas.[1, 2, 3] Affecting millions of predominantly women worldwide, lipedema is often misdiagnosed or overlooked, and can lead to significant physical and emotional distress.[4] Symptomatically, lipedema can cause tenderness, pain, heaviness, and even mobility issues, which can secondarily contribute to the development of obesity.[2, 5] Obesity, one of the scourges of modern health, can, in turn, lead to further generalized health problems, such as osteoarthritis, diabetes, and cardiovascular and metabolic disease.[6]

Lipedema can lead not only to functional impairment but also to severe psychological challenges due to body image issues and social stigma.[7] Many patients recount years of frustration stemming from misdiagnoses, ineffective treatments, and a lack of understanding from healthcare providers.[8] Patients with lipedema may be repeatedly told that their disease is simply a result of being overweight, and has a profound emotional toll, often leading to a sense of isolation and hopelessness.[1, 2] A lifetime of 'fat-shaming,' misdiagnosis, and discrimination often leaves patients with lipedema feeling desperate for someone who will listen, understand, and treat them with respect, as well as offer care that leads to real, lasting improvements in both the form and function of their bodies.[8, 9] Unlike typical obesity, however, lipedema itself is resistant to diet and exercise, often causing significant emotional distress and body image issues among those affected.[5, 10] When patients with lipedema achieve weight loss, the lipedematous areas of the body often display refractory tendencies and typically remain only partially reduced in volume.

The exact cause of lipedema is still unknown,[11, 12] but hormonal factors, genetic predisposition, and connective tissue diseases have all been implicated.[13, 14, 15] As practitioners and researchers continue to unravel the complexities of lipedema, a clearer understanding of its nature, progression, and potential treatments is emerging.[11, 16, 17] As awareness of lipedema grows, there has been an increased focus on developing effective treatment strategies, specifically surgical options.[18] In the meantime, treatment for lipedema has mirrored the poor understanding of the disease itself. In years past, generic liposuction-based debulking was performed by non-dedicated practitioners, who were isolated from both an understanding of the disease biology and the requisite multi-disciplinary teams with nuanced and specialized knowledge of the disease.

As knowledge of lipedema biology expands,[19] it is critical to explore the surgical treatment pathways for lipedema, focusing on the experiences of patients, the disease biology, and the interplay of the related disease entities as a vicious cycle (see Figure 16.1), and the evolving landscape of both non-surgical and surgical approaches.[3, 20] The key diseases related to the lipedema journey include adipose accumulation and obesity, lymphatic dysregulation and lymphedema, connective tissue and joint disease. Through enhanced understanding gained from research, we can glean insights into the multifaceted nature of lipedema and its optimal surgical management, and most importantly, when not to treat surgically, and how to be a holistic thinker and doctor.

Regardless of stage and severity, lipedema requires a multifaceted approach to patient care. Similarly, never before has attention to ongoing advocacy and research in lipedema been of more importance in raising funds and awareness to facilitate further research and clinical understanding. The understandable frustration experienced by patients with lipedema can make them vulnerable to incomplete or unsatisfactory treatments that fail to deliver the benefits they hope for, either in terms of body shape or physical function.[10]

Ultimately, to effectively help patients who have suffered in silence – or worse, have been poorly managed – we must stratify them based on their specific disease manifestations, functional impairments, genetic or acquired co-morbidities, and surgical fitness. This requires assigning treatment pathways that consider which patients need adjunct preparatory interventions, all within the framework of a cohesive, multidisciplinary care team. This chapter outlines the foundation of the authors' system, which places strong emphasis on individual biology and genetic predisposition. The goal is to ensure that patients are well-informed, supported, and empowered to make meaningful decisions about their health.

The need for surgical treatment pathways

The first detailed description of lipedema was published in 1940,[21] but it was only in recent years that the medical community began to recognize its distinct pathology.[5, 13] Physiologically, lipedema has been thought to involve dysregulation of adipose tissue and the lymphatic system. More recently, we have begun to learn that lipedema is driven by dysregulated adipose tissue pathways.[11, 14, 15]

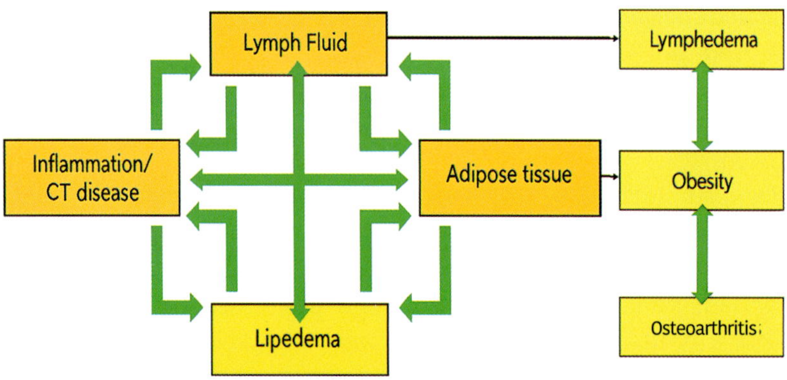

Figure 16.1: The vicious cycle of lipedema. Illustration by authors.

Lipedema is not merely a cosmetic concern; it is a complex disease characterized by an abnormal distribution of fat that does not respond to diet or exercise.[10] It typically presents as a progressive disease that often begins during hormonal changes, such as puberty, pregnancy, or menopause.[16] Patients often report symptoms such as pain, tenderness, and a sense of heaviness in the affected limbs.[7] The psychological impact of lipedema can also be profound, as individuals may find themselves grappling with decreased mobility, social isolation, and low self-esteem due to their body image. Lipedema is, therefore, a multifaceted disease characterized by variable presentations and requires a holistic approach to treatment (see Table 16.1).

Many patients have spent years in frustration, seeking answers and often receiving inadequate care. Patient testimonies are plagued with anecdotes describing dismissive consultations, where symptoms are attributed solely to being overweight rather than addressing the underlying cause of lipedema. As a consequence of confusion among both patients and health professionals regarding lipedema, patients have often attended practitioners with inadequate training, understanding, and facilities to properly diagnose, assess, or treat patients with lipedema. The profound sense of desperation that some patients feel can leave them vulnerable to exploitation by clinicians offering unproven or inappropriate interventions. In some cases, ill-advised surgeries have caused significant harm, harm that is not only costly and more difficult to treat but that may also permanently limit the possibility of achieving optimal outcomes due to damaged or scarred tissue.

Table 16.1: Lipedema treatment and research are motivated by both form and function.

Why do we treat/research lipedema?	
Form	Stigmatization and social acceptance 'Fat shaming' through ignorance Self-esteem (becoming your 'best self') Clothing/activity limitations (avoid limb exposure) Aesthetic concerns
Function	Mobility Pain ECM/connective tissue disease Easy bruising Emotional/psychological distress, depression Multiple lipomata syndrome Lymphedema

ECM = extracellular matrix.

This narrative underscores the importance of raising awareness among healthcare providers and the general public about this often-overlooked disease. Given the chronic nature of lipedema and its resistance to conventional weight loss methods, and an increasing desire for quick-fix solutions across all fields of medicine, surgical intervention has become a focal point of treatment strategies. It is important to remember the most critical surgical pathway, which is identifying patients for whom surgery is not appropriate.

A patho-morpho-metric pathway to holistic care

The authors have developed an algorithmic approach to assessing lipedema, aimed at guiding appropriate management, prioritizing clinical concerns, and identifying suitable candidates for a range of complementary surgical and non-surgical interventions (see Figure 16.2).

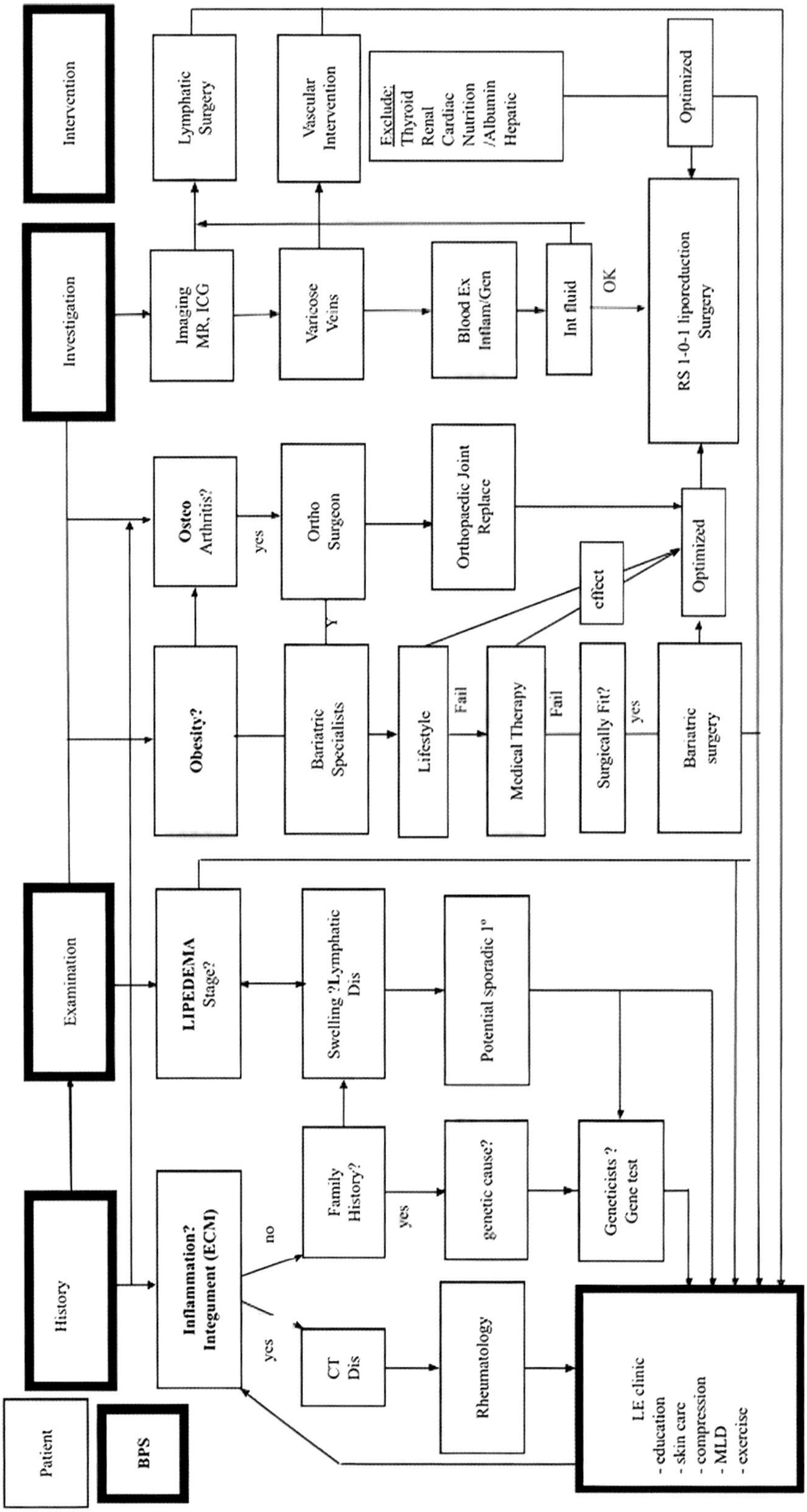

Figure 16.2: The patho-morpho-metric model for assessment and management of patients with lipedema.

Table 16.2 lists the key components in the 'BIOLOGIE' model, a patho-morpho-metric pathway to holistic lipedema care. Each of these components will be discussed in detail. As with all areas of medicine, this process relies on a thorough patient history, a focused physical examination, appropriate diagnostic investigations, and collaboration within a multidisciplinary team. Crucially, all decisions should be guided by a treatment plan tailored to the individual patient and the specific stage of their disease.

Surgical interventions alone cannot provide truly holistic care;[18] effectively meeting the needs of patients with lipedema requires the integrated expertise of a multidisciplinary healthcare team.[22] One of the key strengths of this collaborative approach is its ability to optimize surgical outcomes and improve patient selection for surgery by addressing the complex, multifactorial nature of the disease.

Table 16.2: The 'BIOLOGIE' model: a patho-morpho-metric pathway to holistic lipedema care.

BIOLOGIE model	
B	io-psycho-social
I	nflammation/integument (ECM)
O	besity
L	ymphatic dysfunction
O	steoarthritis
G	enetics/general medical concerns
I	ntervention/surgery
E	valuation (both short and long term)

One key concept in the treatment of lipedema, therefore, is the acknowledgment that 'it takes a village' to prepare a patient for surgery – the importance of a multidisciplinary approach when designing lipedema management pathways cannot be overstated. The complexity of the disease necessitates collaboration between the patient and their surgeons, physicians, dietitians, physiotherapists, psychologists, and patient support groups.[22] Surgeons play a critical role, but pre- and post-operative support from other healthcare professionals is integral to significantly enhance patient outcomes .[22, 23] For instance, dietitians can provide valuable nutritional advice tailored to help patients maintain their weight and overall health post-surgery. Physiotherapists can offer rehabilitation strategies to aid recovery and prevent complications.[4]

Additionally, the psychological support provided by mental health professionals throughout the patient journey is critical. Many patients grapple with body image issues stemming from lipedema, and addressing these concerns can lead to a more holistic treatment experience.[10] This interplay of multiple organ systems necessitates integrative care models that emphasize collaboration and communication across specialties.[4, 8] Furthermore, a more established baseline relationship with one's body image facilitates a more mature adaptation to the new body shape when it arises post-operatively.

Bio-psycho-sociological support

An often-overlooked aspect of surgical treatment pathways for lipedema is the need for psychological support.[7] Patients may experience a range of emotions, including anxiety, depression, and body image issues, both before and following surgery. Providing a dedicated support system is crucial for the patient's overall recovery and satisfaction with surgical outcomes.[18] Mental health professionals can offer counseling and cognitive-behavioral therapy to help patients navigate the emotional challenges associated with their disease and its treatment. Psychological counseling can help process feelings of anxiety related to impending surgery and foster a more positive self-image post-operatively.

Reflecting on the broader context surrounding

lipedema, it is evident that advocating for increased awareness and research is paramount. For too long, lipedema has been underreported and often mischaracterized within the healthcare community and the public. Many patients remain unaware of their disease or the available treatment options. Organizations such as Lipoedema Australia, Lipedema Foundation, Lipedema Simplified, Lipoedema UK, and various online advocacy groups have played a crucial role in driving awareness initiatives (See Chapter 19 for more information). These groups provide valuable educational resources, support networks, and platforms for sharing personal stories. Advocacy and education, through individual stories of those affected by lipedema, can be powerful catalysts for change. There remains a need for funding for research and training for healthcare providers. This would ensure that lipedema is recognized promptly and treated effectively, ultimately improving the quality of care for individuals affected by this condition.

Inflammation and connective tissue dysfunction in lipedema

Lipedema is increasingly recognized as a disease involving more than abnormal fat accumulation. Chronic inflammation, lymphatic impairment, and connective tissue dysfunction all contribute to its pathophysiology. Pro-inflammatory immune cell activity and cytokine signaling are linked to pain, fibrosis, and vascular changes. At the same time, emerging research suggests a possible overlap with connective tissue diseases such as Ehlers-Danlos syndrome. These factors may underlie both symptom severity and variable response to treatment.

Inflammation

A hallmark symptom of lipedema is disproportionate pain and tenderness in the affected areas of tissue. This discomfort is closely linked to an underlying pro-inflammatory microenvironment. Research has shown that several key inflammatory pathways are upregulated in lipedema tissues, including increased infiltration of CD45- and CD68-positive macrophages, as well as overexpression of VEGFR-3 and the M2 macrophage marker CD163.[4] This inflammatory profile suggests a pro-angiogenic and pro-fibrotic state that may contribute to increased vascular permeability, cellular extravasation, and a self-perpetuating cycle of inflammation. These effects are often intensified during periods of systemic inflammation, partly due to the additional accumulation of lymphatic fluid, which further promotes an inflammatory milieu.[20] Obesity, a common comorbidity, also contributes to chronic inflammation,[24, 25] potentially amplifying nociceptor activation and worsening the characteristic pain of lipedema.

Given this inflammatory context, many patients report symptom relief through anti-inflammatory strategies – whether pharmacological (oral or topical agents) or dietary (anti-inflammatory nutrition). This supports the importance of addressing inflammation as a central component of lipedema management.

Controlling the persistent inflammation commonly observed in newly diagnosed patients with lipedema may help explain why some individuals respond well to non-surgical treatments targeting both lymphedema and obesity. Clinically evident lymphedema can occur alongside lipedema, classifying the disease as advanced or severe stage 3. However, subclinical lymphatic dysfunction may also be present in earlier stages and can be detected through advanced diagnostic tools such as indocyanine green (ICG) lymphography or lymphatic bioimpedance analysis. In a study by Buso et al.,[26] 25 out of 45 patients (56%) demonstrated sluggish lymphatic drainage to the groin on ICG imaging and were recommended for manual lymphatic drainage therapy, despite no visible anatomical abnormalities in their lymphatic vessels. This contrasts with an earlier retrospective study by Mackie et al.,[27] which found that 85% of 40 patients had normal lymphatic function.

Connective tissue and extracellular matrix (ECM)
Ehlers-Danlos syndrome (EDS) is a connective tissue disease characterized by hypermobility, a feature recognized in patients with lipedema.[28] Morgan et. al.[13] described a mutation in two of the genes contained in the Michelini et al.[15] lipedema panel and identified in the Morgan et al. analysis were *STAB1* and tenascin-X (*TNXB*), both of which are closely associated with the ECM, and in line with the overrepresentation of microfibril binding from the GO analysis. TNX is a glycoprotein believed to mediate cell-ECM interaction by binding fibrillary collagen directly, via decorin and cell surface integrin.[29] Classical-like Ehlers-Danlos syndrome type 1, one of the 13 types of EDS,[28, 29] is linked to *TNXB* gene variants. This rare but heterogeneous group of connective tissue diseases has not yet been linked to lipedema; however, this finding, reported across two independent research laboratories, is an exciting association. Nevertheless, further work is needed to validate this finding in downstream expression, ideally in human tissues.

Obesity: nutrition and lifestyle counseling

In addition to psychological care, nutritional and lifestyle counseling play an essential role in the multidimensional treatment of lipedema.[1, 4, 5] While surgery can remove excess fatty tissue, adopting a healthy lifestyle can help maintain results and, in many cases, obviate the need for surgery altogether. As clinicians, we see patients intermittently; the measures that patients themselves can take every day may be disproportionately powerful. Dietitians or nutritionists can work with patients to develop personalized meal plans that emphasize wholefoods while minimizing inflammatory triggers. This approach not only supports weight management but also enhances overall health, an important consideration as many patients with lipedema may struggle with co-morbidities, such as diabetes or cardiovascular issues.

While GLP-1 receptor agonists (GLP-1 RAs) are not specifically approved for lipedema treatment, they are being explored for their potential benefits in managing the disease,[30] particularly concerning weight loss and inflammation. There is limited clinical trial data directly focused on GLP-1 RAs for lipedema, but ongoing research and anecdotal evidence suggest they may help with weight reduction, a common symptom of lipedema. In the author's personal experience, treatment with GLP-1 RAs does achieve excellent weight loss results (Figure 16.3), but even in patients in whom weight loss is not achieved, it enables the reduction of symptoms such as pain, heaviness, inflammatory flares, and tenderness in the legs. GLP-1 RAs have become a critical tool for enabling safe and more efficacious surgery. In some cases, the symptom reduction has been so profound as to obviate the need for surgery altogether. As with all new interventions, however, a trial is needed to separate the effects of the GLP-1 RAs from those of weight reduction alone, as well as the resulting reduction in inflammation and swelling.

Osteoarthritis

Due to the morphology of lipedema, a prolonged altered gait manifests as preferential weight bearing on the medial aspect of the foot, which then leads over time to a typical valgus knee deformity, with lateral pain and medial laxity. In the hips, there is often a Trendelenburg-type gait resulting from a disproportionate overuse of the regular stabilizing muscles of the hips for the legs to effectively 'walk around' one another. Finally, potentially due to the ligamentous laxity and deformity of the knee, patients with lipedema frequently present with arch collapse.

In the authors' experience, it is critical to work closely with an orthopedic colleague who

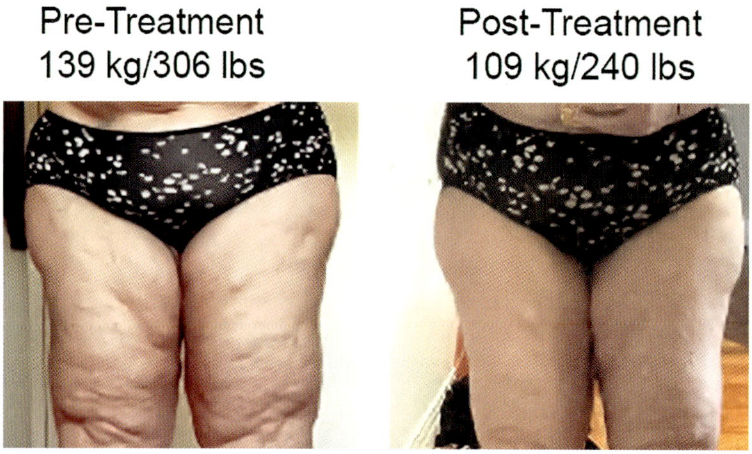

Figure 16.3: Effect on a patient of sustained and supervised use of Ozempic for six months. Before (left) is compared with after Ozempic treatment (right). Photos courtesy of authors.

is familiar with lipedema to enable advanced planning and prioritization of the surgery. In some cases, a significant sub-genicular lipedema tissue deposit, combined with thin skin and lymphedema, may make the access for a total knee replacement unsafe or likely to result in wound breakdown. Mobility is integral to rehabilitation following surgery for lipedema, so it is the authors' practice to treat knees and hips before liposuction. This is particularly true if it is the opinion of the orthopedic colleague that gait is likely to be impaired in the setting of a putative surgical intervention for lipedema. See typical postures of patients with lipedema in Figure 16.4.

Genetics

As outlined in the other chapters of this volume, genetics and gene signaling networks of lipedema are emerging as an exciting new frontier for potential future diagnostics and treatments for lipedema. It is, of course, our collective hope that conversations around surgery for lipedema will one day be redundant. In the meantime, where technology and funding are available, clinicians should take every opportunity to look for hereditary patterns and, when appropriate, offer genetic testing to patients. Every contribution to the collective database is valuable.

General medical health

Maintaining good general medical health is crucial for individuals with lipedema and their co-morbidities. Lipedema can lead to various complications and associated conditions, all of which can both individually form part of a vicious cycle that perpetuates the symptoms of lipedema (Figure 16.1) and also contribute individually to reduced life expectancy and quality of life.

Managing co-morbidities

Consulting with patients about lipedema (see Figure 16.2) also provides an important opportunity to emphasize the importance of managing overall health and strengthening primary health care. This may include managing co-morbidities, discussed further in Chapter 6 in this text, and will have an impact on surgical pathways.

Obesity and metabolic issues

Lipedema can be associated with obesity and metabolic issues like insulin resistance and even diabetes.[8, 31, 32] Together, obesity and diabetes are

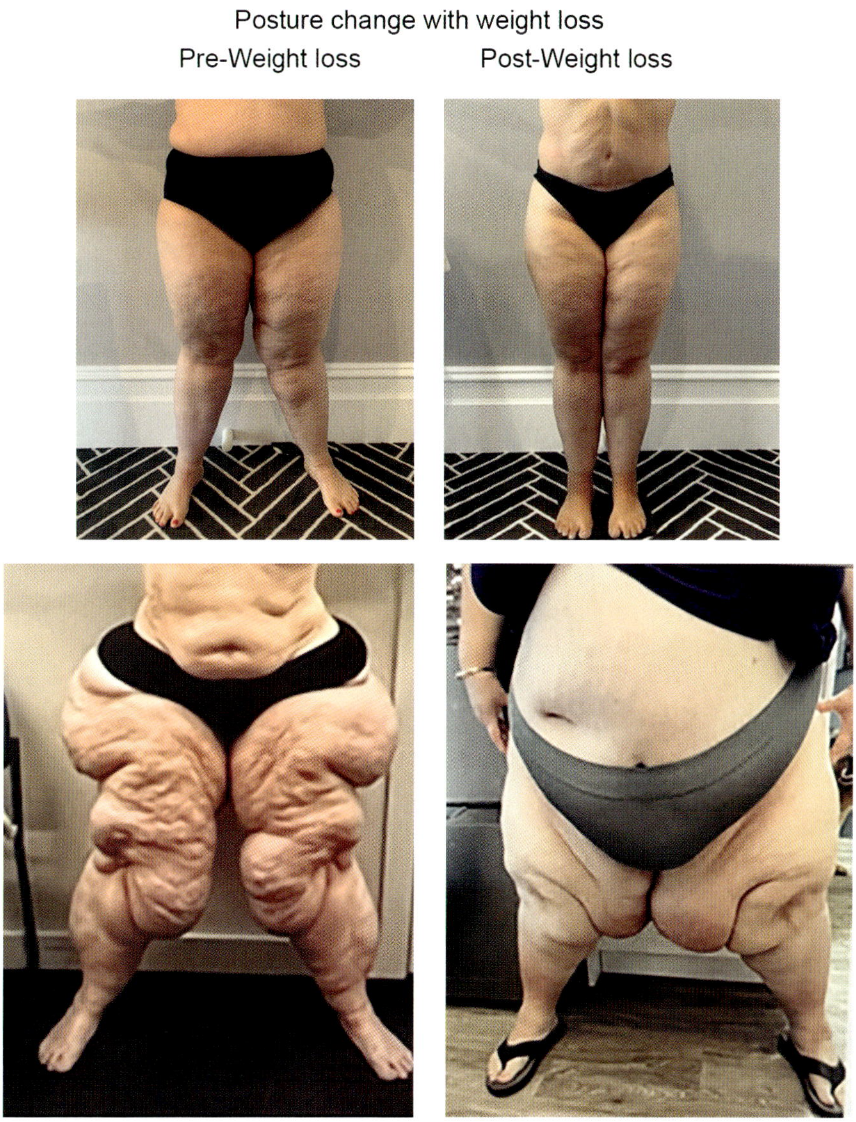

Figure 16.4: Typical posture of lipedema patients (valgus deformity, top left) compared to posture of same patient after weight loss (top right). Posture of other lipedema patients compounded by later stage disease (bottom left), or morbid obesity (bottom right). Photos courtesy of authors used with patient permissions.

two of the major health challenges of modern times. Maintaining a healthy weight and addressing metabolic issues through diet, exercise, and potentially medication (such as metformin) is crucial.[32] In addition, autoimmune diseases are more prevalent in lipedema patient populations,[32] such as atopy, mast cell activation syndrome, and thyroiditis [authors' personal experience]. Finally, the opinion of an endocrinologist, both for thyroid dysregulation and hormonal assessment

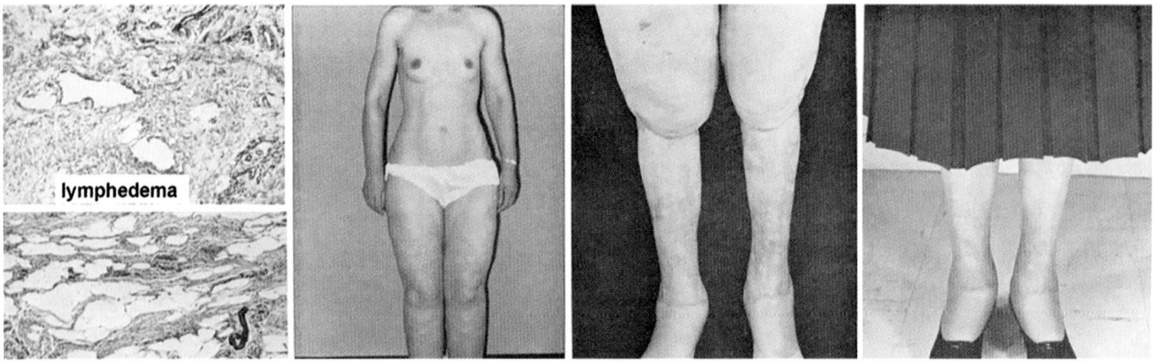

Figure 16.5: 1966 publication by Rank and Wong[33] showing: (A) lymphedema (top left) and lipedema (bottom left) histologic distinctions; (B) pre-operative and (C) and (D) post-operative outcomes in the legs in a patient with lipedema.

can be critical to certain patients,[17] particularly if they have an obvious causal history relating to a period of hormonal change (puberty, pregnancy, IVF, gender reassignment, menopause), or a family history.[19]

Chronic venous disease

Lipedema can be linked to chronic venous disease. Managing venous health through compression stockings, exercise, and other therapies can help alleviate symptoms. However, it is critical to diagnose the exact nature of the venous disease as it may provide clues to any clinical or subclinical lymphatic insufficiency and may also be treated at the time of any skin excision surgery (see below).

Mental health

Individuals with lipedema often experience anxiety and depression due to the disease's impact on body image and physical limitations. Addressing mental health through therapy, support groups, and medication (if needed) is vital, and while beyond the scope of this chapter, a key referral made by the authors is for pre-surgical cases when needed. In Australia, psychological assessment for body dysmorphic disease (BDD) is now mandatory for all patients undergoing cosmetic surgery. The author has found that psychological consultations with patients with lipedema are particularly valuable for identifying pre-operative BDD and for helping manage patient expectations.

Pain and fatigue

Lipedema can cause pain and fatigue, which can be managed through physical therapy, medication, and lifestyle adjustments. A pain specialist is an excellent resource for planning a tailored regimen to facilitate potential future surgery or to reduce pain and promote exercise.

Intervention: overview of surgical pathways

Finally, once all of the above measures are attended to sequentially and diligently, surgery may be considered. Some patients who exhibit multiple complex co-morbidities may take up to two years to prepare for surgery, both physically and mentally. And it is prudent always to remember that the most important surgical pathway is to identify whom NOT to operate on.

History of surgery for lipedema

Comparisons between the limbs of patients with lipedema and those with lymphedema are both natural and understandable. Early surgeons in this field examined the similarities and differences in morphology, histopathology, and treatment approaches for the two diseases. In 1966, Sir Benjamin Rank, Australia's first plastic surgeon, published such a comparison, emphasizing that the primary goals of surgery for most patients are to improve both the form and function of the lower limbs.[33] Rank adapted the Charles procedure, originally developed for lymphedema, for use on the lower limbs of patients with lipedema. To illustrate surgical outcomes, he included a post-operative photograph of a patient wearing shoes and a skirt, a choice that, in the author's view, reflected the patient's priorities and the importance of functional and aesthetic restoration (see Figure 16.5).

Current non-operative treatments for lipedema

Current non-operative treatment options for lipedema include lifestyle modifications such as diet and exercise, manual lymphatic drainage (MLD), complete decongestive therapy (CDT), compression therapy using either tailored or standard garments, and intermittent pneumatic compression (IPC).[5] These interventions have been shown to be safe[22] and may lead to improvements in both the appearance of affected limbs and the severity of pain.[9, 23] However, when symptoms remain inadequately controlled or when patients are dissatisfied with the shape and morphology of their limbs, especially if this affects their function, comfort, or ability to wear certain clothing or footwear, surgical intervention may be a suitable consideration.[33]

Operative management of lipedema

Surgical options for treating lymphedema include tumescent liposuction and, in some cases, lymphatic surgeries.[18] Each pathway presents unique benefits and challenges, making the choice of surgical treatment an individualized process, tailored to the specific challenges faced by each patient.[7] Surgical procedures for lipedema primarily focus on removing the abnormal fat deposits while preserving the surrounding structures, minimizing damage to the lymphatic system, and enhancing the patient's quality of life.[9, 18, 23, 34] Clinicians must consider not only the physical manifestations of the disease but also its psychosocial dimensions to determine the appropriateness, order, and timing of surgeries (see Table 16.2 and Figure 16.2).

Surgical treatment may be appropriate for patients in whom non-operative therapies have failed to alleviate symptoms,[23] for those seeking to improve the shape and function of their limbs, or for individuals who require a more intensive intervention to restore or enhance mobility.[22] The goal of surgery in these cases is often to address the disfiguring effects of lipedema and to support improved functional movement. Even in cases where conservative therapy has not yet failed,[18] there is growing interest in liposuction-based surgical options. This trend has been driven in part by increased investment from device manufacturers, which has expanded the availability and variety of surgical tools, as well as by advocacy groups whose efforts have raised awareness about lipedema and its treatment options.

Most of the surgical methods in use today stem from tumescent liposuction (see below). Variations described include micro-cannular tumescence anesthesia,[35, 36, 37] water jet-assisted liposuction (WAL),[34] and power/vibration-assisted liposuction (PAL).[22] Reports suggest that all of these techniques may be successful in terms of acute and long-term outcomes,[38] and current techniques are based largely on physician preference. Several studies proposed a positive effect on quality of life, pain levels, professional performance, and personal daily life.[1, 6, 35, 37, 38]

Tumescent liposuction

The most common and effective surgical approach for lipedema is tumescent liposuction, whether using power-assisted liposuction (PAL),[18] unassisted liposuction, or water-assisted liposuction (WAL) [3, 34] The tumescent liposuction technique involves injecting a large volume of saline mixed with adrenaline and anesthetic into the affected areas to treat the adipose tissue.[39, 40, 41] The solution causes the fatty tissue to swell, resulting in decreased bleeding and post-operative pain, thus creating a safer and more comfortable procedure for patients.[42] The tumescent fluid creates a swollen, firm state in the fat layer, making the fat cells easier to suction away during the surgery.[42]

Liposuction has undergone an evolution over the years. Schrudde pioneered a fat-removal technique that adapted a sharp uterine curette in 1972,[40] while Illouz described a blunt version that incorporated the suction technique in 1977, to remove a discrete lipomatous lesion with minimal scarring.[43] Blunt subcutaneous tunneling rather than sharp dissection limited local tissue injury to important structures such as nerves, veins, and lymphatic vessels.[43] The concept of a 'wet' technique of liposuction stemmed from Illouz evolving his previous method, and in 1983, reported a series of over 3,000 cases that utilized hypotonic hyaluronidase solution pre-injection to 'emulsify' adipose tissues to facilitate aspiration via suctioning.[41]

In contrast, Fournier preferred dry liposuction as the initial volume of the wet technique would distort the tissues anatomically, in his opinion.[39] The issue of blood loss in early liposuction surgeries was tackled by the use of epinephrine to achieve vasoconstriction. Nevertheless, the volume of adipose tissue removed was proportional to the volume of blood that was lost.[44] Brorson used liposuction to treat a patient with secondary lymphedema in 1987, and in 1993, performed a prospective clinical study that showed this method, combined with controlled compression therapy, to be an effective treatment with minimal recurrence of lymphedema.[42] Liposuction was used by O'Brien et al.[45] to treat 19 patients with primary and secondary lymphedema. Of the 13 patients available for follow-up, he noted subjective improvement in 11 patients, with an average reduction of 23% in excess volume that was sustained at the 9.5-month follow-up.

The application of liposuction to lymphedematous limbs, using tumescent liposuction, has fundamentally changed how lipedema is managed, offering patients improvements in both physical appearance and overall function.[7, 18] Patients frequently report improvements in their daily activities, which positively affect their mental health and quality of life. Many who have undergone this procedure describe a transformative experience, regaining mobility and alleviating pain that had once been a constant part of their lives.

However, while liposuction can provide remarkable results, it is crucial to set realistic expectations. While surgical intervention can provide significant results, complete resolution of symptoms is not guaranteed, and not every patient will achieve the same degree of success. Factors such as the stage of the disease, the patient's overall health, and adherence to post-operative care all play vital roles in outcomes. This variability is seen in patients who, despite experiencing dramatic physical changes after surgery, continue to struggle with the emotional effects of having lived with the disease for years. This highlights the need for comprehensive pre-operative counseling, which can prepare patients psychologically for the changes they will undergo. For many patients with lipedema, undergoing surgery only to have

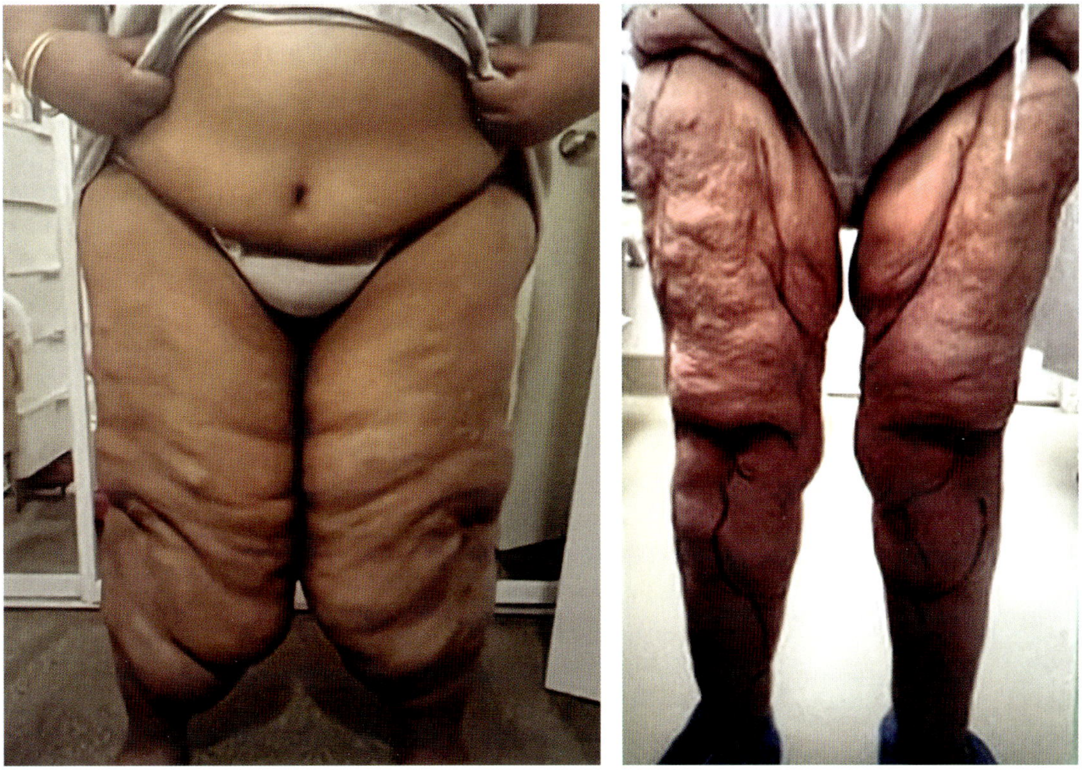

Figure 16.6: Patients attending for revisional surgery for surgery done elsewhere, but in which patients were challenged due to medical PTSD. Patients had not been asked to undertake adequate pre-operative preparation, resulting in outcomes with which they were dissatisfied, at 10 months (left) and twelve months (right) following initial surgery. A resulting additional new diagnosis of 'medical PTSD' potentially presents further challenges for the patient, as it requires psychological counseling/intervention before any consideration of any revision surgery. Courtesy of Dr. Shayan.

their expectations unmet can trigger a profoundly negative emotional response, often intensified by a lifetime of dismissiveness and derision. The author has encountered numerous patients presenting with diagnosable PTSD resulting from previous surgical experiences, making any subsequent attempts at revision especially complex and emotionally charged (Figure 16.6).

While there is a consensus that liposuction is beneficial for lipedema, data collection has been hindered by inherent systemic bias. Some health systems only cover treatment of later-stage disease,[18] while in other systems, there is no insurance coverage at all.[46] Kirstein et al.[18] utilized two validated questionnaires, the World Health Organization Quality of Life BREF (WHOQOL-BREF) and the Patient Health Questionnaire 9 (PHQ-9), to evaluate changes in quality of life in 511 patients with lipedema undergoing liposuction surgery. The post-operative response rate was 11% and, therefore, represents only a small subset of the patients. Further, only 34 patients responded to both questionnaires before and after their surgery, making it difficult to draw definitive conclusions. This low response rate is typical and diminishes the ability to translate results to the entire population of patients with lipedema.[47] Nevertheless, for those participants who responded, there was a significant benefit reported, and the authors concluded that liposuction continued to be a useful treatment for patients with lipedema.

Lymphatic procedures

In addition to tumescent liposuction, other surgical interventions may be suitable for select patients. In combination with or as an alternative to liposuction, lymphatic procedures can also be considered for patients experiencing complications such as lymphedema. Different studies have found 15–56% of patients with lipedema to have some degree of lymphatic dysfunction.[26, 27] A patient suffering from both lipedema and lymphedema may benefit significantly from combined surgical strategies, allowing for a more comprehensive approach. These procedures might include lymphaticovenous anastomosis (LVA) or lymph node transfer, focusing on restoring lymphatic drainage. Although this may be a feature of earlier stages of lipedema, lymphatic impairments are more likely to be a characteristic of stage 4 disease.[19]

It is, therefore, crucial to understand the patient population that may benefit from such procedures. Lymphatic surgeries are more complex and often involve multiple stages, leading to longer overall recovery times. It is therefore important to undertake comprehensive pre-operative counseling to prepare patients for what lies ahead, especially in terms of recovery, potential complications, and the impact on their lifestyle. However, this complexity further underscores the importance of a thorough pre-operative evaluation and collaboration among interdisciplinary teams, including lymphatic specialists, to optimize patient outcomes. At present, LVA surgery is not routinely performed as a treatment for lipedema. However, it may still be utilized in patients with lipedema who develop secondary lymphedema.

Management of integument

Traditional liposuction does not involve the excision of skin from the limbs during the procedure. However, a proportion of patients express a degree of dissatisfaction with the appearance of their post-operative results despite a resolution of symptoms.[18] In these patients, immediate or delayed resection of skin may be possible to reduce seroma risk and the cosmetically unsatisfactory result of abundant loose skin, particularly in younger or more cosmetically sensitive patients. Importantly, both the Michelini and Karnezis groups identified genetic variants associated with the extracellular matrix (ECM).[13, 15] The abnormal connective tissue structure and ECM seen in patients with lipedema, the potential connection to hypermobility, and related diseases such as EDS[29] mean that clinicians have traditionally been hesitant to excise skin and soft tissues in lipedema-affected limbs. Hesitation in resection of the skin has previously been related to the perception that a further surgical insult to a potentially compromised lymphatic system could be problematic.[26, 27] Nevertheless, in carefully screened patients, resection of skin and integument may be safely performed.[2] Early-stage patients do not require removal of excess skin, provided there is no underlying connective tissue disease. However, in the population of later-stage patients, or those who require weight loss, the post-operative skin envelope must be given due consideration. If patients who may require skin excision are uncertain about the resulting scar, it is always preferable to allow the skin envelope to settle on its own accord. However, in patients in whom a resulting skin envelope is unavoidable, a careful process of explanation and informed consent regarding the likely outcome and potential need for further surgery is essential. If the patient is not happy to entertain such a risk, consideration should be given as to whether that particular patient is an appropriate candidate for surgery (see Figure 16.7).

Evaluation – short and long-term

It is critical to evaluate patients with lipedema in the tenets of plastic surgery reconstruction:

1. *Form* – the form of the human body is also part of the function of the body, for self-esteem, communication, socialization, viable employment, and partnering.
2. *Function* – participation in work, family, recreation, exercise, mobility, and the ability to wear clothing and footwear that is comfortable/compatible with the desired recreational activity.

There has been a tendency to suggest that patients with lipedema should simply be grateful for any outcome of a debulking procedure. However, addressing the interconnected aspects of both form and function is essential to truly help patients regain a sense of hope and dignity. Standardized assessment tools, despite their notoriously low response rates,[47] are critical for ensuring the reproducibility of findings and for evaluating the validity of applying those conclusions to broader populations.[18] Blinded, controlled studies are essential in advancing clinical research on lipedema, particularly for evaluating the efficacy of both non-surgical and surgical treatments.[7, 18, 22] By combining large patient cohorts across multicenter studies, more robust and meaningful conclusions can be drawn.[2]

Future perspectives in surgical treatment pathways

Ongoing research into the etiology and mechanisms of lipedema will be necessary to elucidate optimal treatment strategies and methods. Future surgical pathways will be enhanced by innovation and patient-centered care. Emerging technologies, such as bioinformatics, machine learning, and bioengineering, promise to provide deeper insights into the pathology of lipedema, allowing

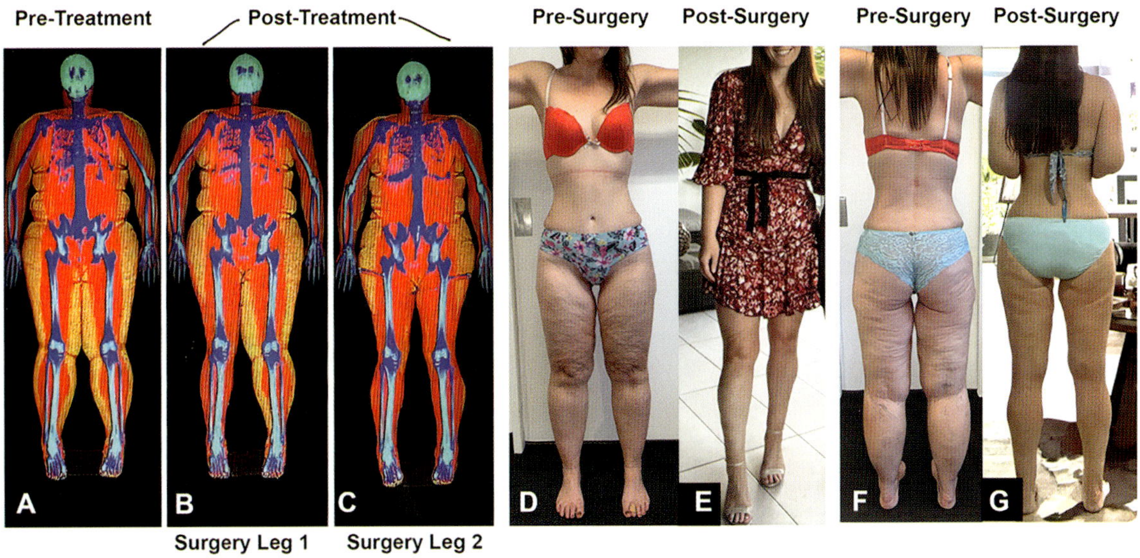

Figure 16.7: Surgery for lipedema: (A)-(C) show changes between stages of surgery (Shayan) on DEXA scan readout (yellow, adipose tissue; red, muscle; blue, bone). Clinical images of preoperative (D, F) and 12-month postoperative (E, G) results showing enhanced form and function of the lower limbs in a 40-year-old patient. Courtesy of Dr. Shayan.

for personalized treatment strategies.[2]

Furthermore, increased awareness and advocacy surrounding lipedema are crucial. As healthcare systems advance, practitioners need to receive training on recognizing and treating lipedema appropriately. Future efforts must focus on increasing access to education and collaborative training programs for surgeons and allied healthcare providers to help ensure that patients, regardless of their geographic location, receive appropriate evaluation and management. Remote and telehealth consultations promise to enhance this capacity.

Nevertheless, the limitations of current surgical techniques still highlight the need for continued research. Recently, it has been shown that lipedema is driven by a unique population of stem cells,[11] on a background of varied genetic predisposition to abnormal adipose morphology and connective tissue biology.[12, 13, 14, 15] Understanding the pathophysiology of lipedema at a molecular and genetic level could lead to innovative treatment options *beyond* surgical intervention, such as targeted therapies or regenerative medicine strategies.

The authors remain optimistic about the future of lipedema care, buoyed by the growing interest within the scientific community and the notable advancements made in recent years. With continued momentum, emerging research and clinical developments have the potential to significantly shorten the time to accurate diagnosis and effective treatment, dramatically improving patient experiences and altering the course of their lives. This hopeful outlook stands in stark contrast to the all-too-common stories of medical neglect, dismissal, and misdiagnosis that many patients have faced.

While the establishment of surgical treatment pathways represents a major step forward, significant challenges persist. Chief among them is the uneven access to specialized surgical care. In many parts of the world, trained clinicians remain scarce, and not all surgeons possess the expertise needed to manage lipedema comprehensively. A holistic understanding is essential – not only for performing lipedema surgeries effectively, but also for addressing the interconnected 'mini-cycles' of co-morbidities that perpetuate and complicate the disease.

Conclusion

In conclusion, the surgical treatment of lipedema is a complex, deeply personal journey shaped by a wide range of clinical, psychological, and social factors. While procedures such as tumescent liposuction can offer substantial relief from pain, mobility limitations, and emotional distress, surgical intervention alone is not sufficient. Optimal outcomes require an integrated approach that includes medical and psychological support, management of co-morbid diseases such as obesity, lymphedema, and autoimmune diseases, as well as lifestyle counseling and patient advocacy.

Through their dual roles as clinicians and researchers, the authors have come to appreciate the importance of comprehensive patient education, multidisciplinary collaboration, and a compassionate, individualized framework of care. As our understanding of lipedema continues to evolve, so must the models through which surgical treatments are delivered, placing patient experience, safety, and empowerment at the forefront.

Ultimately, meaningful progress in lipedema care will depend on continued research, increased awareness, and a sustained commitment to collaborative, empathetic healthcare. The resilience of those living with lipedema is both inspiring and instructive, and it is the responsibility of healthcare professionals to support their journey with knowledge, respect, and unwavering advocacy.

References

1. Bauer AT, von Lukowicz D, Lossagk K, Aitzetmueller M, Moog P, Cerny M, et al. New insights on lipedema: the enigmatic disease of the peripheral fat. *Plast Reconstr Surg.* 2019 Dec;144(6):1475–84. DOI: https://doi.org/10.1097/PRS.0000000000006280
2. Kruppa P, Crescenzi R, Faerber G, Forner-Cordero I, Cornely M, Shayan R, et al. *Lipedema World Alliance Delphi-based Consensus on the Definition and Management of Lipedema: Results from the 2023 Lipedema World Congress in Potsdam.* Potsdam, Germany: Lipedema World Congress; 2023 Oct. Available from: https://lipedemaworldalliance.com/event/lipedema-world-alliance-delphi-consensus-based-position-paper-on-the-definition-and-management-of-lipedema-interim-results/
3. Wold L, Hines EA, Allen EV. Lipedema of the legs: a syndrome characterized by fat legs and edema. *Ann Intern Med.* 1951;34(5):1243–50. Available from: https://klosetraining.com/wp-content/uploads/2021/03/1940-Lipedema-of-the-Legs.pdf
4. Poojari A, Dev K, Rabiee A. Lipedema: insights into morphology, pathophysiology, and challenges. *Biomedicines.* 2022 Dec;10(12):3081. DOI: https://doi.org/10.3390/biomedicines10123081
5. Buck DW, Herbst KL. Lipedema: a relatively common disease with extremely common misconceptions. *Plast Reconstr Surg – Glob Open.* 2016 Sep;4(9):e1043. DOI: https://doi.org/10.1097/GOX.0000000000001043
6. Ghods M, Georgiou I, Schmidt J, Kruppa P. Disease progression and comorbidities in lipedema patients: a 10-year retrospective analysis. *Dermatol Ther.* 2020;33(6):e14534. DOI: https://doi.org/10.1111/dth.14534
7. Hamatschek M, Knors H, Klietz ML, Wiebringhaus P, Aitzetmueller M, Hirsch T, et al. Characteristics and patient reported outcome measures in lipedema patients – establishing a baseline for treatment evaluation in a high-volume center. *J Clin Med.* 2022 May 17;11(10):2836. DOI: https://doi.org/10.3390/jcm11102836
8. Beltran K, Herbst KL. Differentiating lipedema and Dercum's disease. *Int J Obes* 2005. 2017 Feb;41(2):240–5. DOI: https://doi.org/10.1038/ijo.2016.205
9. Tuğral A, Bakar Y. An approach to lipedema: a literature review of current knowledge of an underestimated health problem. *Eur J Plast Surg.* 2019 Dec 1;42(6):549–58. DOI: https://doi.org/10.1007/s00238-019-01519-9
10. Humenikova L, Gates GE. Body image perceptions in Western and post-communist countries: a cross-cultural pilot study of children and parents. *Matern Child Nutr.* 2008 Jul;4(3):220–31. DOI: https://doi.org/10.1111/j.1740-8709.2007.00133.x
11. Ishaq M, Bandara N, Morgan S, Nowell C, Mehdi AM, Lyu R, et al. Key signaling networks are dysregulated in patients with the adipose tissue disease, lipedema. *Int J Obes.* 2022 Mar;46(3):502–14. DOI: https://doi.org/10.1038/s41366-021-01002-1
12. Klimentidis YC, Chen Z, Gonzalez-Garay ML, Grigoriadis D, Sackey E, Pittman A, et al. Genome-wide association study of a lipedema phenotype among women in the UK Biobank identifies multiple genetic risk factors. *Eur J Hum Genet.* 2023 Mar;31(3):338–44. DOI: https://doi.org/10.1038/s41431-022-01231-6
13. Morgan S, Reid I, Bendon C, Ishaq M, Shayan R, Pope B, et al. A family-based study of inherited genetic risk in lipedema. *Lymphat Res Biol.* 2024 Apr 1;22(2):106–11. DOI: https://doi.org/10.1089/lrb.2023.0065
14. Michelini S, Chiurazzi P, Marino V, Dell'Orco D, Manara E, Baglivo M, et al. Aldo-keto reductase 1C1 (AKR1C1) as the first mutated gene in a family with nonsyndromic primary lipedema. *Int J Mol Sci.* 2020 Jan;21(17):6264. DOI: https://doi.org/10.3390/ijms21176264
15. Michelini S, Herbst KL, Precone V, Manara E, Marceddu G, Dautaj A, et al. A multi-gene panel to identify lipedema-predisposing genetic variants by a next-generation sequencing strategy. *J Pers Med.* 2022 Feb 11;12(2):268. DOI: https://doi.org/10.3390/jpm12020268
16. Kaftalli J, Bonetti G, Marceddu G, Dhuli K, E Maltese P, Donato K, et al. AKR1C1 and hormone metabolism in lipedema pathogenesis: a computational biology approach. *Eur Rev Med Pharmacol Sci.*2023;27(6 Suppl.):137-47; Available from:

https://usiena-air.unisi.it/handle/11365/1261114
17. Katzer K, Hill JL, Link to external site this link will open in a new window, McIver KB. Lipedema and the potential role of estrogen in excessive adipose tissue accumulation. *Int J Mol Sci*. 2021;22(21):11720. DOI: https://doi.org/10.3390/ijms222111720
18. Kirstein F, Hamatschek M, Knors H, Aitzetmueller-Klietz ML, Aitzetmueller-Klietz M, Wiebringhaus P, et al. Patient-reported outcomes of liposuction for lipedema treatment. *Healthcare*. 2023 Jan;11(14):2020. DOI: https://doi.org/10.3390/healthcare11142020
19. Child AH, Gordon KD, Sharpe P, Brice G, Ostergaard P, Jeffery S, et al. Lipedema: an inherited condition. *Am J Med Genet A*. 2010;152A(4):970–6. DOI: https://doi.org/10.1002/ajmg.a.33313
20. Hossain L, Gomes KP, Safarpour S, Gibson SB. The microenvironment of secondary lymphedema. The key to finding effective treatments? *Biophys Acta Mol Basis Dis*. 2025 Mar;1871(3):167677. DOI: https://doi.org/10.1016/j.bbadis.2025.167677
21. Allen EV, Hines EA. Lipedema of the legs: A syndrome characterized by fat legs and orthostatic edema. *Proc Staff Meet Mayo Clin*. 1940;15(15):184–7. Available from: https://klosetraining.com/wp-content/uploads/2021/03/1940-Lipedema-of-the-Legs.pdf
22. Podda M, Kovacs M, Hellmich M, Roth R, Zarrouk M, Kraus D, et al. A randomised controlled multicentre investigator-blinded clinical trial comparing efficacy and safety of surgery versus complex physical decongestive therapy for lipedema (LIPLEG). *Trials*. 2021 Oct 30;22(1):758. DOI: https://doi.org/10.1186/s13063-021-05727-2
23. Szolnoky G, Borsos B, Bársony K, Balogh M, Kemény L. Complete decongestive physiotherapy with and without pneumatic compression for treatment of lipedema: a pilot study. *Lymphology*. 2008 Mar;41(1):40–4. Available from: https://journals.librarypublishing.arizona.edu/lymph/article/id/3645/
24. Fuster JJ, Ouchi N, Gokce N, Walsh K. Obesity-induced changes in adipose tissue microenvironment and their impact on cardiovascular disease. *Circ Res*. 2016 May 27;118(11):1786–807. DOI: https://doi.org/10.1161/CIRCRESAHA.115.306885
25. Farooqi IS, Drop S, Clements A, Keogh JM, Biernacka J, Lowenbein S, et al. Heterozygosity for a POMC-null mutation and increased obesity risk in humans. *Diabetes*. 2006 Sep;55(9):2549–53. DOI: https://doi.org/10.2337/db06-0214
26. Buso G, Favre L, Maufus M, Honorati M, Lessert C, Depairon M, et al. Indocyanine green lymphography as novel tool to assess lymphatics in patients with lipedema. *Microvasc Res*. 2022 Mar 1;140:104298. DOI: https://doi.org/10.1016/j.mvr.2021.104298
27. Mackie H, Thompson BM, Suami H, Heydon-White A, Blackwell R, Tisdall Blake F, et al. Differentiation of lipoedema from bilateral lower limb lymphoedema by imaging assessment of indocyanine green lymphography. *Clin Obes*. 2023 Jun;13(3):e12588. DOI: https://doi.org/10.1111/cob.12588
28. Demirdas S, Dulfer E, Robert L, Kempers M, van Beek D, Micha D, et al. Recognizing the tenascin-X deficient type of Ehlers-Danlos syndrome: a cross-sectional study in 17 patients. *Clin Genet*. 2017;91(3):411–25. DOI: https://doi.org/10.1111/cge.12853
29. van Gurp JE, Lechner RL, Micha D, Maugeri A, Dulfer E, van Dijk FS, et al. Tenascin-X deficiency causing classical-like Ehlers-Danlos syndrome type 1 in humans is a significant risk factor of gastrointestinal and tracheal ruptures. *Clin Transl Gastroenterol*. 2025 Mar;16(3):e00821. DOI: https://doi.org/10.14309/ctg.0000000000000821
30. da Costa Viana D, Câmara L. Metabolic therapy for lipedema: can tirzepatide overcome the treatment gap? *J Pharm Res Int*. 2025;37(3):21–8. DOI: https://doi.org/10.9734/jpri/2025/v37i37664
31. Brenner E, Forner-Cordero I, Faerber G, Rapprich S, Cornely M. Body mass index vs. waist-to-height-ratio in patients with lipohyperplasia dolorosa (vulgo lipedema). *J Dtsch Dermatol Ges J Ger Soc Dermatol JDDG*. 2023 Oct;21(10):1179–85. DOI: https://doi.org/10.1111/ddg.15182
32. Forner-Cordero I, Szolnoky G, Forner-Cordero A, Kemény L. Lipedema: an overview of its clinical manifestations, diagnosis and

treatment of the disproportional fatty deposition syndrome – systematic review. *Clin Obes*. 2012;2(3–4):86–95. DOI: https://doi.org/10.1111/j.1758-8111.2012.00045.x
33. Rank BK, Wong GS. Lipoedema. *Aust N Z J Surg*. 1966 Feb;35(3):166–9. DOI: https://doi.org/10.1111/j.1445-2197.1966.tb06053.x
34. Stutz J. Liposuction in lipedema to prevent later joint complications. *Vasomed*. 2011 Jan;23. Available from: https://lipedema.net/wp-content/uploads/2024/12/liposuction20of20lipedema20to20prevent20later20joint20complications.pdf
35. Baumgartner A, Hueppe M, Schmeller W. Long-term benefit of liposuction in patients with lipoedema: a follow-up study after an average of 4 and 8 years. *Br J Dermatol*. 2016 May;174(5):1061–7. DOI: https://doi.org/10.1111/bjd.14289
36. Dadras M, Mallinger PJ, Corterier CC, Theodosiadi S, Ghods M. Liposuction in the treatment of lipedema: a longitudinal study. *Arch Plast Surg*. 2017 Jul;44(4):324–31. DOI: https://doi.org/10.5999/aps.2017.44.4.324
37. Wollina U. Lipedema – an update. *Dermatol Ther*. 2019;32(2):e12805. DOI: https://doi.org/10.1111/dth.12805
38. Witte T, Dadras M, Heck FC, Heck M, Habermalz B, Welss S, et al. Water-jet-assisted liposuction for the treatment of lipedema: standardized treatment protocol and results of 63 patients. *J Plast Reconstr Aesthet Surg*. 2020 Sep 1;73(9):1637–44. DOI: https://doi.org/10.1016/j.bjps.2020.03.002
39. Fournier PF, Otteni FM. Lipodissection in body sculpturing: the dry procedure. *Plast Reconstr Surg*. 1983 Nov;72(5):598–609. DOI: https://doi.org/10.1097/00006534-198311000-00002
40. Hait P. History of the American Society of Plastic and Reconstructive Surgeons, Inc. 1931–1994. *Plast Reconstr Surg*. 1994 Sep;94(4):1A–109A. Available from: https://pubmed.ncbi.nlm.nih.gov/8066127/ and https://journals.lww.com/plasreconsurg/toc/1994/09001
41. Illouz YG. Body contouring by lipolysis: a 5-year experience with over 3000 cases. *Plast Reconstr Surg*. 1983 Nov;72(5):591–7. DOI: https://doi.org/10.1097/00006534-198311000-00001
42. Brorson H. From lymph to fat: complete reduction of lymphoedema. *Phlebology*. 2010 Oct 1;25(1_suppl):52–63. DOI: https://doi.org/10.1258/phleb.2010.010s08
43. Illouz YG. History and current concepts of lipoplasty. *Clin Plast Surg*. 1996 Oct;23(4):721–30. DOI: https://doi.org/10.1016/S0094-1298(20)32567-0
44. Hetter GP. The effect of low-dose epinephrine on the hematocrit drop following lipolysis. *Aesthetic Plast Surg*. 1984;8(1):19–21. DOI: https://doi.org/10.1007/BF01572780
45. O'Brien BM, Khazanchi RK, Kumar PA, Dvir E, Pederson WC. Liposuction in the treatment of lymphoedema; a preliminary report. *Br J Plast Surg*. 1989 Sep;42(5):530–3. DOI: https://doi.org/10.1016/0007-1226(89)90039-8
46. Shayan R. Developing better lipedema surgery through molecular and genetic understanding: our basic science and clinical results. Presentation presented at *Lipedema World Congress*; 2023 Oct 5; Potsdam, Germany. Available from: https://www.lipedema-world-congress.com/on-demand/session-3-basic-science-1-sequencing-stem-cells-genetics-video/
47. Reid I, Hansen J, Karnezis T, Shayan R, Shukla L. Autologous fat grafting: current state of clinical practice in the Australian setting. *Australas J Plast Surg*. 2023 Mar 29;6(1):1–9. DOI: https://doi.org/10.34239/ajops.70236

Chapter Seventeen
Alternative and supplementary surgical approaches to lipedema

Corrado Cesare Campisi, Michele Maruccia and Zoe-Theodora Kolonelos

Introduction

Lipedema is a chronic and progressive adipose tissue and lymphatic disease that primarily affects women, characterized by disproportionate accumulation of subcutaneous adipose tissue (SAT) in the lower body, associated with pain and impaired mobility (Figure 17.1). While conservative treatments such as complete decongestive therapy (CDT), manual lymphatic drainage (MLD), and compression therapy can help manage symptoms, they do not address the pathological adipose tissue deposition. Lipedema reduction surgery (LRS) via liposuction remains the most effective long-term management intervention. Still, not all surgical techniques provide equal benefits, particularly for patients with advanced disease or lymphatic impairment.

In addition to traditional liposuction, alternative and supplementary surgical approaches have been developed to optimize outcomes, minimize complications, and preserve lymphatic integrity. Various state-of-the-art liposuction systems and techniques offer enhanced fat removal with reduced trauma to surrounding tissues. Lymphatic preservation in surgical lipedema treatment is becoming the new gold standard. Lymph-sparing practices, such as the fibro-lipo-lymph aspiration with lymph vessel sparing procedure (FLLA-LVSP), are recommended for lipedema reduction surgery (LRS). Additionally, microsurgical interventions such as multiple lymphatic-venous anastomosis (MLVA) provide a critical adjunct for patients with concurrent lymphatic dysfunction, improving postsurgical lymphatic drainage and reducing the risk of secondary lymphedema.

A tailored, multidisciplinary approach that integrates lymphatic-sparing surgical techniques with preoperative decongestive therapies is essential for optimizing both functional and aesthetic outcomes. As surgical strategies for lipedema continue to evolve, adopting advanced methodologies ensures safer and more effective long-term results for patients.

Pathophysiology

The pathophysiology of lipedema remains poorly understood; however, it has significant implications for surgical considerations. Emerging evidence suggests that the development of lipedema may involve a combination of polygenic susceptibility, hormonal influences, and dysfunctions in the microvascular and lymphatic systems. Consequently, adipose tissue enlargement in affected patients may not represent the initial pathological event, but rather a secondary consequence of lymphangiopathy or

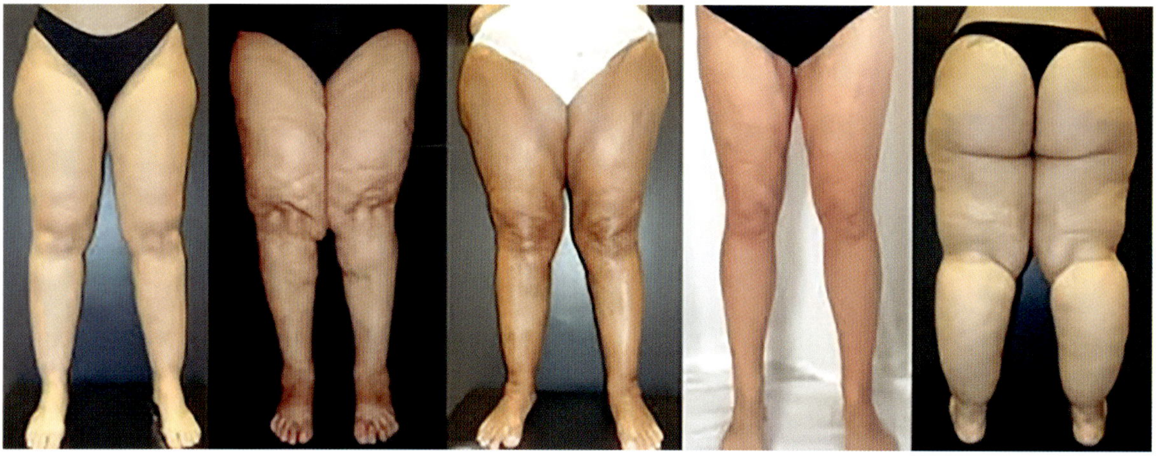

Figure 17.1: Examples of lower limb lipedema. Courtesy of Dr. Campisi.

microvascular impairment.[1]

Disruptions in capillary integrity and impaired lymphatic drainage can lead to increased interstitial fluid retention, which promotes adipocyte hypertrophy and inflammation. Chronic tissue hypoxia and low-grade inflammation further exacerbate fibrotic remodeling, contributing to progressive tissue stiffness and pain. These interconnected pathophysiological mechanisms underscore the complexity of lipedema and highlight the need for targeted therapeutic strategies that address both adipose tissue dysfunction and lymphatic insufficiency.

Stages of lipedema

The progression of lipedema can be divided into three or four stages, as described in Chapter 1. Of importance here is that the surgical treatment of lipedema is most promising when performed before the condition escalates into later stages, which often have severe and debilitating effects on the patient's body and daily life. At the Campisi Clinic, we use four stages as follows:

- **Stage 1**: The skin surface is smooth, but subcutaneous tissues display nodular fat deposition. Patients often report heaviness, discomfort, and pain in the affected areas.
- **Stage 2**: The skin begins to develop an uneven texture with indentations resembling 'mattress-like' dimpling. The subcutaneous fat becomes harder and more fibrotic, reflecting progressive tissue changes.
- **Stage 3 moderate**: Nodular fat deposits grow larger, forming lobules that significantly distort body shape. Skin laxity and overhanging folds become more pronounced. At this stage, mobility may be impaired, and quality of life declines.
- **Stage 3 severe**: This stage involves the coexistence of lipedema with secondary lymphedema, characterized by significant swelling, skin changes, fat deposition, and lymphatic insufficiency.

Types of lipedema

The five types that show the location of lipedema fat are seen in Figure 17.2. Type I is often combined with Type II or III.

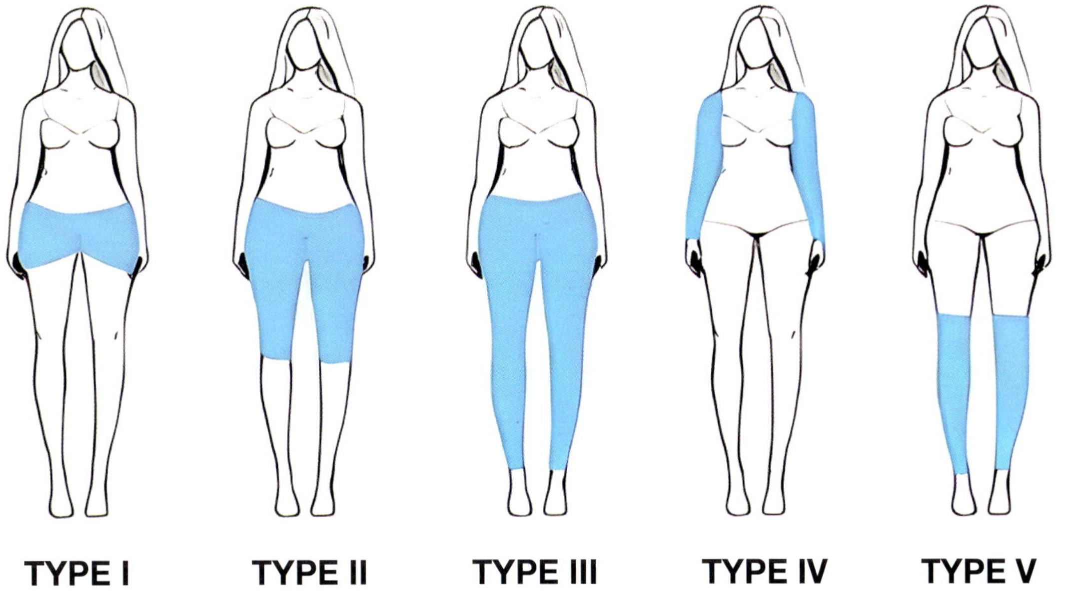

Figure 17.2: Type I: Pelvis, buttocks, and hips (saddle bag phenomenon); Type II: Buttocks to knees, with the formation of folds of fat around the inner side of the knee; Type III: Buttocks to ankles; Type IV: Arms; Type V: Lower leg. Courtesy of Dr. Campisi.

Diagnosing lipedema

Accurate diagnosis of lipedema and any comorbid diseases is critical before referral for surgery. Diagnosis is rarely made in the initial visit with a physician. Even after diagnosis, a patient may experience a significant delay, sometimes several years, before specific treatment is initiated. As lipedema is a chronic disease, patients should seek out medical professionals who have experience recognizing the disease and the related conditions. A thorough and systematic approach combining patient history, clinical examination, and advanced diagnostic technologies, as described in previous chapters, is crucial for accurate identification and staging of the disease.

Technologies used for detecting and assessing lipedema

The diagnostic process for lipedema primarily relies on clinical features. Still, modern technologies provide invaluable adjuncts to aid in confirming the diagnosis, assessing the disease state, and suggesting potential treatment options. If a surgical option is being explored, imaging technologies can be invaluable in the decision-making process (Figure 17.3). A more in-depth discussion of these imaging techniques can be found in Chapters 9 and 10. Key diagnostic tools include:

- **Ultrasound imaging**: High-frequency ultrasound has become a cornerstone in evaluating lipedema tissue. It allows visualization of the characteristic thickened hypodermis with hypoechoic nodular patterns, distinguishing lipedema fat from normal adipose tissue or lymphedema-associated changes.
- **Bioimpedance spectroscopy (BIS)**: This non-invasive method measures extracellular fluid volumes and can be helpful to differentiate lipedema from lymphedema,

particularly when there is suspicion of overlapping diseases. BIS detects subtle increases in fluid accumulation, which are typically absent in pure lipedema but present in the later stages of secondary lymphedema.

- **MRI and CT scans**: Advanced imaging modalities such as magnetic resonance imaging (MRI) or computed tomography (CT), can provide a more detailed view of tissue composition, offering insights into fat distribution and distinguishing lipedema from other conditions, including lipohypertrophy or obesity.
- **Lymphoscintigraphy**: While traditionally prescribed as a means to diagnose lymphedema, a lymphoscintigraphy exam provides valuable insight into the body's lymphatic function. It can analyze beyond the superficial lymphatic network into the deeper lymphatic channels. The profound analysis is more accurate and complete than other exams. Lymphoscintigraphy should be performed as part of every lipedema diagnosis. If impaired lymphatic function is detected, it must be carefully evaluated and cautiously factored into the patient's treatment plan from the beginning. This is especially important in patients who fall into more advanced stages of lipedema and/or patients who are eager to undergo surgery early on.
- **Indocyanine green (ICG) lymphography**: This technique allows real-time visualization of lymphatic vessels and their functionality. It is beneficial in cases where lipedema coexists with lymphatic insufficiency, enabling the tailoring of surgical and other treatment approaches.

The importance of a comprehensive diagnosis

Distinguishing lipedema from lymphedema or a phlebo-hybrid variation of the two is critical for the effective management of these diseases, both in the acute and long-term settings. Conservative treatment and/or surgical intervention should only be prescribed after a complete and comprehensive evaluation performed by a suitable specialist. Lipedema and diseases related to either venous or lymphatic insufficiencies often manifest alongside each other in hybrid forms, or consecutively, one triggering the other.

A lipedema diagnosis should be given only when definitively ruling out the presence of a lymphatic insufficiency. Physicians mustn't confuse a lymphedema, venous, or combination diagnosis with that of lipedema. It can be extremely dangerous, especially if the patient is to undergo surgery. If lymphatic impairment cannot be ruled out initially, the lymphatic system must be investigated more thoroughly to reach a definitive conclusion. If lipedema exists in conjunction with a lymphatic issue, the clinical management of the patient should address both conditions simultaneously, as significant risks could arise otherwise. Any surgical procedure or sequence of surgical procedures should be performed by a plastic surgeon well-versed in lymphology to avoid compromising or complicating the situation.

The interplay between lipedema and the lymphatic system

The lymphatic system serves as a vital drainage network, transporting interstitial fluid, proteins, and immune cells. Emerging evidence suggests a significant interplay between the SAT of lipedema and the lymphatic system. Lipedema's pathological adipose tissue exerts profound alterations on the lymphatic system and needs to be explored when surgical options are being considered. As SAT accumulates in the body, it places a significant mechanical and inflammatory strain on the underlying lymphatic vessels, particularly in advanced stages.[2] The resulting constriction

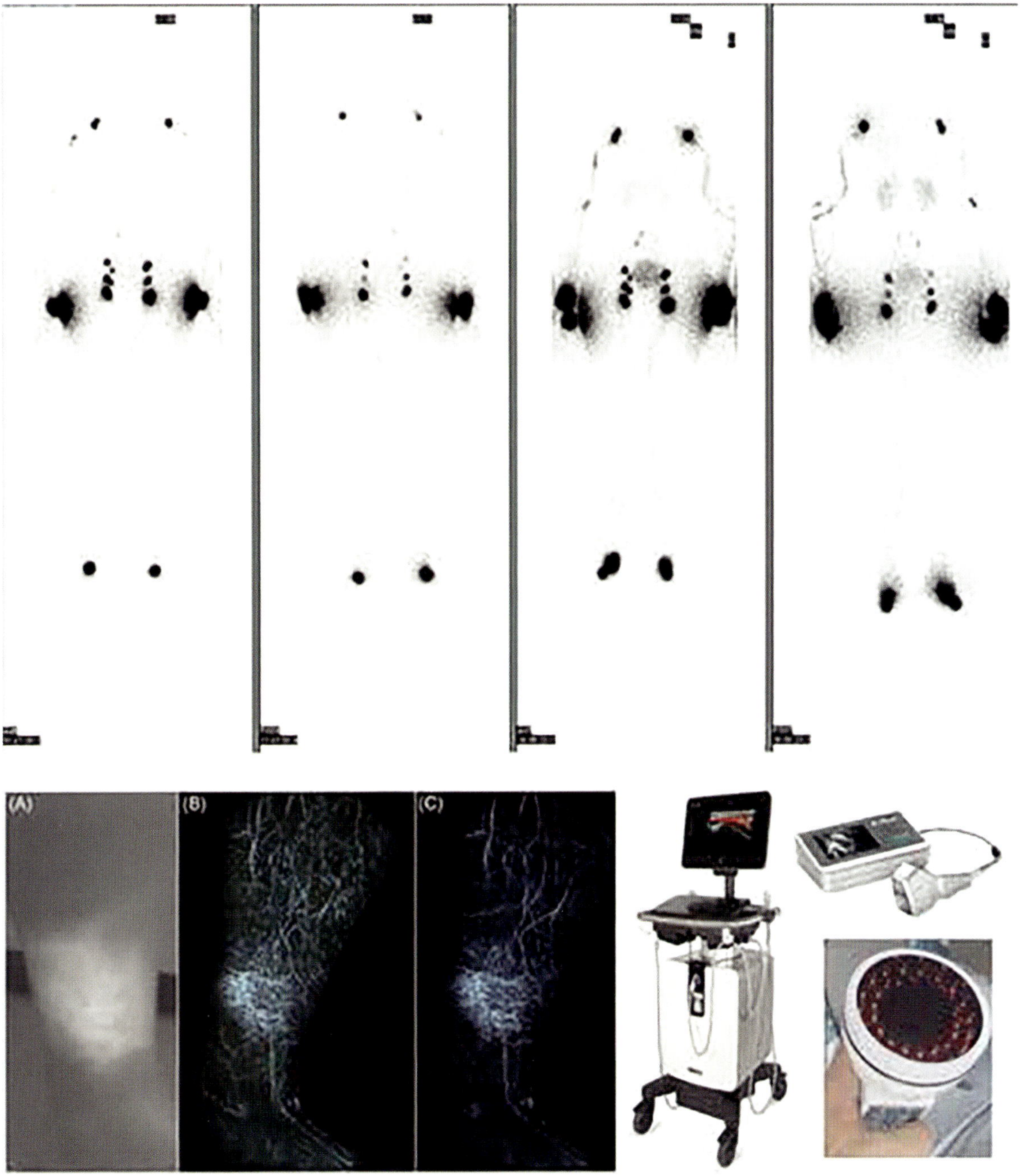

Figure 17.3: Imaging technologies used in the diagnostic process and treatment of lymphedema, lipedema, and all variations of both diseases. Top: lymphoscintigraphy exam results. Bottom left: (A) ICG fluorescent micro-lymphography; (B) photoacoustic lymphangiography of veins and lymphatic vessels; (C) Photoacoustic lymphangiography of lymphatic vessels only. Bottom right: IC flow and ultrasonic devices. Courtesy of Dr. Campisi.

and added pressure can impair lymphatic flow, leading to localized fluid retention and reduced lymph transport efficiency. This altered microenvironment can lead to compromised lymphatic capillaries, reduced contractility of lymphangions, and eventual lymphatic overload. If this occurs, treatments need to be redesigned with an expert lymphologist.[2, 3]

Microvascular dysfunction may lead to increased capillary permeability, promoting interstitial fluid accumulation and subsequent low-grade inflammation. This chronic inflammatory state can impair lymphatic contractility and transport capacity, contributing to fluid stasis and tissue fibrosis. Lymphatic dysfunction often exacerbates lipedema's progression, leading to secondary lymphedema (see Figure 17.4). This bidirectional relationship highlights the importance of early intervention strategies that optimize lymphatic function while addressing the pathological adipose hypertrophy characteristic of lipedema.[2]

Lymphedema vs. lipedema

Lymphedema is a chronic disease caused by impaired lymphatic drainage, leading to the accumulation of lymphatic fluid in the tissues. Unlike lipedema, which is primarily characterized by disproportionate fat accumulation, lymphedema presents as persistent swelling, most commonly affecting one or both limbs. This swelling results from the lymphatic vessels' inability to transport fluid efficiently back into the circulatory system. The swelling observed in patients with lipedema is usually non-pitting. Either disease can become a comorbidity of the other. When both diseases exist simultaneously, it is sometimes referred to as lipolymphedema.[3]

Lipedema with secondary lymphedema

The risk of developing secondary lymphedema is significantly increased in individuals with lipedema.[4, 5] Patients with lipedema may display features of lymphedema, particularly in advanced stages,[1, 6] and can present through multiple pathological pathways. It may arise when primary lymphedema predisposes an individual to the development of lipedema, when longstanding lipedema leads to secondary lymphatic dysfunction, or when both diseases emerge concurrently, contributing to a complex interplay of adipose and lymphatic dysfunction. Patients with co-occurring lipedema and lymphedema exhibit characteristics of both diseases: fat distribution and tenderness typical of lipedema, combined with lymphedema-like swelling that

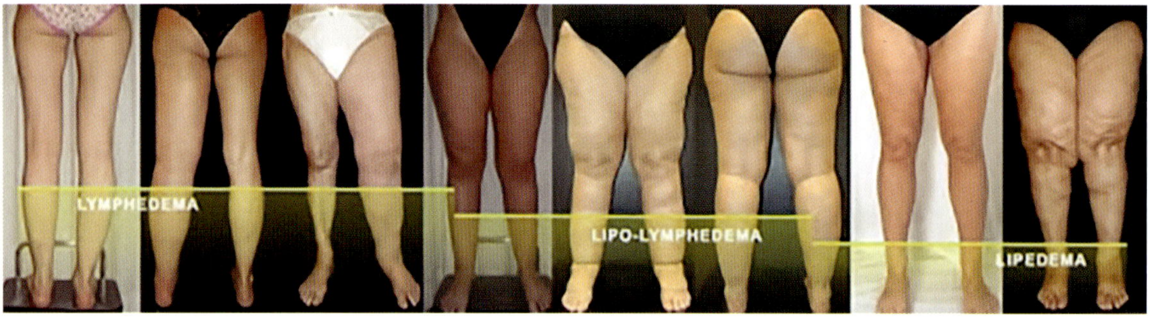

Figure 17.4: Examples of similarities and differences in the lower limbs. Visual overlap of lymphedema, lipo-lymphedema (lipedema with secondary lymphedema), and lipedema. Courtesy of Dr. Campisi.

begins in the feet or hands and advances upward.

Studies suggest that the pathological fat in lipedema is metabolically and hormonally active,[1, 6] secreting pro-inflammatory cytokines and adipokines. These signals can also exacerbate the lymphatic system's dysfunction, thereby compounding the symptoms. The lymphatic impairment, in turn, disrupts the body's ability to clear waste products and inflammatory molecules from the tissues, further fueling the disease's progression. Patients with undiagnosed lipedema, especially in its advanced stages, face a significantly high risk of progressing into secondary lymphedema. This convergence of adipose and lymphatic pathology can have a profound impact on the patient's quality of life.

The coexistence of adipose and lymphatic dysfunction presents a uniquely challenging surgical environment, requiring careful preoperative management. Given the heightened risk of complications, patients should undergo intensive conservative decongestive therapy before surgery to maximize lymphatic drainage and reduce tissue congestion (see Figure 17.5). This approach helps optimize surgical outcomes and minimize postoperative risks.[3]

Treating lipedema: multimodal strategies

Therapy for lipedema includes both conservative and surgical measures to prevent the progression and alleviate existing symptoms. The current gold standard in conservative treatment is complete decongestive therapy (CDT),[3, 7, 8] a conservative treatment involving manual lymphatic drainage (MLD) and compression therapy (CT), as described extensively in Chapter 12. Lipedema management should encompass conservative,

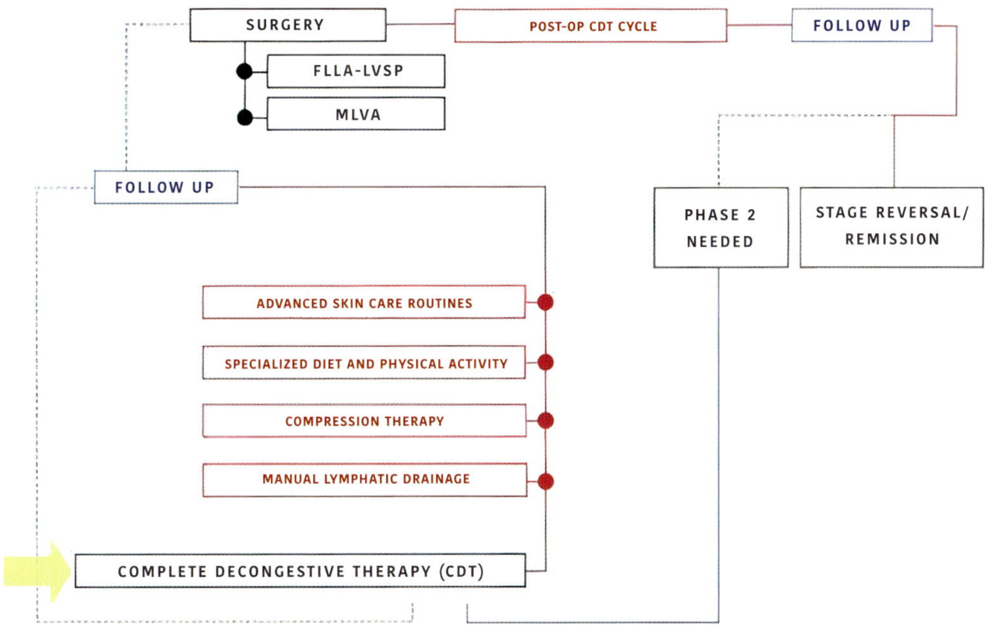

Figure 17.5: Flowchart for the Campisi Clinic treatment of lipedema. Multi-modal treatment diagram; from complete decongestive therapy (CDT) to stage reversal and/or remission.

interventional, and surgical approaches, each tailored to the stage of the disease and the patient's specific needs. Comprehensive guidelines for these treatment modalities should follow the International Society of Lymphology (ISL) consensus document for clinical best practices.[2] Conservative and interventional treatment protocols should be initiated immediately after diagnosis. CDT treatment cycles can aid in alleviating symptoms and preventing disease progression, and should be coupled with specific diet, exercise, and skin care programs to maximize the quality of life (QoL) and overall well-being of patients with lipedema.[3, 4] However, if the patient is not reporting a significant decrease in symptoms after a few months of CDT, the treatment regimen should be adjusted to prepare for surgical intervention.

Manual lymphatic drainage

A cornerstone of CDT, MLD is a specialized physiotherapeutic technique designed to stimulate lymphatic flow and reduce fluid accumulation. When performed by trained practitioners, MLD follows structured protocols, employing precise, rhythmic, and directional hand movements to facilitate lymphatic drainage while minimizing tissue strain. These techniques are tailored to the patient's situation and can enhance preparation for and recovery from surgery.

Compression therapy

Compression therapy is the second pillar of conservative treatment for lipedema, aimed at reducing edema, improving lymphatic flow, and alleviating discomfort. Two primary modalities are compression garments and/or bandages, as well as sequential pneumatic compression pumps. Multilayered compression bandaging applied by trained professionals or medical-grade compression garments (flat-knit is recommended) provides continuous external pressure to support tissue integrity, enhance venous return, and prevent fluid accumulation. Sequential pneumatic compression pumps, on the other hand, deliver controlled, rhythmic pressure to stimulate lymphatic drainage and mobilize interstitial fluid. When incorporated into a comprehensive treatment regimen, the combined use of these therapies can significantly improve symptom management, slow disease progression, and enhance overall patient well-being. Compression therapy can also be a powerful adjunct to surgical intervention.

Specialized diet and physical activity

Targeted exercises and tailor-made diet plans are optimal at helping patients increase lymphatic drainage, promote circulation, manage weight, and enhance surgical outcomes. Lifestyle changes should be paired with and designed in tandem with CDT cycles. Low-impact activities like yoga, Pilates, aerobics, rebounding, walking, and swimming naturally activate the body's muscle pumps, promoting passive lymph transport. Gentle, tailor-made workout routines are recommended to maintain joint mobility and muscle tone while avoiding excessive stress on affected limbs.

Skin care

Daily skin care routines are an indispensable practice in conservative treatment for edema-related pathologies. As the natural skin barrier is often compromised with lipedema, leaving the skin significantly more susceptible to infections, especially via furrows and/or rhagades. Germs may penetrate the body through these minor tears in the skin, potentially causing a serious infection. Compromised lymphatics and poor metabolic function in the region allow bacteria to spread more easily, making it more difficult to fight infections.[3] Meticulous skin care practices, both before and after surgery, aid in optimizing surgical outcomes.

Additional therapeutic technologies for the treatment of lipedema

A multidisciplinary approach typically yields the most advantageous and long-lasting results for patients. Additional technologies exist that can significantly curb the progression and alleviate the symptoms of lipedema as well as complement surgical intervention. See Chapter 13 for a discussion of further complementary interventions. Campisi Clinic supplementary technologies and protocols for lipedema treatment include:

LPG

A mechanical massage technique for cellular stimulation through reproducible mechanical massage. It is highly effective in rejuvenating the body's connective tissues, including the skin, muscles, blood, and lymphatic circulation systems. The machine employs suction and rollers to mobilize tissues, reduce fibrosis, and enhance circulation. This treatment may alleviate discomfort while improving tissue pliability and elasticity.

Shockwave therapy

Acoustic waves are utilized to stimulate local circulation, break down fibrotic tissues, reduce pain, and enhance lymphatic drainage. This type of treatment is a game-changer for patients, as the non-invasive therapy provides symptomatic relief while improving skin texture. The technology, which increases circulation and reduces inflammation, is a powerful tool in curbing the progression of pain and discomfort in patients' affected body parts while also positively impacting body image and confidence by reducing the fibrotic appearance of the skin.

Vacuum therapy

Vacuum technology is a non-invasive therapeutic method that employs negative pressure to enhance blood and lymphatic circulation, thereby facilitating the reduction of fluid accumulation in tissues. By promoting lymphatic drainage, vacuum therapy can help alleviate swelling and discomfort associated with diseases such as lymphedema and lipedema. Incorporating vacuum therapy into CDT may improve outcomes by complementing MLD, compression therapy, and exercise regimens.

Alternative supplementary surgical approaches for lipedema

Achieving optimal results often requires patients to dedicate significant time and effort to treatment regimens, including prolonged sessions of MLD, compression, and other therapies, usually extending over weeks, months, and even years. The long-term practicality of this is generally very limited. This extensive commitment is not always feasible or a welcomed reality for many patients as it comes with its own set of physical, emotional, and financial drawbacks. These circumstances may influence patient decision-making regarding surgical intervention.

Liposuction for lipedema reduction surgery (LRS)

While conservative and interventional treatments play a crucial role in symptom management and enhancing the quality of life for individuals diagnosed with lipedema, they may not be sufficient in curbing the chronic, long-term progression of the disease. When consistent cycles of CDT are insufficient in managing the progression or symptoms of lipedema, surgical intervention becomes a critical option. The most sustainable and effective long-term management for lipedema involves integrating a structured conservative treatment cycle with surgical intervention.

Resective procedures are used to treat patients with lipedema surgically. Lipedema reduction surgeries (LRS) will involve some form of tissue removal, either employing liposuction and/or excision. Supplementary procedures may be required to treat lymphatic dysfunction and/or excess skin that can result from large-volume liposuction. Surgery should be evaluated as a treatment option promptly, as in most cases, the best time for surgical intervention is as soon as possible.

There are many benefits that those suffering from lipedema may achieve after undergoing one or multiple successful liposuctions; firstly, the mass reduction itself from the aspiration of adipose tissue will greatly relieve the patient's chronic and often debilitating sensations of heaviness in their affected body parts. The push-pull motion of the cannula not only helps reduce lipedema through aspiration but also breaks up the very dense and fibrotic SAT. This can eventually lead to reductions in pain and related symptoms post-operatively, while also improving skin quality, texture, and appearance.

Pre- and post-operative protocols

Meticulous pre- and post-operative care is critical for patients with lipedema to ensure the most viable outcomes and long-standing results after surgery. Patients should complete a rigorous series of CDT before and after surgery. A comprehensive approach, incorporating manual and mechanical lymphatic drainage, compression therapy, a specialized diet, targeted physical activity, and skin care, is recommended. The patient should undergo LRS in the most optimal conditions possible to maximize success and decrease the need for follow-up surgical intervention. When the edema is reduced to a manageable minimum, the surgeon can more easily target only the SAT, promoting a more suitable outcome overall (see Figure 17.6). Compression garments should be worn consistently post-operatively. The timeline for such treatment should be determined by the doctor on a case-by-case basis, with specific reference to staging and the patients' overall clinical and pathological indications before and

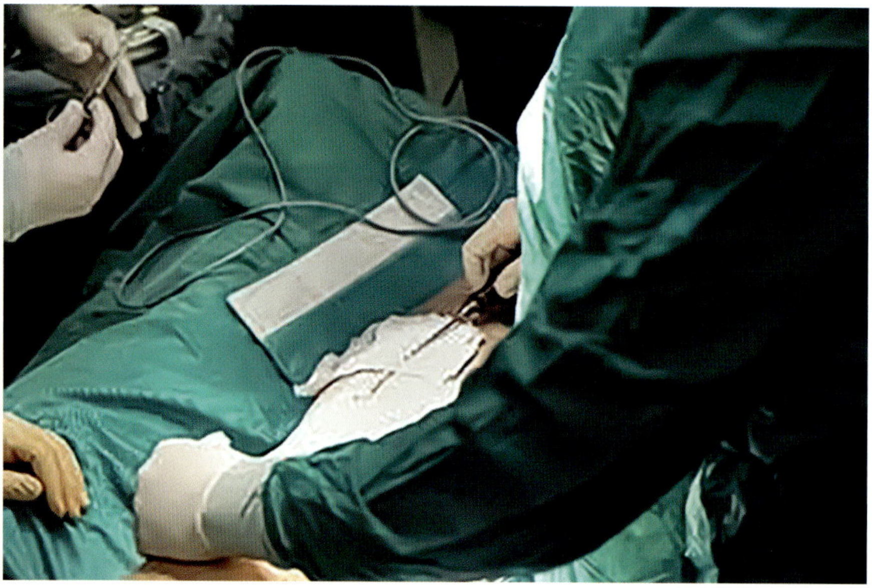

Figure 17.6: Dr. Corrado Campisi performing lipedema reduction surgery via fibro-lipo-lymph aspiration with lymph vessel sparing procedure (FLLA-LVSP). Courtesy of Dr. Campisi.

after surgery. A CDT cycle should always be administered post-operatively (for a minimum of a week) to maximize healing and optimize the surgical outcomes.

Liposuction as treatment for lipedema

Liposuction is typically used for cosmetic purposes. However, because lipedema SAT is associated with pain, lymphedema, obesity, venous disease, hypermobile joints, and dysmobility, LRS by way of liposuction is medically necessary to reduce SAT when not reduced by usual measures.[4] Standard liposuction, which aims to remove excess adipose tissue through suction-assisted techniques for purely aesthetic indications, is not recommended for patients with complex adipose tissue diseases and edema. Even in strictly aesthetic interventions, there are significant risks of consequential damage to the lymphatic system while undergoing liposuction. When the thin, hollow cannula is inserted beneath the skin and the aggressive push-pull motions needed to aspirate fat and reshape specific areas are performed, there is a significant potential threat to the delicate lymphatic matrix in that area. While liposuction is most commonly performed for aesthetic purposes, various specialized liposuction techniques and technologies are used in the medical treatment of lipedema.

Liposuction with tumescent fluid injection

Tumescent fluid injection is a critical preparatory step in liposuction for lipedema, designed to enhance patient safety and optimize fat removal. This technique involves the infusion of a specialized solution into the targeted adipose tissue before the actual liposuction procedure begins. The solution consists of a combination of lidocaine (a local anesthetic), epinephrine (a vasoconstrictor), and a saline or lactated Ringer's solution to expand the fat layer and minimize trauma.

The tumescent technique is strongly recommended as it serves multiple essential purposes in lipedema liposuction, significantly enhancing both the safety and efficacy of the procedure. The inclusion of lidocaine provides localized anesthesia, reducing the need for general anesthesia and improving post-operative comfort. Additionally, epinephrine induces vasoconstriction, which minimizes intraoperative blood loss and post-surgical bruising. By infiltrating the fat layer with fluid, the procedure facilitates the separation and removal of adipose tissue while minimizing trauma to surrounding structures. This technique also enhances overall safety by reducing complications such as excessive fluid loss and hematoma formation, making it a cornerstone of modern liposuction approaches for treating lipedema.

Lymphatic vessel sparing liposuction

Liposuction for lipedema should be performed in synchronicity with a lymph-sparing procedure and standard lymph-conscious practices. Fibro-lipo-lymph aspiration with lymph vessel sparing procedure (FLLA-LVSP) is the gold standard for lymphatic conservation in patients with lymphedema and lipedema with secondary lymphedema. It can also be applied to patients with lipedema alone. This procedure will be explained in greater detail later in this chapter.

Contrary to aesthetic liposuction, which often employs the so-called criss-cross technique for aspiration, LRS should be executed in a direction parallel to the lymphatic vessels to avoid the risk of damage and complications (see Figure 17.7). Caution should also be exercised regarding the cannula shape and sharpness, as these may pose a significant threat when positioned near lymphatic pathways. Finally, the negative pressure required for suctioning fatty tissue should also be well balanced. Sufficient pressure should be applied to achieve the desired debulking goals while prioritizing the conservation of surrounding tissue.

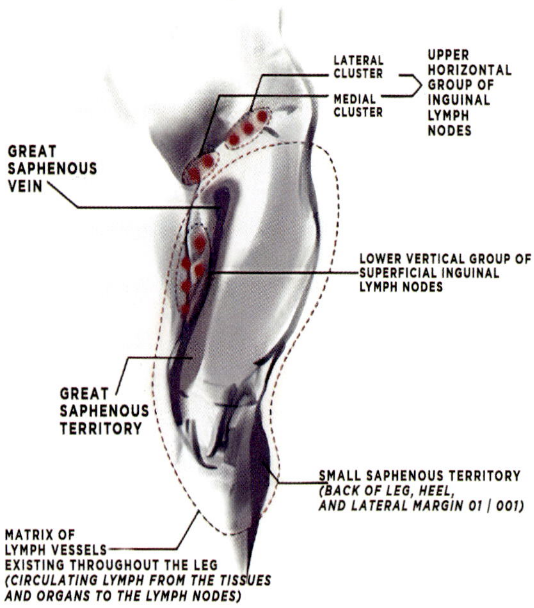

Figure 17.7: Diagram of the vein and lymphatic areas of importance in the lower limb. Courtesy of Dr. Campisi's Lab.

Very high negative pressure aspirates more fat cells more quickly, which consequently creates a higher risk of injury to tissue and lymphatic vessels.[3] A harmonious balance between manual dexterity and technological tools is of utmost importance.

Liposuction systems for lipedema reduction surgery

There are many forms of liposuction modalities used in LRS that are all great at precision SAT removal. Aside from the circumferential reduction of the patient's affected limbs, significant associated improvement of function and overall aesthetics are observed. LRS via liposuction is known to decrease symptoms and significantly elevate QoL. All of the following liposuction technologies used for LRS should be performed in combination with wet or tumescent methods. The dry methods (liposuctions without fluid) are strongly advised against; they can cause severe tissue trauma and often leave unnatural or unsightly dents, divots, or rippling on the body.[3]

The integration of ultrasound, laser, radiofrequency (RF), water-assisted, and power-assisted technologies in liposuction has significantly improved surgical outcomes for patients with lipedema, as well as for the general population. These methods enhance fat emulsification, reduce trauma to surrounding tissues, and promote better skin retraction. No technique is clinically proven to be superior to the others. The effectiveness of the selected technology relies heavily on the surgeon's capabilities and preferences.[3] Each technique offers its own unique set of advantages, including improved fat removal, minimized tissue trauma, and enhanced post-operative recovery. The modality is secondary; more important is the surgeon's training and overall experience with edema.

Based on our own experience at Campisi Clinic, hybrid systems are most promising overall. Ultrasound-assisted liposuction devices that incorporate aspects of power-assisted and suction-assisted technology, along with tumescent fluid injection, are considered the gold standard for LRS. This style of hybrid technology offers optimal results both functionally and aesthetically for patients, while dramatically reducing physical fatigue for the surgeon, particularly regarding the more strenuous efforts required to aspirate fibrotic SAT. Our opinion on this type of system is based on the post-operative results of more than 300 patients over 2 years (see Figure 17.8).

Ultrasound-assisted liposuction

Ultrasound-assisted liposuction (UAL) employs high-frequency ultrasonic waves to liquefy adipose tissue before aspiration. This minimally invasive technique facilitates fat removal while decreasing the risk of mechanical trauma, making it particularly advantageous for fibrotic lipedema tissue. The precision targeting of fat deposits is a key feature of this technology and technique. With ultrasound imaging, surgeons may identify and selectively remove lipedema fat, ensuring the preservation of healthy tissue and minimizing disruption to lymphatic vessels. The integration of ultrasound energy allows for the emulsification of fibrotic and diseased adipose tissue, facilitating its removal with less force and strain. The material contents of the extracted matter reveal predominantly fibrotic components, showing no injury to adipocytes, a minimal blood cell component, and no tissue distortion. The technique is safer and less aggressive, resulting in reduced post-operative pain, bruising, and swelling compared to traditional liposuction techniques. Additionally, the cavitation effect of ultrasound can promote lymphatic preservation and decrease post-operative swelling.

The downsides of the UAL method are few in respect to the advantages gained for both the patient and the surgeon. A prolonged operative time due to the ultrasonic fragmentation phase could be an initial deterrent for surgeons, and the technology carries a risk of thermal injury if not carefully controlled. As with all other methods of liposuction, a shallow learning curve is expected. When all this is compared to the incredible results and material characteristics of the aspirated matter, it's easy to see why UAL is the liposuction method of choice in all Campisi Clinics' surgical centers.

Laser-assisted liposuction

Laser-assisted liposuction (LAL) utilizes laser energy to break down and destroy fat cells while simultaneously sparing the surrounding tissue, stimulating collagen production, and thereby promoting skin shrinkage with associated tightening effects. This method is particularly beneficial for patients with mild skin laxity, as it can help enhance post-surgical contouring. Furthermore, laser energy has a coagulative impact, reducing intraoperative bleeding and post-operative bruising. Despite these advantages, LAL may generate excessive heat, posing a risk of burns or prolonged inflammation. This method especially requires an experienced surgeon who is an expert in the technology. There are significant risks of unsightly scars, dents, or defects after burns caused by laser. The effectiveness of LAL

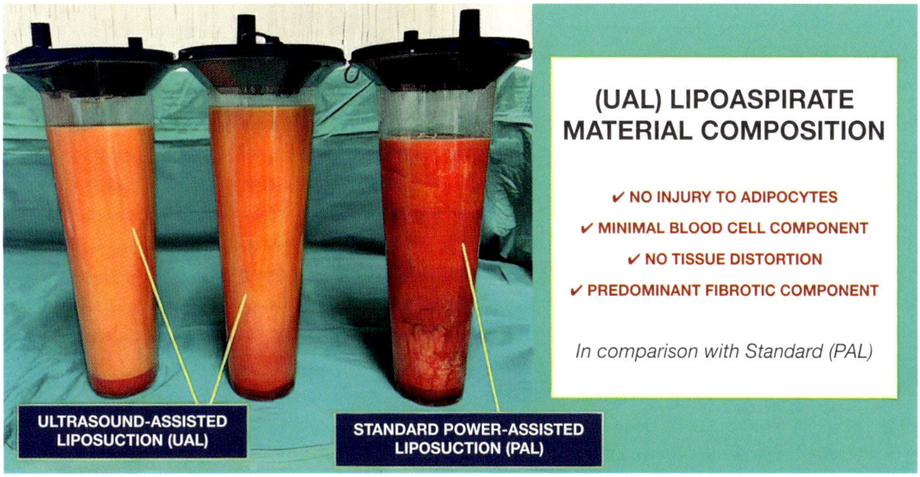

Figure 17.8: Precision aspiration of ultrasound-assisted liposuction (UAL). Material composition: UAL vs. standard power-assisted liposuction (PAL). Courtesy of Dr. Campisi.

in treating extensive lipedema deposits remains debated. Tissue shrinkage promoted by LAL should not be the primary criterion for choosing this technique, since comparable results can be achieved with specialized cannulas or adjunctive skin tightening devices.

Radiofrequency-assisted liposuction

Radiofrequency-assisted liposuction (RFAL) applies RF energy to heat and emulsify fat while simultaneously tightening the surrounding skin. This dual effect makes it particularly useful for patients with more advanced lipedema, who may experience significant skin laxity following fat removal. RF energy also enhances vascular coagulation, reducing blood loss during surgery. However, similar to laser techniques, excessive thermal exposure can increase the risk of burns, and the procedure requires precise temperature monitoring to avoid complications.

Water-assisted liposuction

Water-assisted liposuction (WAL) utilizes a pulsating jet of tumescent solution to dislodge fat gently, reducing mechanical trauma and preserving lymphatic structures. WAL is particularly advantageous for patients with lipedema due to its tissue-sparing properties, which help maintain vascular and lymphatic integrity. Additionally, this technique minimizes post-operative swelling and discomfort, leading to a smoother recovery. However, WAL may require longer operative times compared to energy-based liposuction techniques, and its efficacy in managing fibrotic tissue can be limited.

Power-assisted liposuction

Power-assisted liposuction (PAL) utilizes a rapidly vibrating cannula to facilitate fat removal, thereby reducing the physical effort required by the surgeon and enhancing procedural efficiency. This method is beneficial for treating fibrotic or advanced-stage lipedema, where fat deposits are denser and more resistant to manual extraction. PAL allows for precise fat removal while minimizing tissue trauma. However, it does not offer the skin-tightening benefits of energy-based liposuction techniques, which may necessitate additional post-operative interventions for optimal contouring.

Fibro-lipo-lymph aspiration with lymph vessel sparing procedure

The lymph vessel-sparing procedure, known as fibro-lipo-lymph-aspiration with a lymph vessel sparing procedure (FLLA-LVSP), is a surgical technique developed to treat advanced stages of lymphedema and any stage of standard lipedema. This minimally invasive method focuses on removing excess fibrotic and fatty tissue while meticulously preserving the integrity of lymphatic vessels to prevent or cause further lymphatic damage. The procedure begins with preoperative mapping of the lymphatic vessels using imaging techniques, such as indocyanine green (ICG) lymphography and ultra-high-frequency ultrasound (UHFUS) mapping of the superficial lymphatics (see Figure 17.9). This mapping allows surgeons to identify and avoid lymphatic channels during the aspiration process. The ISL emphasizes the importance of lymphatic-sparing techniques to preserve lymphatic integrity during fat removal. This procedure significantly reduces pain, restores mobility, and improves quality of life when performed by experienced surgeons.[2]

During surgery, specialized liposuction cannulas are used to aspirate the pathological adipose and fibrotic tissue, carefully sparing the lymphatic vessels identified during pre-operative mapping. This approach ensures that the removal of excess tissue does not compromise existing lymphatic function. See Figure 17.10 for a tissue comparison of standard liposuction versus FLLA-LVSP. FLLA-LVSP is the gold standard procedure in lymph-sparing for LRS and/or the debulking of lymphedema-related fibrotic tissue. It is suitable and safe to apply in conjunction with lymphatic microsurgery.[3, 9, 10]

Clinical outcomes of the FLLA-LVSP have been promising. Studies have reported significant reductions in limb volume and improvements in symptoms, such as heaviness and discomfort. For instance, in one study, patients experienced an average reduction in excess limb volume from 20.19% to 2.68% in the upper limbs and from 21.24% to 2.64% in the lower limbs after undergoing the procedure.[9] The surgery is efficient, with the entire leg being completed within approximately 90 minutes. Patients often benefit from immediate cosmetic improvements and a short recovery time.

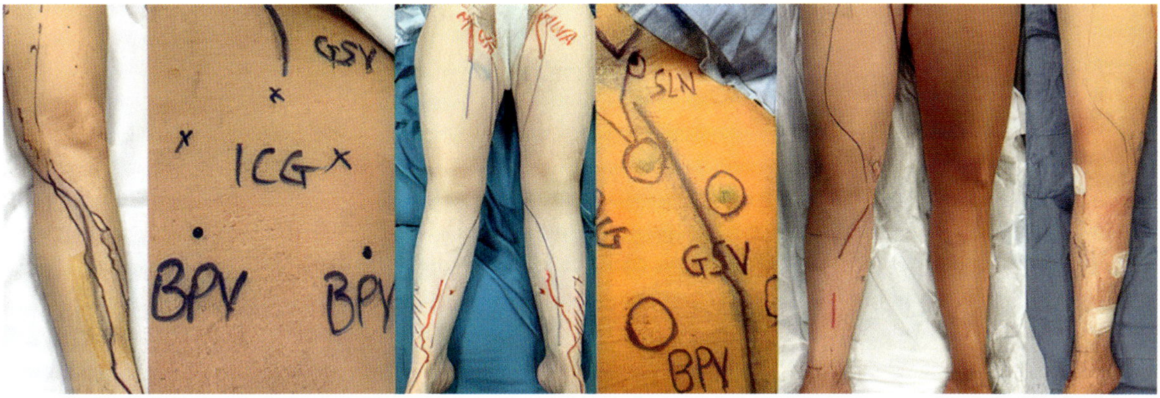

Figure 17.9: Perioperative lymph vessel sparing mapping techniques. Courtesy of Dr. Campisi.

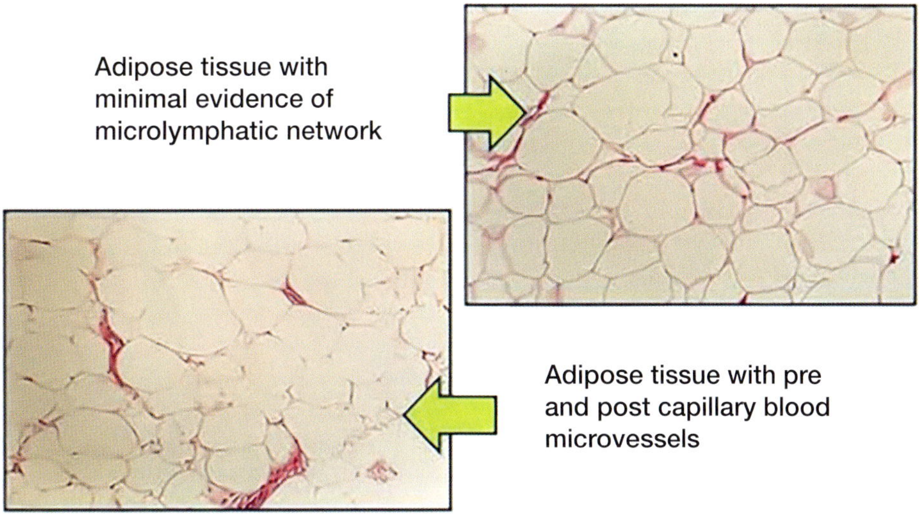

Figure 17.10: Tissue analysis comparing the standard liposuction method (top) with the fibro-lipo-lymph aspiration lymph vessel sparing procedure (FLLA-LVSP) technique. Courtesy of Dr. Campisi's Lab.

For patients with impaired lymphatic function, such as those with diagnosed lipedema with secondary lymphedema, FLLA-LVSP should be performed in conjunction with or after other lymphatic surgeries, such as multiple lymphatic-venous anastomoses (MLVA). This combined or consecutive surgical approach offers a comprehensive treatment strategy by first restoring lymphatic flow through MLVA and subsequently removing residual fibrotic and fatty tissue with FLLA-LVSP.[11,12]

Surgical indications for lipedema with lymphatic insufficiency

The progression of lipedema into more advanced stages causes significant strain on the lymphatic system, potentially triggering a secondary lymphedema. This may arise conversely, in that lymphedema is the initial pathology, and as a result of lymph stagnation, deposits of fibrotic tissue manifest throughout the affected body parts. In some cases, both pathologies (lymphedema and lipedema) have a simultaneous onset. These complex pathologies ultimately involve both disproportionate adipose deposition and lymphatic dysfunction, and this presents a unique challenge in treatment. Surgical intervention, when conservative management has been optimized yet remains insufficient, provides a pathway to meaningful improvement in symptoms and quality of life. Among the available techniques, MLVA (Figure 17.11) and FLLA-LVSP have emerged as the most promising procedures, offering targeted solutions for addressing the multifaceted aspects of these diseases with long-term success rates.

Multiple lymphatic-venous anastomosis

Multiple lymphatic-venous anastomosis (MLVA) is a derivative microsurgical technique designed to restore lymphatic circulation by creating anastomoses between lymphatic vessels and veins. MLVA is an advanced refinement of the lymphatic-venous anastomosis (LVA) technique. LVA and lymphatic-venous bypass (LVB) are often used interchangeably to describe the same super microsurgical procedure used to treat lymphedema. LVB is sometimes used in a broader sense, including cases where multiple anastomoses are performed in a single procedure, whereas LVA and MLVA are considered distinct procedures. As the name suggests, MLVA involves

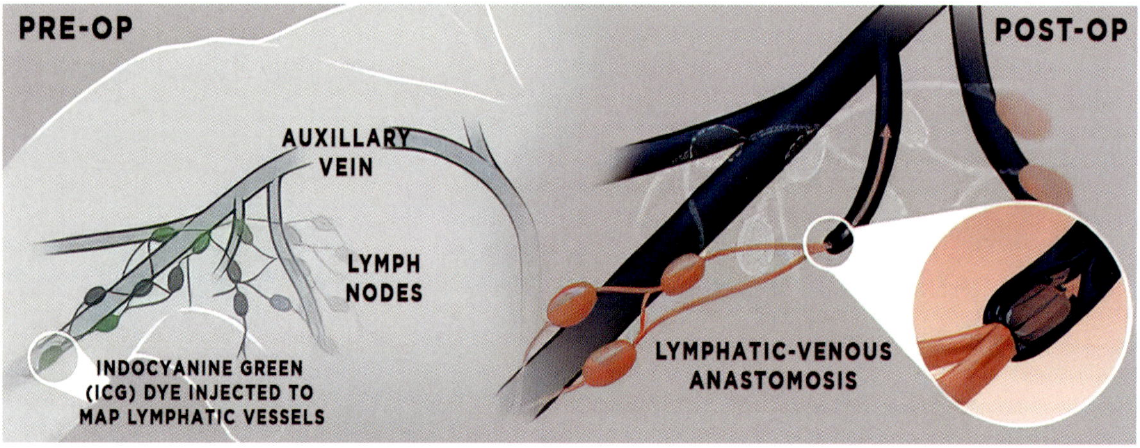

Figure 17.11: Diagram of multiple lymphatic-venous anastomosis (MLVA) of the upper limb. Courtesy of Dr. Campisi.

the creation of multiple anastomoses within a single incision site (see Figure 17.12), whereas LVA consists of a singular connection. The MLVA approach enhances lymphatic drainage efficiency by facilitating multiple pathways for lymphatic outflow, which may improve long-term surgical outcomes. The procedure directly addresses lymphatic dysfunction, which is almost always the root or adjunct cause of chronic swelling and tissue fibrosis seen in lipedema with secondary lymphedema.

The surgery involves meticulous identification of functional lymphatic vessels using indocyanine green (ICG) lymphography or fluorescein dye mapping, followed by their connection to adjacent venous structures. The careful selection of lymphatic vessels and a suitable collateral branch of a main vein is of major importance. Poor selection and/or execution may lead to a thrombosis, risking the compromise of the entire intervention. The joining of two circulatory systems stimulates a new consistent and natural flow of lymphatic fluid by employing the kinetic perpetual pumping of the venous counterpart. The highly sophisticated and particularly minuscule microsurgical procedure was developed as a treatment for lymphedema by way of surgically rerouting blocked or damaged lymphatic pathways. MLVA involves creating multiple connections, or anastomoses, between lymphatic vessels and nearby veins (see Figure 17.13 A and B). This bypass alleviates lymphatic stasis, reducing swelling and improving tissue oxygenation. Before microsurgery, the patient must complete a rigorous cycle of CDT to enter the operating room in the most optimal condition with as little edema as possible. This is critical, as the surgeon will be able to assess and work with the microscopic lymphatics more easily in a decongested limb or body part.[2, 3, 11, 12]

Key advantages of MLVA include:

- Physiological restoration: Promotes natural lymphatic drainage.
- Minimally invasive nature: Reduces downtime and allows for faster recovery compared to other invasive procedures.
- Durable outcomes: Significantly decreases limb circumference and improves skin texture over time.

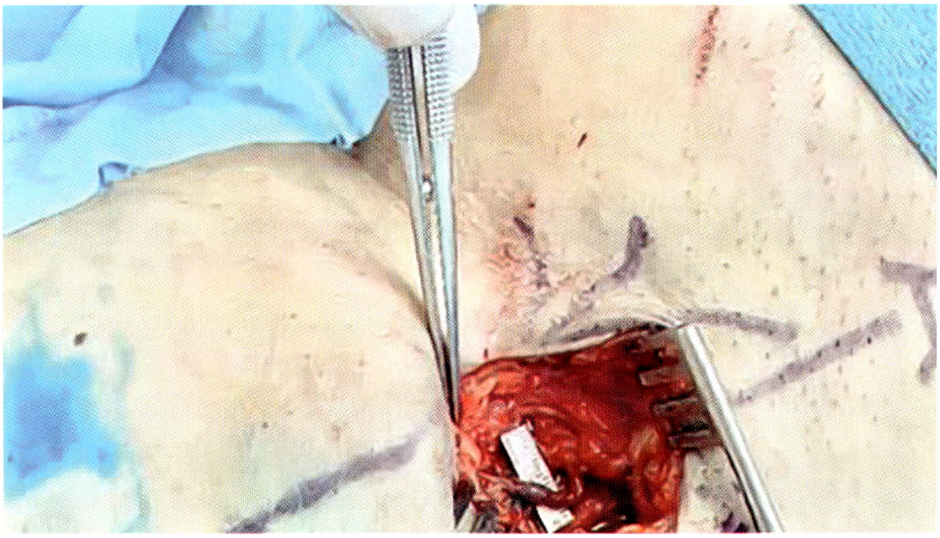

Figure 17.12: Inguinal incision point showing successful MLVA, as performed by Dr. Corrado Campisi.

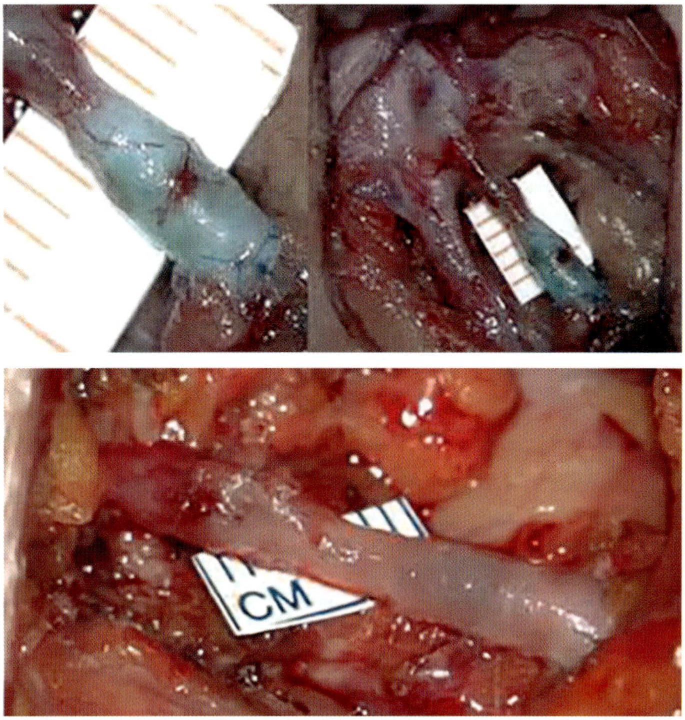

Figure 17.13: Multiple lymphatic-venous anastomosis (MLVA) by Dr. Corrado Campisi.

The success of MLVA depends on the surgeon's expertise in microsurgical techniques, particularly in identifying and preserving fragile lymphatic structures. When MLVA is performed successfully, the volumetric reductions are astonishing and long-lasting, successfully achieving remission of lymphatic dysfunction.

Synergy between MLVA and lymph sparing lipedema reduction surgery

In cases where lipedema exists alongside lymphatic dysfunction, and even in advanced lipedema with secondary lymphedema, combining MLVA and LRS can yield superior results (see Figure 17.14). While MLVA addresses lymphatic flow dysfunction, LRS reduces adipose tissue volume, which can exacerbate lymphatic compromise. Together, these techniques offer a comprehensive approach, targeting both structural and functional components of both diseases. MLVA should always be done first, even when both interventions are programmed to be done perioperatively. FLLA-LVSP is the most recommended LRS technique due to its overall safety. Surgeons unfamiliar with lymphatic mapping and/or lacking the technology to do so successfully should employ alternative lymph vessel sparing protocols to protect the lymphatic system.[11, 12]

By integrating these procedures into a tailored treatment plan, the dual goals of symptom relief and long-term management can be achieved. The precision of MLVA, coupled with lymphatic preservation protocols, underscores the importance of a specialized approach – one that is best carried out by expert lymphatic surgeons with a deep understanding of both diseases, such as those at the forefront of lymphological advancements.

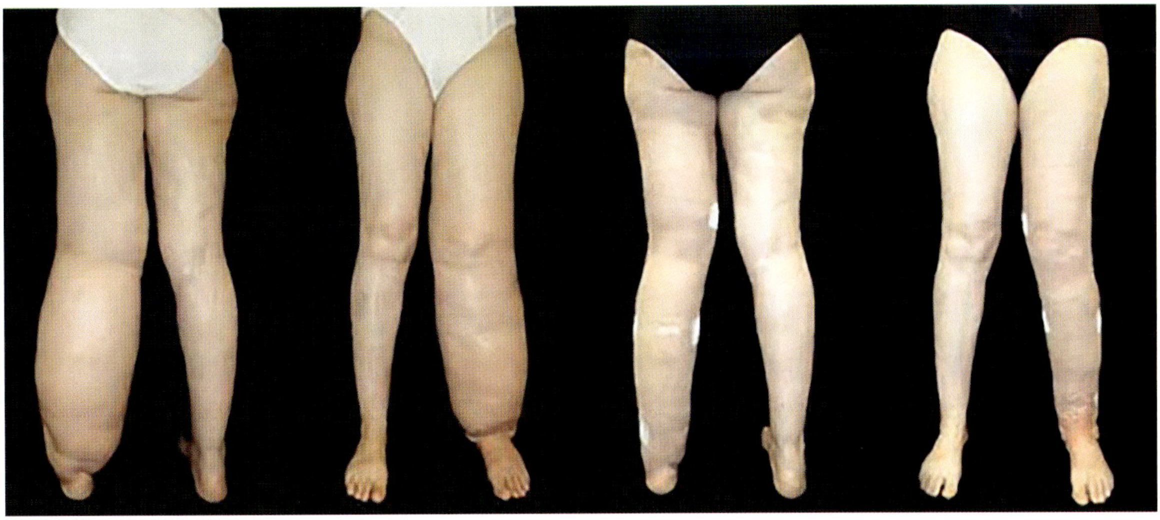

Figure 17.14: Post-op results from multiple lymphatic-venous anastomosis (MLVA) and fibro-lipo-lymph aspiration with lymph vessel sparing procedure (FLLA-LVSP). Courtesy of Dr. Campisi.

Skin tightening surgery

The best practices for LRS are to remove SAT gradually, either through multiple interventions or by first performing an MLVA if necessary. Large-volume aspirations or excisions in a single sitting are outdated and strongly recommended against.[3] Patients, especially those suffering from advanced stages of lipedema, should exercise caution when choosing a surgeon. It is essential to look for a practitioner who is not only well-versed in liposuction for LRS but also an expert lymphologist and plastic surgeon who can also perform skin tightening surgeries if needed. This is particularly important with conserving and/or ameliorating lymphatic function post-operatively. Thigh lift and arm lift procedures are particularly risky as they can trigger a secondary lymphedema. These skin-lifting procedures, when performed without careful consideration of the lymphatic system and its abundant vessel matrix and node clusters located in those same areas, pose a substantial risk of major complications.

When a patient suffers from pronounced lipedema, the volume reduction should be divided into smaller volumetric debulking phases to achieve a more natural final body contour. A surgeon should prioritize minimizing the risk of complications by avoiding damage to the lymphatic system and preventing the need for supplementary skin tightening surgeries. Multiple surgical interventions may seem economically and/or psychologically more strenuous for the patient, but the effects achieved are far more desirable. The healing process is also smoother and less traumatic when approached in a stepped process. Skin elasticity has its limitations. A staged debulking allows for the skin to contract and adjust itself gradually with each circumferential change. Extra-large volumetric aspirations do not yield satisfactory functional and aesthetic results, nor are they justified when considering overall risk.[3]

When skin removal is necessary, procedures such as thigh lifts and arm lifts can address excess skin issues post-operatively. However, it's imperative to perform these surgeries with meticulous care to preserve the lymphatic structures inherent in these regions. A surgeon with a thorough

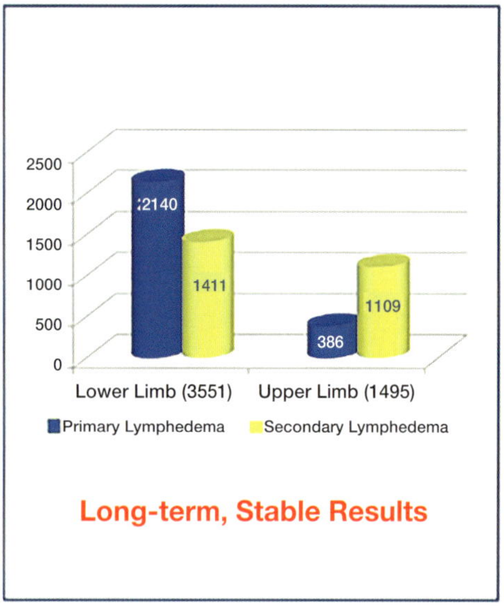

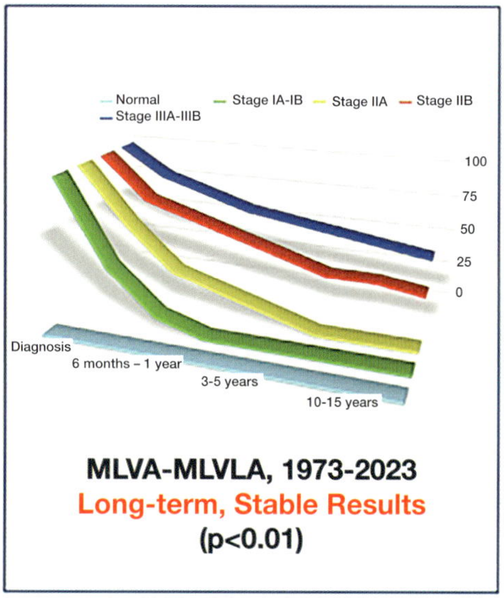

Figure 17.15: Campisi Clinic surgical data, 1973–2023. Over 5000 cases treated with microsurgery, MLVA / MLVLA (follow up: 5 to 20 plus years). Courtesy of Dr. Campisi's Lab.

understanding of lymphatic anatomy and the use of lymph-sparing surgical approaches is essential to minimize the risk of post-operative lymphatic complications. Collaborating with a surgical team experienced in both lipedema management and lymphatic preservation is crucial for optimizing patient outcomes and maintaining lymphatic health.[13]

Patient reported outcomes after lipedema reduction surgery

Most notably, there is decreased swelling and less need for compression. Sensations of pain, discomfort, and bruising also diminish. Mobility is improved, and QoL is boosted. Weight loss, weight control, and long-term weight management all become easier. Significant improvements are also observed with body image and emotional responses. Many patients experience stage reversal.

Patients with or at risk for lymphatic impairment experience significant volumetric changes when having MLVA surgery before or in conjunction with lymph vessel sparing LRS, such as FLLA-LVSP. Results are sustainable in the long term, and most patients reduce their need for CDT and compression garments after surgery. Stage reversal or remission is achievable through this method.

Patients with lipedema who undergo surgery experience a significant reduction in spontaneous pain, pressure sensitivity, feeling of tension, bruising, and general impairment.[4] Almost all patients experience improved mobility.[14] Increased mobility correlates with significant increases in patient overall QoL. Patient-reported postoperative outcomes show reduced pain and improvements in walking speed, stair climbing, and sit-to-stand functions, which in turn enhance emotional and social well-being. LRS results in tissue changes that are consistent with stage regression in some patients.[15] See Figure 17.15 for Campisi Clinic surgical outcomes data. Notable improvement in lymphatic function is also observed after surgery. Tissue injury during surgery could result in connections between lymphatic vessels and veins, allowing lymph to be delivered directly to the bloodstream. Injuries to the respective muscle fascia could promote drainage of the lymph from the superficial to the deep lymphatic vascular system.[3]

The physical effects of surgery manifest across both major and minor aspects of patients' daily functioning. Enhanced mobility and reduced symptom burden are among the most significant improvements, contributing to downstream benefits in overall QoL. Patients frequently report increased energy levels and greater ease in achieving or maintaining weight loss. Additionally, we have observed successful stage reversal of lipedema in many cases, particularly among patients who undergo surgical intervention during the earlier stages of the disease.

The emotional toll of the disease is also known to be significantly reduced after LRS. Patients who suffer from profuse psychological duress from the complications of lipedema report feeling happier post-operatively. Simple daily activities that lipedema rendered taxing for patients become more enjoyable again. Restrictions on the types of clothing and/or shoes they can wear may diminish after debulking. A single surgical procedure can help reduce clothing sizes by 1 to 3 sizes.[4] The significant reduction in the need for complete decongestive therapy after LRS is a major motivation for those considering surgical intervention as a treatment.

Conclusion

Exploring innovative and adjunctive surgical techniques that enhance patient outcomes beyond traditional liposuction is of utmost importance, given the complex pathophysiology of lipedema. These alternative approaches aim to improve lymphatic function, reduce fibrotic tissue, and optimize contouring while mitigating disease progression. Comprehensive, patient-centered treatment is necessary to advance the disease's treatment further towards a cure. By integrating the supplementary strategies discussed in detail, clinicians can provide a more holistic and effective approach to managing lipedema, addressing both functional and aesthetic concerns to improve patients' quality of life.

References

1. Buso G, Depairon M, Tomson D, Raffoul W, Vettor R, Mazzolai L. Lipedema: a call to action! *Obesity*. 2019 Oct;27(10):1567–76. DOI: https://doi.org/10.1002/oby.22597
2. Consensus 2023. The diagnosis and treatment of peripheral lymphedema: 2023 Consensus document of the International Society of Lymphology. *Lymphology*. 2024 Aug 27;56(4). Available from: http://journals.librarypublishing.arizona.edu/lymph/article/id/6372/
3. Jandali Z, Jiga LP, Campisi C, editors. Lipedema: A Practical Guidebook. Cham: Springer International Publishing; 2022. Available from: https://link.springer.com/10.1007/978-3-030-86717-1
4. Herbst KL, Hansen EA, Cobos Salinas LM, Wright TF, Larson EE, Schwartz JS. Survey outcomes of lipedema reduction surgery in the United States. *Plast Reconstr Surg – Glob Open*. 2021 Apr;9(4):e3553. DOI: https://doi.org/10.1097/GOX.0000000000003553
5. Rasmussen JC, Aldrich MB, Fife CE, Herbst KL, Sevick-Muraca EM. Lymphatic function and anatomy in early stages of lipedema. *Obesity*. 2022;30(7):1391–400. DOI: https://doi.org/10.1002/oby.23458
6. Herbst KL. Rare adipose disorders (RADs) masquerading as obesity. *Acta Pharmacol Sin*. 2012 Feb;33(2):155–72. DOI: https://doi.org/10.1038/aps.2011.153
7. Bejar-Chapa M, Rossi N, King N, Hussey MR, Winograd JM, Guastaldi FPS. Liposuction as a treatment for lipedema: a scoping

review. *Plast Reconstr Surg – Glob Open*. 2024 Jul;12(7):e5952. DOI: https://doi.org/10.1097/GOX.0000000000005952

8. Witte T, Dadras M, Heck FC, Heck M, Habermalz B, Welss S, et al. Water-jet-assisted liposuction for the treatment of lipedema: standardized treatment protocol and results of 63 patients. *J Plast Reconstr Aesthet Surg*. 2020 Sep 1;73(9):1637–44. DOI: https://doi.org/10.1016/j.bjps.2020.03.002
9. Campisi CC, Ryan M, Boccardo F, Campisi C. Fibro-lipo-lymph-aspiration with a lymph vessel sparing procedure to treat advanced lymphedema after multiple lymphatic-venous anastomoses: the complete treatment protocol. *Ann Plast Surg*. 2017 Feb;78(2):184. DOI: https://doi.org/10.1097/SAP.0000000000000853
10. Campisi CC, Ryan M, Boccardo F, Campisi C. Prevention of lymphatic injuries with lymphatic mapping: the combined technique. *J Plast Reconstr Aesthet Surg*. 2016 Aug 1;69(8):e164–5. DOI: https://doi.org/10.1016/j.bjps.2016.04.025
11. Campisi CC, Molinari L, Campisi CS, Villa G, Fulcheri E, Campisi C, et al. Surgical research, staging-guided technical procedures and long-term clinical outcomes for the treatment of peripheral lymphedema: the Genoa Protocol. *J Surg Surg Res*. 2020 May 28;6(1):041–50. DOI: https://doi.org/10.17352/2455-2968.000096
12. Villa G, Campisi CC, Ryan M, Boccardo F, Di Summa P, Frascio M, et al. Procedural recommendations for lymphoscintigraphy in the diagnosis of peripheral lymphedema: the Genoa Protocol. *Nucl Med Mol Imaging*. 2019 Feb 1;53(1):47–56. DOI: https://doi.org/10.1007/s13139-018-0565-2
13. Vitorasso C de SR, Silva ACB, Batista BP de SN, Kamamoto F. Lymphatic Improvement after suction-assisted lipectomy in a lipedema patient. Plast Reconstr Surg – Glob Open. 2023 Jun;11(6):e5097. DOI: https://doi.org/10.1097/GOX.0000000000005097
14. Wollina U, Heinig B. Treatment of lipedema by low-volume micro-cannular liposuction in tumescent anesthesia: results in 111 patients. *Dermatol Ther*. 2019;32(2):e12820. DOI: https://doi.org/10.1111/dth.12820
15. Wright T, Babula M, Schwartz J, Wright C, Danesh N, Herbst K. Lipedema reduction surgery improves pain, mobility, physical function, and quality of life: case series report. *Plast Reconstr Surg – Glob Open*. 2023 Nov;11(11):e5436. DOI: https://doi.org/10.1097/GOX.0000000000005436

VII
Self-care and resources: tools and support

Chapter Eighteen
Self-care strategies for lipedema

Kate Forster

Introduction

As a chronic and often misunderstood disease, lipedema presents unique challenges that extend beyond medical management alone. For individuals living with lipedema, self-care plays a critical role in maintaining physical function, managing symptoms, and enhancing quality of life. However, the effectiveness of self-care is closely tied to the level of understanding and support offered by healthcare practitioners. This chapter examines how practitioner knowledge, or lack thereof, can influence patient outcomes and engagement in self-management. It also explores structured self-care programs developed in various countries, highlighting diverse approaches to education and empowerment. Finally, the chapter provides a detailed review of evidence-based self-care practices tailored to lipedema, offering practical guidance to support individualized, sustainable, and informed strategies for daily living with this complex disease.

Defining self-care

A key initial challenge in practicing self-care for lipedema is understanding what self-care truly entails – what it includes, and just as importantly, what it does not. Because lipedema primarily affects women, many patients are already exposed to a wide range of self-care messaging in popular media. These messages often emphasize relaxation-oriented practices such as gentle exercise, eating healthy foods, lighting candles, taking baths, and engaging in mindfulness or meditation. While these activities may offer general benefits, self-care for individuals living with lipedema requires a more targeted and structured approach.

In Germany, the importance of patient-centered self-management is formally recognized in the S2 Guidelines for Lipedema,[1] following its initial inclusion in the earlier S1 Guidelines.[2] Recommendation 9.1 of the S2 guidelines underscores the centrality of active patient engagement:

'Effective self-management is an important component of health literacy. It shall be promoted, and the patient shall be encouraged to take an active role. Problem-solving strategies and specific therapeutic aims shall be developed together to promote the increase of self-efficacy.'[1]

The authors further emphasize the patient's essential role in their care:

'...Apart from the caregiver, the woman affected by lipedema herself might then be the person with the greatest influence on treatment success.'[1]

This emphasis on agency and active participation reflects a broader shift in global health systems toward supporting self-care as a vital component of managing chronic diseases. As the World Health Organization (WHO) notes, self-care is not a new concept, but its advancements in technology increasingly shape its modern evolution:

'The ability of individuals, families, and communities to … cope with illness and disability with or without the support of a health worker, is nothing new. But new products, information, and technologies are changing – and have the potential to change – how people access healthcare, as well.'[3]

Together, these perspectives underscore the importance of empowering individuals with lipedema to take an informed and proactive role in their care, supported by evidence-based guidance, community resources, and emerging technologies.

The role of healthcare services in self-care

An essential first step in implementing effective self-care strategies for lipedema is obtaining an accurate and timely diagnosis. Unfortunately, due to widespread lack of awareness about the disease among healthcare professionals, diagnosis is often delayed by several decades. An accurate diagnosis not only validates the individual's lived experience but also allows for appropriate differential diagnosis, helping to distinguish lipedema-related symptoms from those caused by other medical conditions. This distinction is critical, as not all symptoms experienced by someone with lipedema necessarily originate from the disease itself.

The average age of diagnosis is approximately 44, although symptoms often begin during puberty.[4] This long diagnostic delay means that many individuals spend years not understanding why their bodies respond differently from those of their peers. For instance, others may experience more flexibility in weight gain or loss and do not report the same lower-body pain or discomfort. In the absence of a diagnosis, people with lipedema frequently receive self-care advice from family, friends, or even clinicians that directly conflicts with their own bodily experiences. This may include persistent recommendations for calorie restriction, skepticism about reports of pain or hypersensitivity, or even misdiagnoses that result in ineffective or inappropriate treatments.

Such diagnostic delays are not unique to lipedema; they are also common in other diseases that develop gradually and do not prompt urgent medical intervention. For example, international research on diseases like celiac disease reveals that well-being often improves substantially after an accurate diagnosis and the initiation of symptom-relieving treatment.[5]

Similarly, responses from participants in the *Lipoedema UK Big Survey*[4] highlight the emotional and psychological relief that comes with finally receiving recognition and appropriate care from healthcare professionals:

'To be spoken to as a patient with an illness made a huge difference, and to be helped to manage the condition made me look at my own body in a different way for the first time in possibly 45 years. The nurse I saw was excellent, and she told me to love my legs because they were my legs. This was life-changing for me.'

'…It was wonderful to be listened to and be taken seriously and to be treated with compassion, caring, and dignity after being ignored and dismissed for fifty years. Even writing this is making me tearful.'

'It was great to have a name to put to my symptoms finally. It all fell into place, and I didn't feel like I was going mad anymore. Also happy that my fat legs weren't 'my fault'…'

Receiving a diagnosis helps individuals reframe symptoms previously considered 'normal' or inevitable as medically significant. Pain, in particular, is often misunderstood or underrecognized. As shared by a representative of a Dutch patient advocacy organization during the 2023

Lipedema World Congress in Potsdam, patients usually only recognize sensations as pain when others point out that their experiences are not typical. Nootenboom[6] relayed several poignant patient reflections:

'Only after someone told me they didn't experience the same sensation, I realized it was pain.'

'You don't know something is painful until you experience it differently'.

This lack of awareness often extends across generations. Many patients report having family members, especially mothers or daughters, with undiagnosed lipedema who, similarly, had not realized that symptoms like pain or swelling were abnormal until receiving a diagnosis:

'Because my mom and I both have it, I didn't know that other people did not experience the same discomfort as we did'.[6]

Anecdotal reports from other countries echo these insights underscoring the transformative role of diagnosis, not only in individual care but also in raising awareness within families. Effective self-care, therefore, often begins with a profound re-evaluation of long-held beliefs about health and bodily norms. Diagnosis can prompt a necessary 'reset' in how individuals understand their symptoms and can also lead to earlier identification and support for affected family members. Healthcare practitioners play a pivotal role in initiating this process, reinforcing the importance of clinical awareness, empathy, and timely intervention.

Impact of healthcare providers on self-care

Engaging with healthcare providers for education and support in managing lipedema is often challenging due to significant variability in professional knowledge about the disease. Unlike patient advocacy organizations, which typically offer more focused and up-to-date resources, many healthcare professionals lack adequate training or awareness of lipedema. A 2022 survey of 600 patients with lipedema in Norway revealed that four out of six respondents felt disappointed or disillusioned during their initial consultation with a healthcare provider.[7] Many reported being advised simply to lose weight or being told that their pain was normal. Alarmingly, only about one-third of respondents were referred to a physiotherapist or specialist. These findings highlight a persistent gap in primary care services and underscore the need for greater access to specialized care if healthcare providers are to play an effective role in supporting patient self-management.

Lipedema self-care programs

Learning about self-care for lipedema can vary significantly from person to person. Many individuals turn to the internet, which offers access to the latest information and emerging practices. While this accessibility can be beneficial, it also presents challenges. Without a clear understanding of research methodology or the ability to critically evaluate sources, individuals may struggle to differentiate between evidence-based guidance, commercial marketing, and anecdotal reports. As a result, reliance on unverified information may lead to confusion or the adoption of ineffective or even harmful interventions. For this reason, guidance from a knowledgeable and experienced healthcare practitioner is strongly recommended whenever possible.

There are numerous advantages to having informed healthcare professionals engage in conversations with patients about self-care and self-management. One key benefit is the encouragement of ongoing self-assessment and reflection, an approach supported in the literature on chronic disease management. Recognizing that self-motivation can fluctuate and that personal priorities often shift over time reinforces the importance of integrating self-care into routine clinical discussions and reviews. As de Iongh[8] notes:

'Understanding what is important to the patient at the time is vital, and often this means quality of life rather than clinical markers. I apologise if what is important to me – being able to socialise, drive, or wear nice shoes without orthotics – doesn't fit with what doctors need to achieve clinically. Still, hopefully we can work towards both of these with a shared agenda and mutual respect and understanding.'

The availability and quality of self-care education vary widely across healthcare systems, often limited by provider training, healthcare infrastructure, and funding constraints. A comprehensive overview of global programs would exceed the scope of this chapter; instead, the following section highlights a few representative examples available at the time of writing. Each program has been in operation for approximately five years or more and was selected to illustrate a range of educational and delivery approaches.

Germany

In Germany, the organization Lymphselbsthilfe e.V. has developed a structured self-help education program known as GALLiLy. This acronym loosely translates to 'living a healthy and active life with lipedema and lymphedema'.[9] This program, delivered in four-day sessions, is funded through Germany's self-help support system and reflects a culturally embedded approach to self-management education.

Initially, Lymphselbsthilfe focused its educational content on lymphedema, but more recently, it has expanded to include individuals with lipedema. Importantly, the program does not offer generalized guidance on obesity management, maintaining instead a condition-specific focus. The sessions are designed to empower participants by helping them recognize and build upon their existing self-care strategies, particularly about nutrition, physical activity, and symptom management. A key feature of the program is its emphasis on a 'slow and steady' approach to goal setting, encouraging participants to focus on one topic at a time.

This incremental model contrasts with the urgency often seen among newly diagnosed individuals seeking advice in online forums. These individuals frequently express a desire to enact sweeping changes rapidly, in the hope of quickly improving their quality of life. The GALLiLy program, by contrast, is grounded in the belief that a lack of confidence in one's ability to succeed, rather than a lack of motivation, is often the primary barrier to sustained behavior change. It acknowledges the common fear that managing lipedema will require overwhelming effort and sacrifice, and instead offers a supportive, paced environment where sustainable progress is prioritized.

United Kingdom

In the United Kingdom, the patient advocacy organization Lipoedema UK offers a more flexible and open-ended approach to self-care education through its Members' Webinars (see page 277 for links and further details). These weekly online sessions cover a wide range of topics relevant to those living with lipedema. Each session lasts approximately one hour and is available to all members, both in real-time and as recorded content for later viewing. The sessions are organized into four primary categories:

1. **Expert presentations** by international healthcare professionals, sharing current research and clinical findings relevant to lipedema management.
2. **Monthly clinical advisor sessions**, facilitated by healthcare professionals in the UK (including nurses, manual lymphatic drainage (MLD) therapists, and lipedema specialists) who volunteer with Lipoedema UK. These sessions employ a question-and-answer format to address a wide range of topics tailored to participant needs. They are particularly beneficial for individuals who are newly diagnosed,

experiencing difficulty accessing local support, or seeking tailored guidance on specific aspects of self-care.

3. **Emotional support and mental well-being**, including motivational tools and strategies for psychological resilience, stress reduction, and self-management.
4. **Personal stories and peer inspiration**, often focusing on daily life with lipedema. While the central theme is lipedema, sessions may occasionally explore related diseases or broader topics of interest to the community.

Unlike structured educational programs, this model has no attendance requirements or prescribed pathways. It allows individuals to self-direct their learning, choose topics based on personal relevance, and implement changes at their own pace. Participants are free to engage as frequently or selectively as they wish, fostering a sense of autonomy and personalization in the self-care process.

The regular frequency of these sessions offers additional benefits. Not only do they provide opportunities to engage with the most up-to-date information and clinical perspectives, but they also allow individuals to revisit and reinforce key concepts over time. Moreover, the sessions create a consistent space for connection with others affected by lipedema, fostering community, shared experience, and mutual support.

Programs in other countries

Self-directed education is not unique to Germany and the United Kingdom. ABRALI in Brazil, for instance, offers monthly educational sessions to its members. Please refer to Chapter 19 for a list of organizations, along with their contact information.

Self-care interventions for lipedema

A wide range of interventions may be considered as part of a self-care approach to lipedema (see Figure 18.1), although the strength of evidence supporting their efficacy is often limited. Many of these interventions overlap with established treatment strategies, but when performed independently by patients, they are considered forms of self-care. This section explores several of the most common and accessible options.

A key principle of effective self-care for lipedema is the need for individualized assessment; patients must determine for themselves whether a particular intervention yields meaningful improvement in their symptoms. However, this process can be challenging, as there is currently no standardized self-assessment tool specifically designed for lipedema. A thoughtful, incremental approach, where one change is implemented at a time and sufficient time is allowed to evaluate its impact before introducing another, can be illuminating, though it requires patience and discipline. Moreover, there is no fixed timeframe in which the benefits of a given intervention can be expected to manifest fully. The effectiveness of various strategies may also change in response to significant life transitions, such as menopause or post-surgical recovery. A previously unsuccessful intervention may prove beneficial under different physiological or emotional circumstances.

Despite the variability in individual responses, there is consensus around several core self-care strategies for lipedema:

1. **Ways of eating** While Chapter 14 provides a detailed discussion of nutritional approaches and their potential to reduce inflammation, pain, and limb volume, our focus here is on the role of eating behaviors within the context of self-care. Self-care involves not only managing

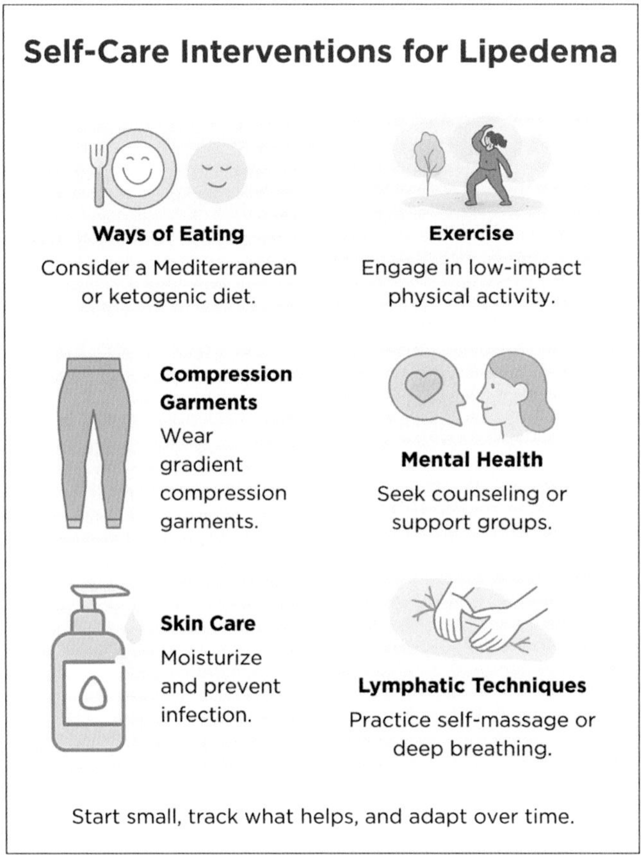
Self-Care Interventions for Lipedema
Ways of Eating
Consider a Mediterranean or ketogenic diet.
Exercise
Engage in low-impact physical activity.
Compression Garments
Wear gradient compression garments.
Mental Health
Seek counseling or support groups.
Skin Care
Moisturize and prevent infection.
Lymphatic Techniques
Practice self-massage or deep breathing.
Start small, track what helps, and adapt over time.

Figure 18.1: Six categories for self-care.

dietary changes but also navigating complex emotional relationships with food, including self-judgment or fear of external criticism. Many individuals with lipedema report long-standing struggles related to body image and eating, often shaped by repeated advice to lose weight without adequate understanding of their disease. As the author's mother poignantly expressed: 'I wished it were possible to give up eating and live', reflecting the emotional toll of navigating food choices while living in a stigmatized body.

2. **Exercise** Physical activity recommendations for lipedema typically emphasize low-impact forms of exercise, although these should be tailored to an individual's overall health status. Importantly, the most beneficial type of exercise is one that can be performed consistently and sustainably. A personalized approach, tailored to physical capacity, preferences, and lifestyle, is essential for achieving long-term adherence and optimal benefits. A further discussion of exercise for lipedema is below.
3. **Compression garments** Although compression does not reduce lipedema fat, it can offer several benefits, including improved support for tissues, reduced

discomfort, and facilitation of daily physical activity. One of the primary challenges lies in obtaining well-fitting garments, especially given the disproportionate limb shape often seen in lipedema (e.g. larger thighs tapering to smaller ankles). Lipoedema UK clinical advisors frequently recommend multi-part compression systems, such as separate socks or stockings paired with capri leggings or shorts. This modular approach enhances the fit and functionality while also improving the practicality of donning and removing garments.

4. **Mental health** The psychological impact of living with lipedema can be significant. Delayed diagnosis, limited public and professional awareness, and the stigma associated with unexplained weight gain or pain can contribute to feelings of frustration, isolation, and despair. Addressing mental health is a vital aspect of comprehensive self-care for any chronic condition, and, therefore, access to psychological support should be part of the core offering for patients.
5. **Skin care** Individuals with lipedema often face unique dermatological challenges, including the need for compression garments, ongoing limb enlargement, and the development of skin folds. Regular moisturizing and skin inspection are crucial to prevent irritation, breakdown, and infection.
6. **Dry brushing, self-lymphatic drainage, and manual lymphatic drainage (MLD)** Although the evidence supporting these techniques for lipedema-specific outcomes is limited, many patients report subjective benefits, including improved comfort and a sense of care. For some, the therapeutic relationship with an MLD practitioner is as valuable as the physical treatment itself. While MLD may not lead to significant changes in fat tissue or limb volume, it can meaningfully enhance quality of life.

Tracking and measuring: tools and confidence

One of the most practical and empowering strategies in lipedema self-care is encouraging individuals to regularly monitor their symptoms and track changes in their quality of life. This process may involve collecting both objective data (e.g. limb measurements, body weight, or waist-to-height ratio) and subjective assessments (e.g. pain, discomfort, energy levels). Developing confidence in one's ability to test new self-care strategies is essential, but it must be accompanied by reliable methods for evaluating their effects, both positive and negative.

Given the wide array of self-care options available, individuals may be influenced by anecdotal reports, online trends, or testimonials from prominent figures. While such sources may offer inspiration, they should not replace attentive listening to one's own body or personal symptom patterns. Unfortunately, there is currently no standardized tool for lipedema-specific self-assessment, though general principles and suggestions can guide the process. In this context, support from an experienced healthcare professional can be invaluable, helping patients interpret their data and make informed, individualized decisions.

Suggested metrics for tracking include weight, waist-to-height or waist-to-hip ratio, and limb circumference measured at consistent anatomical landmarks (often the same points used for fitting compression garments). Although lipedema is distinct from obesity, the frequent overlap and the routine practice of weighing patients in medical settings mean that weight remains a common data point. For some, incorporating additional measurements, such as limb volume or changes in specific circumferences, can provide a more comprehensive and less emotionally charged picture of progress.

Mobile applications offer additional tools for tracking diet, physical activity, symptom severity, and other health indicators. These range from general wellness apps to specific platforms (e.g. those designed for individuals with diabetes). However, the use of tracking technologies must be approached thoughtfully. For individuals with a history of disordered eating, such as orthorexia nervosa, a condition marked by an obsessive focus on healthy eating, monitoring food intake, or exercise data may exacerbate compulsive behaviors or emotional distress. Therefore, the appropriateness of any tracking method should be evaluated in the context of an individual's psychological history and current well-being.

Collaborating with a qualified practitioner can help ensure that data tracking serves as a constructive self-care tool, rather than a source of stress or obsession. With proper guidance, patients can build confidence in interpreting their own experiences, making adjustments, and developing sustainable habits that support long-term health and quality of life.

Lipedema-specific self-care: exercise

As noted earlier in this chapter, much of the general guidance on self-care, such as engaging in gentle exercise and practicing self-compassion, is broadly applicable to many chronic diseases. However, for individuals with lipedema, specific anatomical and physiological factors must be taken into account when designing an exercise routine. Activities that combine relaxation and movement, such as yoga or meditation-based practices, can be especially beneficial as they often incorporate deep breathing and mindfulness, which are helpful not only for physical health but also for emotional regulation and well-being.

Anatomical considerations and precautions

Several features of lipedema anatomy may affect exercise choice and performance, for example, many individuals with lipedema experience hypermobility, which can compromise joint stability. While practices like yoga or Pilates are often recommended for their low-impact nature, they may require modification for those with hypermobile joints. Therefore, it is advisable to seek medical guidance before beginning any stretching-based regimen and inform instructors about the disease. Patient advocacy organizations such as The Lipedema Foundation, Lipedema Simplified, or Lipoedema UK offer educational resources that can be shared with instructors to support appropriate adaptations.

Yoga and Pilates

There are numerous styles of yoga, each with different intensities and goals. One lipedema-specific approach is Lymphatic Yoga®, developed by Edely Wallace.[10] This style emphasizes diaphragmatic breathing and slow, deliberate movements without the prolonged static holds common in yin yoga. Wallace has led sessions at conferences hosted by the Fat Disorders Research Society and Lipoedema UK, and recordings are available on both her website and those of the respective organizations (see reference list and Chapter 19 for links).

While lymphatic yoga classes are not widely available, many individuals find benefit in more commonly offered styles such as 'gentle yoga,' 'restorative yoga,' or 'yin yoga,' provided that instructors can modify poses and advise on appropriate duration of holds. Chair yoga is another accessible option, offering both gentle and challenging routines that do not require balance in a standing position. Similarly, Pilates, with its focus on core strength, stability, and controlled movement, can be highly beneficial, particularly when tailored to accommodate joint alignment and body awareness (see Chapter 13).

Aquatic exercise

Water-based exercise is frequently recommended for individuals with lipedema due to its joint-sparing qualities and enhanced range of motion. The water's resistance provides proprioceptive feedback, which is especially helpful for those with hypermobility, while hydrostatic pressure mimics the effects of compression garments by promoting fluid return.[11, 12]

However, water's buoyancy may present both advantages and challenges. Individuals with lipedema often have a disproportionate amount of lower-body adipose tissue, resulting in greater buoyancy compared to others of similar weight but with different fat distribution. As a result, those with lipedema may find it more difficult to maintain stable footing in deeper water. For these reasons, exercising in shallower water may offer better stability and comfort. Submerging affected limbs also maximizes the benefits of hydrostatic pressure, particularly for those with coexisting lymphedema.

Although some individuals report anxiety related to changing room environments or physical exposure, feedback from participants in the *Lipoedema UK Big Survey*[4] overwhelmingly supports aquatic exercise as a valuable and enjoyable form of symptom management.

Evidence and emerging research

Although research on exercise in lipedema is still in its early stages of development, existing studies provide valuable insights into the unique physiological features of the disease. For instance, van Esch-Smeenge et al.[13] found that individuals with lipedema exhibited significantly reduced leg muscle strength compared to individuals with obesity. Sharing such findings can be validating for patients, helping to counter misconceptions and offering useful evidence to present to personal trainers or instructors. It also reinforces the potential of exercise to improve muscle strength, enhance postural control, and reduce the risk of falls.

Practical guidance and individualization

One common question among individuals with lipedema is whether high-impact exercise is safe or beneficial. Further research is needed in this area, particularly regarding the interaction between weight, joint health, and fat distribution, as well as various types of activity. Standard medical advice for starting a new exercise regimen, such as consulting a physician and being aware of delayed-onset muscle soreness, also applies in this case.

Special attention should be given to gait and alignment. Lipedema can alter biomechanics by displacing fat in ways that shift the hips, knees, and ankles out of alignment, potentially contributing to pronation of the feet.[14] A gait assessment and properly fitted footwear or orthotics may be essential components of a safe and sustainable exercise plan.

Ultimately, the most effective exercise is the one an individual feels confident performing, can maintain regularly, and derives a sense of accomplishment from. Supporting patients in identifying and committing to such activities is central to long-term self-care and overall well-being.

Mental health self-care

The psychological toll of living with a chronic disease is well-documented in the scientific literature. It should be a core component of any comprehensive self-care plan for individuals with lipedema. Chronic illnesses often require ongoing self-management, which can be mentally and emotionally taxing. As with other long-term diseases, the cumulative burden of symptoms, delayed diagnosis, and limited public and clinical understanding can significantly affect mental well-being. For example, individuals diagnosed with diabetes are two to three times more likely than the general population to experience depression.[14] As Joseph Gallo, MD, MPH, Professor of mental health at the Johns Hopkins Bloomberg School of Public Health, has noted:

'There is ample clinical and epidemiologic evidence that shows the risk of depression is higher amongst those who suffer from chronic illnesses… much of managing multiple diseases requires self-care on the part of the person, and depression can make caring for oneself difficult.'[15]

Lipedema is no exception. As discussed in Chapter 8, lipedema has been shown to impair quality of life significantly. Findings from the *Lipoedema UK Big Survey*[4] revealed that only 12% of respondents reported no negative impact on their quality of life, and just 1% described the condition as having a positive effect on their quality of life. In stark contrast, 87% of participants reported that lipedema negatively affected their well-being. While it may seem unrealistic to expect a complete reversal of these figures, there is nonetheless considerable opportunity for improvement through targeted mental health support and structured self-care interventions.

One promising avenue lies in group-based psychosocial support. Research suggests that participation in peer support groups, regardless of specific diagnosis, can be highly effective in improving coping strategies and emotional resilience. In the United Kingdom, the National Health Service (NHS) has implemented group support programs for individuals living with various chronic conditions. These initiatives have been shown to enhance adherence to self-management plans and reduce the frequency of hospital admissions.[16] Similar models could be beneficial when tailored for the lipedema population.

Incorporating mental health self-care into the broader lipedema management plan is not only evidence-based but essential. Strategies may include access to mental health professionals, participation in support groups, mindfulness practices, and fostering a compassionate inner dialogue, particularly in light of the stigma, misdiagnosis, and frustration often experienced by those with lipedema. Building emotional resilience can significantly improve quality of life and, notably, support greater consistency in physical and medical self-care behaviors.

The role of community in self-care

In the *Lipoedema UK Big Survey*[4] many people discussed the impact of being validated through participation in lipedema groups. The internet has brought many people together into formal and informal self-help groups. Care must always be taken when recommending online or in-person self-help groups that are not part of a formally recognized organization or part of a healthcare clinic or service provider. Less formal groups may lack oversight mechanisms and may not have access to the most comprehensive and current information. Joining a local or national not-for-profit organization that supports people living with lipedema can help people by providing access to information about various self-care methods and also serve as an outlet to help others and contribute to improving the lives of future generations. Please refer to Chapter 19 for a list of organizations dedicated to supporting and caring for individuals with lipedema.

Conclusion

In the absence of a definitive cure for lipedema, individuals are encouraged to cultivate a personalized approach to living well with the disease. Developing effective self-care strategies is a dynamic and empowering process that is often enhanced by engagement with a supportive community. Collaboration with knowledgeable healthcare practitioners, along with proactive exploration of both in-person and virtual resources, can foster a sense of agency and resilience. Remaining informed about emerging research, evidence-based interventions, and educational opportunities further supports physical and emotional well-being, providing a hopeful and proactive path forward in managing lipedema.

References

1. Faerber G, Cornely M, Daubert C, Erbacher G, Fink J, Hirsch T, et al. S2k guideline lipedema. *JDDG J Dtsch Dermatol Ges.* 2024;22(9):1303–15. DOI: https://doi.org/10.1111/ddg.15513
2. Reich-Schupke S, Schmeller W, Brauer WJ, Cornely ME, Faerber G, Ludwig M, et al. S1 guidelines: lipedema. *J Dtsch Dermatol Ges.* 2017;15(7):758–67. DOI: https://doi.org/10.1111/ddg.13036
3. WHO. World Health Organization. *Putting people first in managing their health: new WHO guideline on self-care interventions.* Available from: https://www.who.int/news/item/23-06-2021-putting-people-first-in-managing-their-health-new-who-guideline-on-self-care-interventions
4. Fetzer A, Fetzer, Sharie. *Lipoedema UK Big Survey 2014 Research Report.* Lipoedema UK; 2016 Jul p. 1–8. Available from: https://lipoedema.co.uk/wp-content/uploads/2024/05/LATEST-LUK000-UK-Big-Survey16-Mar24-web.pdf
5. Majsiak E, Choina M, Golicki D, Gray AM, Cukrowska B. The impact of symptoms on quality of life before and after diagnosis of coeliac disease: the results from a Polish population survey and comparison with the results from the United Kingdom. *BMC Gastroenterol.* 2021 Mar 4;21(1):99. DOI: https://doi.org/10.1186/s12876-021-01673-0
6. Nootenboom K. Pain in lipedema: patient representative talk. *Lipodema World Congress*; 2023 Oct; Potsdam, Germany. Available from: https://www.lipedema-world-congress.com/on-demand/
7. Madsen E. Patient representative talk: patient survey feedback (NLLF). *Lipedema World Congress*; 2023 Oct; Potsdam, Germany. Available from: https://www.lipedema-world-congress.com/on-demand/
8. de Iongh A. Patients need support to self manage their long term conditions. *BMJ.* 2014 Apr 28;348:g2973. DOI: https://doi.org/10.1136/bmj.g2973
9. Helmbrecht S. Self-management program: 'Healthy and active living with lipoedema and lymphoedema (GALLiLy) . Lipedema World Congress; 2023 Oct; Potsdam, Germany. Available from: https://www.lipedema-world-congress.com/on-demand/
10. Wallace E. *Lymphatic Yoga® Online Studio.* Available from: https://lymphaticyoga.net/
11. Maccarone MC, Venturini E, Menegatti E, Gianesini S, Masiero S. Water-based exercise for upper and lower limb lymphedema treatment. *J Vasc Surg Venous Lymphat Disord.* 2023 Jan 1;11(1):201–9. DOI: https://doi.org/10.1016/j.jvsv.2022.08.002
12. Keane L. What happens to the body when it is immersed in water. Aquatic Rehabilitation & Exercise Academy (AREA). https://www.youtube.com/watch?v=c1DruV04lJw&t=18s
13. van Esch-Smeenge J, Damstra RJ, Hendrickx AA. Muscle strength and functional exercise capacity in patients with lipoedema and obesity: a comparative study. *J Lymphoedema.* 2017;12(1):27–31. Available from: https://woundsinternational.com/wp-content/uploads/2023/02/jol_12-1_27-31_vanesch.pdf
14. Forner-Cordero I, Perez-Pomares MV, Forner A, Ponce-Garrido AB, Munoz-Langa J. Prevalence of clinical manifestations and orthopedic alterations in patients with lipedema: a prospective cohort study. *Lymphology.* 2021;54(4):170–81. DOI: https://doi.org/10.2458/lymph.4838
15. Fernandez, G. *The Intersection of Mental Health and Chronic Disease.* John Hopkins/Bloomberg School of Public Health. 2021. Available from: https://publichealth.jhu.edu/2021/the-intersection-of-mental-health-and-chronic-disease
16. Gruber J, Lordan G, Pilling S, Propper C, Saunders R. The impact of mental health support for the chronically ill on hospital utilisation: evidence from the UK. *Soc Sci Med 1982.* 2022 Feb;294:114675. DOI: https://doi.org/10.1016/j.socscimed.2021.114675

Chapter Nineteen
Resources for managing lipedema: empowerment for every stage of the journey

Catherine Seo and Leslyn Keith

Introduction

Resources matter when living with and navigating a chronic disease like lipedema. It is not just a medical journey – it's an emotional, social, financial, and logistical one. Lipedema is a progressive and often painful fat and lymphatic disease that affects millions of people, primarily women, yet remains underdiagnosed and misunderstood in both medical and public spheres. For many, the path to diagnosis is filled with confusion, mislabeling, and dismissal from healthcare providers. This not only delays appropriate care but also contributes to stigma and a deep sense of isolation.

Because lipedema is often mistaken for obesity or lifestyle-related weight gain, patients may carry not only physical symptoms but also the emotional burden of stigma, self-blame, and frustration. The lack of widespread clinical awareness places a significant burden on patients, many of whom are left to research their symptoms, advocate for recognition, and navigate fragmented healthcare systems without adequate support. At the same time, providers seeking to support their patients may find themselves without clear guidelines, resources, or professional networks to draw upon.

This chapter serves as a guide for both patients and healthcare professionals, offering curated, evidence-informed resources from around the world to assist in understanding lipedema and its underlying disease science, building an effective care team, identifying appropriate therapeutic garments, connecting with peer and professional support networks, and addressing the psychological, social, and financial challenges that often accompany lipedema.

Whether you are a patient newly confronting the possibility of lipedema, someone further along in their management journey, or a provider committed to offering informed, compassionate care, the resources presented here are intended to empower, educate, and invite connection. With the right tools and support, lipedema management becomes not only more effective but also more humane, and no one has to navigate it alone. Healing, support, and hope are possible.

Educational and clinical resources

Educating oneself about lipedema is a powerful step in managing the disease effectively. Understanding the condition helps individuals recognize symptoms early, advocate for accurate diagnosis, and make informed choices about treatment options.

Knowledge empowers patients to navigate medical systems with confidence, identify supportive healthcare providers, and adopt lifestyle strategies, such as compression, exercise, and a balanced diet, that can reduce pain, improve mobility, and enhance overall quality of life. Educational resources in this section include guidelines for lipedema treatment from various countries, reputable websites and organizations, as well as training and certification programs for lipedema care.

Lipedema treatment guidelines

Lipedema treatment guidelines provide expert-informed, evidence-based recommendations for diagnosis and management, covering conservative therapies, surgical options, and multidisciplinary care. Developed by national and international experts, these tools support accurate diagnosis, enhance access to treatment, and contribute to advancing research and informing policy. The most current guidelines are listed below in chronological order, with the most recent first.

- **Brazilian lipedema guidelines**
  Amato et al. (2025). Brazilian Consensus Statement on Lipedema using the Delphi methodology. *Jornal Vascular Brasileiro* 2025; 24: e20230183. https://www.scielo.br/j/jvb/a/BjWVDJpPcdTPKx5MqJQ9NRs/?lang=en
- **German S2k guidelines for lipedema**
  Faerber et al. S2k guideline lipedema. *Journal der Deutschen Dermatologischen Gesellschaft*, 2024; 22(9): 1303–1315. https://onlinelibrary.wiley.com/doi/10.1111/ddg.15513
- **US standard of care document**
  Herbst et al. Standard of care for lipedema in the United States. *Phlebology* 2021; 36 (10): 779-796. https://journals.sagepub.com/doi/ full/10.1177/02683555211015887
- **Dutch guidelines**
  Halk AB, Damstra RJ. First Dutch guidelines on lipedema using the International Classification of Functioning, Disability and Health. *Phlebology* 2017; 32(3): 152–159. https://journals.sagepub.com/doi/abs/10.1177/0268355516639421

Prominent websites and organizations

Well-respected lipedema websites and organizations offer trusted information, education, and support for both patients and healthcare providers. They provide tools for self-care, diagnosis, treatment, and professional development, helping to reduce misdiagnosis and improve care. These resources also foster a sense of community, empower patients, and promote earlier, more effective interventions. See a list of prominent organizations in Table 19.1.

Training and certification programs for lipedema care

Training and certification in lipedema care can equip healthcare professionals to diagnose and treat the condition more accurately, reducing delays and improving patient outcomes. Certified providers offer more personalized, evidence-based care and are better prepared to address both physical and emotional aspects of the disease. This growing area of expertise also strengthens advocacy, reduces stigma, and fosters a more informed and supportive medical community.

Recognized certifications

Several certifications and designations for lipedema and lymphatic care are recognized internationally, providing high-quality, evidence-informed training.

- **Certified lymphedema therapist (CLT)**
  A certified lymphedema therapist (CLT) is a licensed healthcare professional trained in manual lymph drainage and complete decongestive therapy through 135+ hours of specialized instruction, often including lipedema care.

Table 19.1: Prominent lipedema-focused websites and organizations.

Organization	Description	Website
ACVEL (Asociación de la Comunidad Valenciana de Enfermos de Linfedema y Lipedema)	Regional nonprofit in Valencia, Spain, offering support, education, and access to care for individuals with lymphedema and lipedema	acvel.es
Association Lipoedème France	French national association for patient advocacy and public awareness	lipoedeme-france.com
Associação Brasileira de Lipedema	National Brazilian association for awareness, education, and support	doacao.lipedema.org.br
Dutch Lipedema Association	National resource in the Netherlands for awareness and community education	lipoedeem.nl
FDRS (Fat Disorders Resource Society)	Educational conferences, patient support, and advocacy	fatdisorders.org
International Lymphoedema Framework (ILF)	International framework promoting education and best practices in lymphatic care	lympho.org
LE&RN	Advocacy and research for lymphatic diseases	lymphaticnetwork.org
LIO Lipedema Italia	Italian advocacy and support organization for lipedema patients	lioitalia.org
Lipedema Costa Rica (supported by PROSADEH.org)	Costa Rican nonprofit organization dedicated to educational resources, advocacy, peer-to-peer support, and connection to healthcare providers	luminaraspa.com/lipedema-in-costa-rica/
Lipedema Foundation	Research and education network for lipedema and fat disorders	lipedema.org
Lipedema Project	Research, film, and global awareness efforts	lipedemaproject.org
Lipedema Simplified	Patient-centered education, events, and provider resources	lipedema-simplified.org
Lipedema World Alliance	Global collaboration of professionals, patients, and advocates for lipedema	lipedemaworldalliance.com
Lipoedema Australia	National organization supporting awareness, diagnosis, and management in Australia	lipoedemaaustralia.com.au
Lipoedema UK	UK-based patient and clinician education	lipoedema.co.uk
LIPÖDEM Hilfe e.V. (Germany)	Advocacy, legal support, and public awareness in Germany	lipoedem-hilfe-ev.de
Lymf Sverige	Swedish organization for lymphatic and lipedema support and education	lymfsverige.se

- **LANA certification (CLT-LANA)** This certification, offered by the Lymphology Association of North America (LANA), is an advanced credential for certified lymphedema therapists who have completed at least 135 hours of training. It requires passing a standardized national exam and is widely regarded as a gold standard, primarily in the United States and Canada, for professional excellence in lymphatic therapy.
- **Accredited lymphoedema practitioner (ALPP)** The Australasian Lymphology Association's ALPP certification recognizes health professionals in Australia and New Zealand who meet accredited standards in lymphedema and lipedema care through approved training, registration, and ongoing professional development.

Educational providers

Several respected organizations worldwide offer specialized training in the treatment of lipedema and lymphedema. These programs provide evidence-based education for healthcare professionals in essential topics, including manual lymphatic drainage, compression therapy, and complete decongestive therapy (see Table 19.2).

Finding expert diagnosis and care-provider directories

Finding a qualified provider is crucial for accurate lipedema diagnosis and effective care. Patients should seek clinicians who specialize in lymphatic or adipose tissue disorders and who understand the unique challenges of managing a complex, chronic disease like lipedema. Experienced providers may offer both conservative and surgical options tailored to the disease and are committed to collaborative, patient-centered care. This section lists provider directories to identify professionals for diagnosis and treatment, organized alphabetically. For tips on how to use provider directories most effectively, see Figure 19.1.

- **Australasian Lymphology Association (ALA)** – National Lymphoedema Practitioners Register: https://www.lymphoedema.org.au/accreditation-nlpr/find-a-practitioner/ The ALA National Lymphoedema Practitioners Register is a publicly accessible directory of health professionals across Australia and New Zealand who have achieved ALPP accreditation. Providers may also have expertise in lipedema care.
- **Chikly Health Institute** – Find a Therapist: https://chiklyinstitute.com/find-a-therapist The Chikly Health Institute provider directory is a global online tool that helps users locate therapists trained in Chikly's lymph drainage therapy (LDT) and related methods in the US and Canada.
- **Lipedema and Me** – Community-Curated Surgeons Directory: https://findasurgeon.lipedemaandme.com/ Lipedema and Me is an online platform that offers a global 'Find a Surgeon' tool for lipedema reduction surgery.
- **Lipedema Foundation** – Provider Directory: https://www.lipedema.org/provider-directory The Lipedema Foundation Provider Directory is an online tool that helps patients find US-based therapists and clinicians experienced in treating lipedema. The foundation advises combining directory use with their Patient Self-Advocacy Guide to prepare for consultations: https://www.lipedema.org/guide
- **Lipedema Project/Lipedema Simplified** – Provider Directory: https://lipedemaproject.org/lipedema-lipoedema-lipodem-provider-directory/ The Lipedema Project/Lipedema Simplified maintains a global, patient-submitted directory of providers

Table 19.2: Educational providers in lipedema and lymphedema care.

Organization	Focus/certifications	Website
AbralliPro for HealthCare Professionals	The world's first postgraduate medical education program dedicated to lipedema care and management	https://www.instagram.com/abralipedemapro/
Academy of Lymphatic Studies (ACOLS)	CLT and lymphedema management certification; specialized lipedema modules	acols.com
Casley-Smith Lymphoedema Education UK	Specializes in advanced methods of MLD and CDT, based on the internationally recognized Casley Smith approach. Courses are offered in the UK	casle.org.uk/find-a-full-course
Chikly Health Institute	Training in lymph drainage therapy (LDT), developed by Dr. Bruno Chikly. In-person and online courses worldwide, with certification options for healthcare professionals	chiklyinstitute.com
Foeldi College	MLD training. Collaborates with Klose Training & Consulting for advanced therapy concepts and reviews	foeldicollege.com
Klose Training	Comprehensive lymphedema therapy certification (CLT); continuing education in lymphatic disorders in the US and internationally	klosetraining.com
Lymphoedema Training Academy	International education provider based in UK. Certification courses in lymphedema and lipedema	lymph.org.uk
Monarch Consulting & Education	Evidence-based training for healthcare professionals in lymphatic therapy, including CLT and lipedema care. Training in a variety of MLD techniques (Vodder, Chikly, Upledger, and Földi)	monarchce.com
Norton School of Lymphatic Therapy	Provider of CLT training in the US, with a curriculum based on the Vodder method of CDT	nortonschool.com
Vodder School International (Dr. Vodder Akademie)	Original source of MLD training; advanced lymphatic education in Europe & North America	vodderschool.com

who diagnose and treat lipedema, including doctors, surgeons, lymphatic therapists, and compression garment fitters.

- **Lymphatic Centers of Excellence (COE)**: https://lymphaticnetwork.org/centers-of-excellence
  The Lymphatic Education & Research Network (LE&RN) designates select institutions as COEs for meeting high stan-dards in comprehensive, multidisciplinary lymphatic care. These centers offer advanced diagnostics, imaging, conservative therapies, and surgical options, along with services such as genetic counseling and professional education.

- **Lymphatic Education & Research Network (LE&RN)** – How to find a qualified lymphedema therapist: https://lymphaticnetwork.org/living-with-lymphedema/find-a-lymphedema-therapist Links to reliable provider directories are given along with key questions to assess a therapist's credentials and practice focus. Designed for both patients and providers, the resource guides users to qualified therapists. It outlines what to expect from effective complete decongestive therapy (CDT), including education and long-term self-care goals.
- **Lymphology Association of North America (LANA)** – LANA-certified therapist directory: https://www.clt-lana.org/therapists The LANA online directory lists certified lymphedema therapists in the US and Canada who have completed at least 135 hours of accredited training and passed a national certification exam.
- **Manual Lymph Drainage United Kingdom (MLD^UK^)** – Find a Therapist: https://mlduk.org.uk/find-a-therapist/ A professional association offering a public directory of qualified MLD therapists trained in recognized methods and actively engaged in education and best practices in the United Kingdom.
- **National Lymphedema Network (NLN)** – Lymphedema Therapy Directory: https://lymphnet.org/search/ The NLN offers a searchable directory to help patients locate certified lymphedema professionals across the US. Listings include therapists and physicians, searchable by location, and provide access to standardized, evidence-based care. Each provider listed has met specific training requirements, and many hold advanced certifications such as CLT or CLT-LANA.

Lifestyle and self-care resources

Lifestyle strategies play a central role in the daily management of lipedema, offering patients practical tools to reduce symptoms, improve mobility, and enhance overall well-being. While no single approach fits all, individualized plans that include therapeutic nutrition, gentle movement, compression therapy, and self-care practices can make a meaningful difference. This section highlights trusted resources to support sustainable lifestyle adjustments grounded in clinical experience and patient-reported outcomes. By integrating these strategies, patients and healthcare providers can work together to achieve long-term symptom control and an improved quality of life.

Self-care education

- **ABRALI (Brazilian Lipedema Association)**: Instagram @abralipedema The association provides support, resources, and workshops for individuals living with lipedema, helping them navigate the challenges associated with the condition.
- **GALLiLy Self-Empowerment Program**: https://www.lymphselbsthilfe.de/ Self-help groups for individuals with lymphedema and lipedema are offered throughout Germany by Lymphselbsthilfe e.V. (Federal Association for Lymphostatic Diseases).
- **Lipedema Courses by Lipedema Mamas**: https://www.lipedemacourses.com/ Lipedema Mamas' courses offer practical, experience-based guidance on nutrition, movement, self-care, and surgery preparation to help manage lipedema and improve quality of life.
- **Lipedema Simplified/The Lipedema Project Webinars & Heart to Heart Events**: https://lipedema-simplified.org/ The Lipedema Project and Lipedema Simplified offer online courses, webinars,

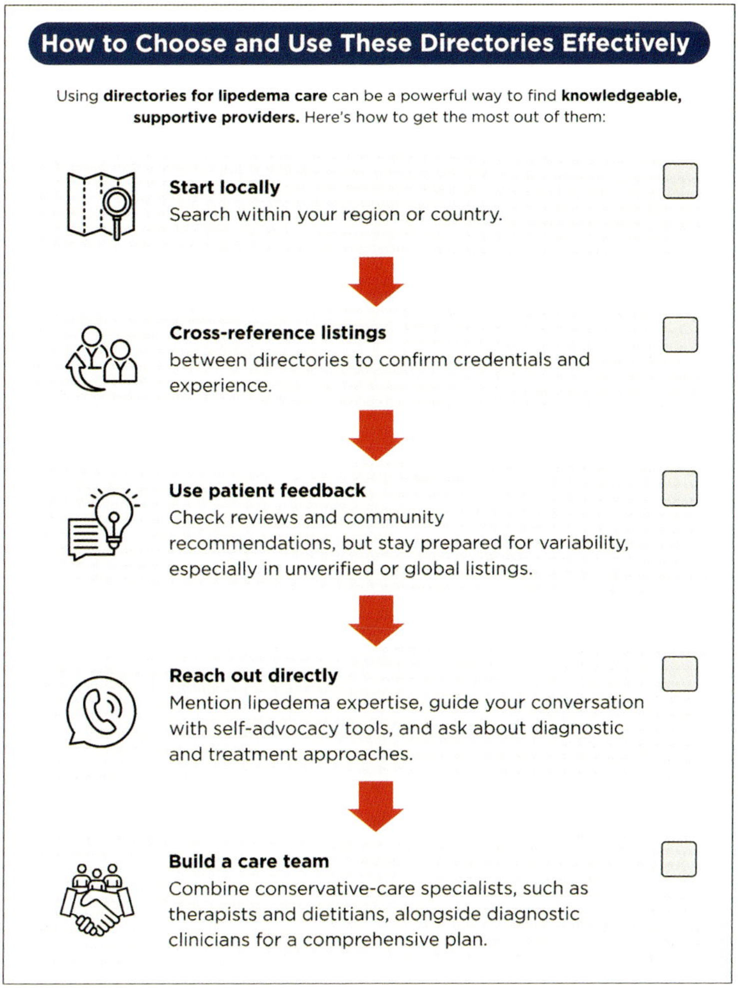

Figure 19.1: Tips for getting the most out of provider directories.

and events covering diagnosis, conservative care, surgery, and recovery. Programs include expert-led sessions and virtual events, such as the 'Heart to Heart' series, providing flexible, evidence-based education for patients and providers.

- **Lipedema World Congress 2023 recordings**: https://www.lipedema-world-congress.com/on-demand/ The Lipedema World Congress held in Potsdam, Germany, in October 2023 featured expert sessions on diagnostics, conservative care, self-care practices, surgery, and emerging therapies. All presentations were recorded and are available for on-demand viewing.
- **Lipoedema UK Health and Wellness program**: https://lipoedema.co.uk/lipoedema-uk-members-webinars/ Lipoedema UK offers educational opportunities for members through webinars and well-being sessions. The *2014 Big Survey* findings and other research projects from Lipoedema UK can be found here: https://lipoedema.co.uk/lipoedema-uk-research-publications/

- **Lymphatic Lifestyle Solutions (LLS)**: https://self-care-therapy.mykajabi.com/ LLS is a clinician-developed, evidence-based program created to help individuals with lipedema and lymphedema manage symptoms through lifestyle changes. It combines ketogenic nutrition, movement, stress reduction, and sleep strategies in a self-paced course accompanied by live meetups.

Compression garments

Compression garments help alleviate pain, swelling, and heaviness associated with lipedema by enhancing lymphatic flow, promoting mobility, and supporting tissue health. They are a key component of comprehensive care. See Chapters 12 and 13 for details. Table 19.3 provides a list of popular compression garment brands and their respective uses.

Providers and individuals are encouraged to reach out to compression garment fitters at local and virtual medical supply practices for guidance on measuring, fitting, and insurance billing. A list of durable medical equipment (DME)/medical suppliers for compression garments is provided in Table 19.4.

Movement and exercise

Regular low-impact exercise, as described in Chapters 12 and 13, helps manage lipedema symptoms by stimulating lymphatic flow, improving circulation, and reducing pain and stiffness. Movement also supports mobility, joint health, and metabolic function, while enhancing mood and independence, making it a vital and sustainable part of lipedema care when tailored to individual needs. Here is a list of local and online resources to consider:

Aqua exercise

- Lynda Keane: https://aquaticacademy.co.uk/team_member/lynda-keane/
- Most swimming pool programs offer water exercise classes suitable for individuals with lipedema. Look for an Arthritis Foundation Aquatic Exercise Program at your local pool.

Chair exercises

Check listings from your local recreation department for senior exercise classes. Here are some suggested online resources:

- Sit and Be Fit: https://www.sitandbefit.org/
- Heart and Soul Fitness: https://hasfit.com/
- Grow Young Fitness: https://www.growyoungfitness.com/

Gentle movement classes

- Tai Chi Foundation online classes: https://www.taichifoundation.org/live-online-courses/
- Movement with Miranda (Lipedema Simplified TRIBE): https://learn.lipedema-simplified.org/tribe

Yoga

- Lymphatic Yoga®, created by Edely Wallace, https://lymphaticyoga.net/
- Lymph Yoga with Babz in Boston – Balance with Babz: https://www.balancewithbabz.com/
- Yoga with Shoosh: https://yogawithshoosh.com/
- Lymphatic Flow Yoga Series with Shoosh Lettick Crotzer: https://www.youtube.com/watch?v=8btp39n5luc
- Cindy Beers – Yoga and Lipedema: https://cindybeers.com/lipedema-and-yoga

Table 19.3: Compression garment manufacturers are offering products specifically designed for patients with lipedema.

Brand	Features	Website
Bioflect	Infrared-emitting compression wear designed for lymphatic support	bioflect.com
Circaid	Adjustable Velcro inelastic compression wraps ideal for managing swelling	circaid.com
CZSalus	Italian-designed compression wear with lymphatic stimulation benefits	czsalus.com
Jobst	Trusted medical compression brand offering a variety of garments and levels of support	jobst.com
Juzo	Durable, medical-grade compression	juzousa.com
Lipoelastic	High-quality post-liposuction compression garments used globally	lipoelastic.com
Lymphe DIVAs	Stylish options with medical functionality	lymphedivas.com
Marena	Post-surgical compression garments with soft fabric design	marenagroup.com
Medi	A comprehensive range of compression options and accessories	mediusa.com
Sigvaris	Offers custom sizing	sigvaris.com
Solidea	Stylish, breathable compression for everyday wear	solideausa.com
Wear Ease	A complete line of post-surgical bras and camisoles, as well as therapeutic pressure garments	Boise, ID (866)251-0076 wearease.com

Table 19.4: Durable medical equipment (DME) and medical suppliers for compression garments.

Company	Products/services	Contact information
Absolute Medical, Inc. absolutemedical.com	Compression garments	Chicago, IL (312) 233-2207 customerservice@absolutemedical.com
Comfort Care Medical comfortcaremd.com	Compression garments, Velcro wraps	Catonsville, MD 888-358-1580
Compression Closet thecompressioncloset.com	Compression garments, Velcro wraps	Crystal Lake, IL (815) 342 0370 or (815) 364 2781 theresa@thecompressioncloset.com
Compression Guru compressionguru.com	Compression garments, Velcro wraps	Franklin, TN 888 550 2709 support@compressionguru.com
D&J Medical dandjmedical.com	Compression garments, reimbursement	Forest Hill, MD 410-893-1116
Luna Medical lunamedical.com	Bandages, compression garments, reimbursement	Chicago, IL 800-380-4339
SunMed Medical Solutions sunmedmedical.com	Compression garments, wound care	Marlton, NJ 800-714-7434

Table 19.5. Compression pump providers.

Device name	What it does	Best for	Website
AIROS 6 & 6P	Six-chamber compression system with programmable pressure; Medicare-covered	Lymphedema, lipedema, and post-surgical swelling	airosmedical.com
AIROS 8 & 8P	Eight-chamber system with adjustable zones and peristaltic mode	Advanced lipedema/ lymphedema needing intensive therapy	airosmedical.com
Bio Compression ENTIREx	High-end clinical system with full-length garments for arms and legs	Clinical settings or intensive therapy programs	biocompression.com
Bio Compression SC-2004	Gradient sequential compression; quiet and user-friendly	Chronic lipedema/ lymphedema for regular home use	biocompression.com
BTL Lymphastim	Large-cuff, adjustable zone compression used in clinics	European-based clinic treatment	btlnet.com
Juzo IPC System	Four-chamber intermittent compression; compact and portable	Lightweight home use	juzousa.com
Lympha Press Optimal Plus	Provides calibrated, sequential compression with lipedema-specific settings and full-body garments	Moderate to severe lipedema and lymphedema; patients needing tailored therapy	lymphapress.com
Lympha Press PCD-51	Offers home-use compression with preset cycles and a simple interface	Mild to moderate symptoms; at-home use	lymphapress.com
NormaTec Pulse Pro 2.0	Pulsed dynamic compression for circulation and recovery	Lipedema patients seeking comfort and relief; also used in sports recovery	hyperice.com
Tactile Medical AffloVest	Wearable airway clearance vest with indirect lymphatic benefits	Patients with lipedema and respiratory co-morbidities	tactilemedical.com
Tactile Medical Flexitouch Plus	Delivers advanced, automated lymphatic drainage with customized sequences and truncal options	Complex cases with fibrotic tissue or truncal involvement	tactilemedical.com

Nutrition approaches

A thoughtful nutritional approach can help manage lipedema by reducing inflammation, supporting lymphatic health, and improving overall well-being. Non-inflammatory, low-carb, or ketogenic-style diets may ease pain, swelling, and tissue fibrosis by addressing insulin resistance and systemic inflammation. Nutrition can also support weight stabilization, energy levels, and gut health, thereby enhancing the effects of treatments such as compression and movement. In general, no single diet works for everyone; many with lipedema benefit from a nutrient-dense, sustainable eating plan tailored to their specific needs. (Please see Chapter 14 for more information.) The following section provides resources to support dietary change.

Lymphatic Education & Resource Network (LE&RN) Symposium Series

- Dr. Eric Westman https://lymphaticnetwork.org/symposium-series/presenters/dr.-eric-westman
- Dr. Leslyn Keith https://lymphaticnetwork.org/symposium-series/presenters/leslyn-keith

Nutrition organizations

- Nutrition Network: https://nutrition-network.org/ is an accredited online education and community platform, founded by The Noakes Foundation, with leading doctors and scientists, offering healthcare practitioners the latest science on Therapeutic Carbohydrate Restriction.
- The Nutrition Coalition: https://www.nutritioncoalition.us/ is a non-profit, non-partisan educational organization that aims to ensure that the U.S. Dietary Guidelines for Americans are evidence-based, to reverse chronic diseases.

Nutrition coaching and classes

- Carrie Reedy BHSc (Nut Med), CPN
  Website: https://carriereedy.com/
  Email: info@carriereedy.com
  Carrie is a functional nutrition practitioner who supports individuals with lipedema through personalized nutrition and lifestyle strategies.
- Eric Westman, MD
  Website: https://www.adaptyourlife.com/
  Dr. Eric Westman's Adapt Your Life program is a virtual, science-based weight management platform co-founded with nutritionist Amy Berger, offering a structured ketogenic and low-carb curriculum designed to help reverse metabolic conditions such as obesity, type 2 diabetes, and heart disease.
- Lymphatic Lifestyle Solutions (LLS):
  https://self-care-therapy.mykajabi.com/Lymphaticlifestylesolutions
  LLS is a clinician-developed, evidence-based program created to help individuals with lipedema and lymphedema manage symptoms through lifestyle changes. It combines ketogenic nutrition, movement, stress reduction, and sleep strategies in a self-paced course accompanied by live meetups.

Books on nutrition

- Ede G. *Change Your Diet, Change Your Mind*. London: Yellow Kite (Hachette), 2024.
  A science-based guide that helps you improve your mental health through nutrition. A Harvard-trained psychiatrist, Dr. Ede challenges conventional dietary advice and demonstrates how food influences brain chemistry, mood, focus, and memory. Backed by research, practical tips, and real-life stories, this book empowers readers to harness the power of food as a powerful medicine for the mind.
- Taubes G. *Good Calories, Bad Calories*. Knopf, 2007.

Challenges the belief that dietary fat is the primary cause of obesity and chronic disease, arguing instead that refined carbohydrates and sugar are to blame. Backed by extensive research, the book reveals how flawed science and politics have influenced dietary guidelines, highlighting the crucial role of insulin and metabolism in weight gain and overall health.

Compression pumps

Pneumatic compression pumps are therapeutic devices that use gentle, rhythmic air pressure to stimulate lymphatic and venous flow, helping to reduce swelling, pain, fluid retention, and heaviness – common symptoms of lipedema. When used regularly, especially in conjunction with MLD, compression garments, and exercise, they can enhance limb contour, mobility, and comfort. These pumps offer a convenient and non-invasive method for extending treatment benefits at home or in clinical settings, playing a crucial role in daily symptom management and post-surgical recovery. Refer to Chapter 13 Complementary therapies in lipedema, for further information. Table 19.5 lists several providers of compression pumps. Contact the provider directly for more information on uses, contraindications, availability, insurance coverage, and necessary documentation.

Community and emotional support

For individuals living with lipedema, the community – especially online – offers vital connection, education, and emotional support. These platforms provide a safe space to share experiences, ask questions, and find validation from others who understand the condition. Many people report feeling seen for the first time, breaking through the isolation often caused by delayed diagnosis and limited medical recognition.

Support groups also provide practical guidance on treatments, compression, nutrition, and daily management, while fostering confidence and self-advocacy. Many members are involved in advocacy, research, and public education, helping to reduce stigma and improve care. These communities serve as essential lifelines for information, empowerment, and hope.

Lipedema communities

- **Lipedema Simplified's TRIBE Community**
  https://learn.lipedema-simplified.org/tribe
  A thriving online membership group offering weekly live sessions, mentoring, Q&A with experts, and peer connection. Members report reduced isolation, emotional support, and practical education.
- **Lipedema.com**
  https://www.lipedema.com/
  A comprehensive platform featuring free support and interest groups, education sessions, and advocacy initiatives. This grassroots effort helps foster local and virtual connections among patients and healthcare professionals.
- **Lympha Press Lipedema & Lymphedema Round Tables**
  https://www.lymphapress.com/roundtables/
  The Lympha Press Lipedema & Lymphedema Round Tables are free monthly virtual forums featuring expert panels, personal stories, and practical advice on managing care. They offer education, support, and connection for patients, caregivers, and clinicians, with sessions archived online for easy access.

Facebook groups

Facebook groups for lipedema provide peer support, symptom management tips, and shared experiences in a safe and understanding

Table 19.6: Lipedema Facebook groups.

Group Name	Region	Description
Global Lipoedema Awareness – Surgeries/Surgeons	Global	A women-only group sharing surgical experiences and recommendations for surgeons
Keto and Fasting for Lymphedema	USA	Support group focused on keto and intermittent fasting for lymphedema management
Keto Lifestyle for Lipedema and Lymphedema	Global	Lifestyle and dietary tips centered around keto for lipedema and lymphedema
Leichter Leben mit Lipödem	Germany	Group focused on daily living strategies and peer encouragement
Lipedema Sisters Italia	Italy	Italian-language peer support and shared lived experience
Lipo for Lipedema in Germany	Germany	German-language discussions on surgery and conservative care
Lipoedema Australia (formerly LASS)	Australia	Australia's largest national group for education, treatment discussions, and community
Lipoedema Events & Groups Space UK	UK	Dedicated to UK events, local providers, and peer networking
Lipoedema Information UK	UK	Provides self-care tips, advocacy updates, and treatment insights
Lipoedema Sisters USA	USA	US-based group focused on shared experiences, resources, and support
Lipoedema Surgery Australia	Australia	Focused on surgical and recovery insights within Australia
Lipoedemaladies (UK)	UK	Private, women-only support network in the UK
Lipoedema Warriors	Global	An international, women-only community for education and empowerment
Lipödem Hilfe Deutschland e.V. (public page)	Germany	Nonprofit page offering information, regional support, and advocacy
Lipödem Hilfe Gruppe	Germany	Peer community covering diagnosis, self-care, and treatment options
Lipedema en Latinoamérica	Latin America	Spanish-speaking regional group focused on self-care and support
Lipedema/ Lipoedema Simplified Support	Global	Official support group from Lipedema Simplified offering research updates, learning, and connection
Lipedema & Lymphedema Heart to Heart Events	Global	Community around the virtual symposiums, conferences, and related lipedema events
Talk Lipoedema	UK	Hosted by a UK charity, this group provides emotional support, expert Q&A, and community events
The Lipedema Project España	Spain	Spanish-language community for education and awareness

space. They provide practical advice, emotional connection, and updates on treatment, making them valuable resources for those living with the condition. See Table 19.6 for an alphabetical list of Facebook groups focused on lipedema.

Podcasts

Podcasts about lipedema offer accessible education, expert insights, and real-life stories that support symptom management and emotional well-being. They foster connection, reduce isolation, and empower both patients and professionals. The following podcasts, listed in Table 19.7, offer a wide range of perspectives – from expert clinical insights to lived experiences – making them valuable resources for both patients and professionals in the global lipedema community.

Health and wellness coaching

- Cindy Beers, MS, 500ERYT, Clinical Hypnotherapist: https://cindybeers.com/lipedema-and-yogo/
- Heddy Pugh, ICC, CMT | Founder and Immersive Coach at Heddy Life: www.heddylife.com Helping clients build confidence and approach their lipedema journey with calm and clarity.
- Emmy's Box of Hope https://learn.lipedema-simplified.org/ Emmy's Box of Hope is a free resource package from Lipedema Simplified crafted to support individuals on their lipedema journey. It includes tools like a downloadable self-care journal, an inspirational coloring book, and playful wellness activities (like 'learning to juggle scarves') designed to uplift mood and stimulate lymphatic movement.

Financial and practical help

The financial burden of living with lipedema can be substantial, encompassing costs for compression garments, therapy, mobility aids, and specialized care, often with limited or no insurance coverage. Many patients also face high out-of-pocket expenses for surgery, travel, and consultations with knowledgeable providers. Lost income due to reduced mobility or time off for medical care can further strain finances. Daily functional support needs, such as assistance with basic tasks, are often overlooked by healthcare systems, further complicating the challenge. Recognizing these financial realities is key to providing more equitable and compassionate care. Several resources for economic and practical support are listed here.

Insurance and disability

- Submit compression prescriptions with supporting medical notes
- Use diagnostic codes: ICD-10 R60.0 (Edema), I89.0 (Lymphedema)
- New ICD-11 code: EF0.2.2 (Lipoedema)

Workplace accommodations

- **Lisa Duerre**, Lipedema Advocate, Speaker and Workplace Consultant for Real Change: www.lisaduerre.com/lipedema-advocacy/
- Discuss protections and accommodations with human resources for employees with chronic illnesses.
- Use flexible schedules and ergonomic support tools.

Financial assistance resources

- **HealthWell Foundation:** https://www.healthwellfoundation.org/ The HealthWell Foundation is a US-based nonprofit dedicated to ensuring that underinsured

Table 19.7: Podcasts focused on topics of interest to the lipedema community.

Podcast name	Region	Description
Lipoedema Surgery	Australia	Hosted by Shell and Tiana Personal stories and expert interviews on conservative care, surgery, and self-empowerment
Lipedema Mamas Podcast	USA	Hosted by Ashley Fisher and Shawn Bigby Weekly episodes with tips on nutrition, mindset, surgery prep, and life with lipedema
Stronger Than Lipedema	USA	Hosted by Cindy Howell and Kristy Dellacroce Uplifting podcast on wellness, inflammation, mindset, and thriving with lipedema
Recognizing & Treating Lipedema	USA	Hosted by Dr. Caroline Fife ft. and Dr. Karen Herbst Clinically focused interview on lipedema diagnosis, treatment, and awareness
Living Well with Lipedema (Flash Briefings)	USA & Global	Hosted by Lipedema Simplified Short daily audio segments with research tips, mindset tools, and self-care guidance
LymphCast	USA & Global	Hosted by various experts Episodes across lymphatic and lipedema topics with researchers, clinicians, and advocates
Dear Body, I'm Listening	USA & Global	Hosted by Donna Piper Interviews and personal stories about women living with chronic illness, including lipedema

patients with chronic or life-altering illnesses can access the treatments they need. Its mission is to reduce financial barriers by covering copays, premiums, deductibles, and other out-of-pocket medical expenses.

- **PAN Foundation**: https://www.panfoundation.org/ The Patient Access Network (PAN) Foundation is a US-based nonprofit organization dedicated to making healthcare more affordable and accessible for underinsured patients facing chronic, serious, or rare conditions. Its mission is to accelerate access to equitable healthcare through financial assistance, advocacy, and education, helping patients cover out-of-pocket treatment costs and navigate healthcare systems. The vision is a future where everyone has equitable access to the care they need.
- **GoFundMe and other fundraising platforms:** Many lipedema patients successfully raise funds for surgery, garments, or travel using fundraising platforms. Here are a few suggestions for funding sources:
  - GoFundMe: https://www.gofundme.com/
  - Ketto (India-based) https://www.ketto.org/
  - HelpHopeLive: https://helphopelive.org/

Compression garment support programs

- Compression Fund: https://compression-fund.org/
- Sigvaris® Compression with a Cause Program: https://www.sigvaris.com/en-us/services/compression-with-a-cause
- National Lymphedema Network (NLN) Garment Program: https://lymphnet.org/page/garment-program

Books and media

Books

- Amato A. *Ketogenic Therapy for Lipedema: Transforming Fat into Energy (The Lipedema Journey)*. Independently published, 2024. A practical guide that explores how a ketogenic diet can help manage lipedema. It combines clinical insights, research, and over 77 recipes to support fat metabolism, reduce inflammation, and improve symptoms through a low-carb, high-fat approach.
- Amato A. *The Essential Guide To Living With Lipedema: Discovering the Truth and Transforming Treatment of a Misunderstood Condition*. Independently published, 2024. This guide is a comprehensive resource that sheds light on this often misunderstood condition. It offers guidance on diagnosis, treatment options, and daily management, empowering readers with knowledge, personal stories, and tools to improve quality of life. Offers a compassionate and comprehensive examination of lipedema, delving into its complexities and providing insights into treatment and management.
- Dayan E, Kim JN, Smith ML, Seo CA, Damstra RJ, Schmeller W, Frambach Y, Carmody MA, Földi E, Rockson SG. (Eds). *Lipedema – The Disease They Call FAT: An Overview for Clinicians*. Boston, MA: Lipedema Simplified Publications, 2017. A concise, illustrated monograph produced by the Lipedema Project and LE&RN for both medical professionals and patients. It covers everything from basic epidemiology and differentiation (e.g. lipedema vs. obesity) to staging, diagnostic criteria, and conservative and surgical treatments. It is highly recommended as a reference for educating both healthcare providers and patients.
- Jandali Z, Jiga LP, Campisi C. (Eds). *Lipedema: A Practical Guidebook*. Cham: Springer; 2022. This book is a user-friendly resource offering clear, evidence-based information on recognizing, diagnosing, and managing lipedema. It provides practical tips, treatment options, and support strategies for patients, caregivers, and healthcare providers.
- Keith L. *The Ketogenic Solution for Lymphatic Disorders: Lose Weight and Dramatically Reduce Lymphatic Swelling*. Cheyenne, WY: Gutsy Badger Books; 2019. Primarily directed toward healthcare providers who wish to integrate ketogenic nutrition into their practice, this book explains how a low-carb, high-fat (ketogenic) diet can support lymphatic health and reduce swelling.
- Keith L. *The Lymphatic Code: Using a Ketogenic Lifestyle to Enjoy a Robust Lymphatic System That Promotes Overall Health and Wellness*. Cheyenne, WY: Gutsy Badger Books; 2022. A broader guide, released in January 2022, explores the function of the lymphatic system and offers practical lifestyle advice for both laypeople and professionals, including information on ketogenic nutrition.
- Lukowicz DD von, Sauter MD, Lipp A-TD,

Fleischmann D. *All about LIPEDEMA*. Kollnburg, Germany: Scout Medien GmbH, 2021. An informative guide that explains what lipedema is, how it's diagnosed, and the best ways to manage it. Designed for both patients and professionals, this resource covers symptoms, treatment options, and daily living tips to support a better understanding and care.

- O'Hara S. *Legs Like Mine: A Whimsical Life With Lipedema*. Independently published, 2023. Offers a bold, heartfelt, and visually vibrant look at life with lipedema. Blending colorful illustrations with personal stories and empowering affirmations, O'Hara challenges the shame and invisibility often surrounding the condition. With humor and honesty, she captures the emotional and social realities of lipedema while celebrating bodies that are rarely seen in mainstream narratives. More than a book, it's a mirror – one that brings comfort, connection, and joy to those who often feel unseen.
- Pitotti G. *Lipedema, it's not your fault!: Nutrition and Management Guide for Lipedema: understanding it, treating it, and accepting it to move beyond the stigma*. Independently published, 2023. This compassionate nutrition and management guide helps readers understand, treat, and accept lipedema. It offers practical advice on care and lifestyle changes while challenging stigma and empowering those living with the condition.
- Seo C. *Lipedema – The Disease They Call Fat*. Boston, MA: Lipedema Simplified Productions; 2015. This is a 55-minute documentary that explores the personal and medical realities of living with lipedema. Featuring interviews with patients, clinicians, and surgeons across the US and Europe, the film highlights the challenges of misdiagnosis, weight bias, and limited treatment options. Produced in collaboration with the Lipedema Project and the Friedman Center, it offers both education and advocacy, raising awareness and giving voice to this long-overlooked condition.

Staying informed and empowered

Staying informed about lipedema is key to effective management and self-advocacy. As research, treatments, and resources evolve, staying current empowers individuals to make informed decisions about their care. Following reputable organizations, attending webinars, and engaging with the community through support groups and podcasts offer both medical updates and real-life insights. In this still-emerging field, knowledge is a powerful tool for personal empowerment and broader advocacy.

- sign up for newsletters from Lipedema Simplified and LE&RN
- follow hashtags like #lipedemaawareness, #lipedemawarrior
- attend conferences and virtual events.

Conferences

These conferences offer a blend of research, education, clinical innovation, peer stories, and global networking – both in-person and virtual – helping advance lipedema care, awareness, and community empowerment. The following are some of the notable global conferences and congresses focused on lipedema.

- **Lipedema World Congress** Organized by the Lipedema World Alliance, this high-profile international event brings together experts – lymphologists, surgeons, therapists, nutritionists, and patient advocates – for multidisciplinary sessions covering the latest developments in science, diagnosis, conservative and surgical treatments, and patient-centered strategies. https://2025-lipedema-world-congress.com/

- **FDRS / Lipedema Foundation Live Research & Annual Conference** A hybrid academic and clinical gathering hosted in partnership with the Fat Disorders Resource Society, featuring a live biobank research component, expert lectures, and discussions on lipedema and related disorders. https://www.fatdisorders.org/events
- **Lipoedema Australia Conference** A national event offering workshops, practitioner-led sessions, advocacy networking, and hybrid participation for clinicians, patients, and caregivers in Australia. https://www.lipoedema.org.au/conference
- **Lipedema Simplified Biannual Heart-to-Heart Events** A three-day 'Heart to Heart' virtual congress hosted by Lipedema Simplified/The Lipedema Project, featuring global experts, patients, and clinicians focusing on diagnosis, genetics, imaging, conservative and surgical care, nutrition, self-care, and holistic strategies. https://learn.lipedema-simplified.org/lipedema-lymphedema-event
- **International Lymphoedema Framework Conference** The International Lymphoedema Framework (ILF) conferences bring together clinicians, researchers, and patients to share knowledge, advance care, and promote global collaboration in the management of lymphedema and related conditions. Through scientific sessions, practical workshops, and patient-centered initiatives, the conferences aim to improve treatment standards, support advocacy, and foster international best practices. https://www.lympho.org/index.php
- **World Congress of the International Society of Lymphology** The World Congress of the International Society of Lymphology (ISL) serves as the premier global forum for lymphatic health. It brings together clinicians, researchers, surgeons, therapists, and industry professionals every two years to share the latest scientific advances, clinical best practices, and emerging therapies for lymphatic and lymph-associated diseases, such as lymphedema and lipedema. https://isl.arizona.edbetter u/

Conclusion

Whether you are a patient newly diagnosed or a healthcare provider seeking to better support those with the disease, know that you are not alone. A growing global network of dedicated researchers, clinicians, advocates, and individuals living with this disease works every day to expand knowledge, improve care, and build a more compassionate and informed future. Resources now exist that offer not only medical guidance but also emotional support, community connection, and practical tools for daily life.

Empowerment begins by connecting with trusted networks, learning from reliable sources, and valuing the lived experiences of those navigating lipedema. Healing starts when patients feel seen. Support grows through compassionate listening. And meaningful progress unfolds when clinicians and patients know where to turn, finding a resilient and informed community that is already paving the way forward, together.

VIII
A look to the future

Chapter Twenty
Lipedema diagnosis and management:
the next chapter

Stanley G. Rockson

It is with a sense of great anticipation that I find myself writing these words. At an unprecedented moment in medical evolution, the world is, at last, ready to acknowledge the pathological diagnosis of lipedema – its natural history, co-morbidities, and the unique medical needs of affected individuals. The preceding chapters in this volume attest to the significant progress achieved in recent years, lending optimism as we look to the future.

It has not always been so. Although lipedema was identified as a distinct disease with unique clinical features over 80 years ago,[1] it has remained relatively neglected by the majority of healthcare providers. By way of stark contrast, we can examine the fate of a similarly common human pathology, namely, cardiovascular disease (Figure 20.1). With widespread general recognition among modern practitioners at nearly the same point in medical evolution, this disease has been the beneficiary of aggressive attempts to reverse its impact. As shown in the figure, just three medical advances – among many – have dramatically altered its course and nearly eradicated its mortality burden.[2]

Until recently, lipedema has not been quite so fortunate. While, thankfully, the diagnosis of lipedema does not usually threaten survival, it can be readily acknowledged that the impact on function and quality of life is profound (see Chapters 2 and 8).[3]

The content of the preceding chapters gives testament to the changing face of lipedema management. The advances of the last decade provide a template for the future of this disease (Figure 20.2).

While the distinctions among lipedema, lymphedema, and constitutional obesity can be challenging (Chapters 6–9), the educational process for both the public and health care professionals increasingly provides a meaningful context for diagnostic clarity that facilitates the needed and appropriate care for each of these entities.[4] Education at all levels is key, but this educational effort must continue to be sustained by the insights derived from focused epidemiology and public health initiatives.

The research community has become aware of the complex and exciting biology of lipedema; burgeoning investigative advances in human genetics and other disciplines are increasingly yielding results that will foster precise, objective criteria for establishing diagnoses and refining both personalized therapeutic approaches and prognostic categorization.[5, 6, 7, 8] For decades, the diagnosis of lipedema has relied on physician-driven pattern recognition; the inability to substantiate the diagnosis using objectively measured parameters has hampered both healthcare delivery and the development of targeted therapeutic interventions. The recent advances detailed in this volume attest

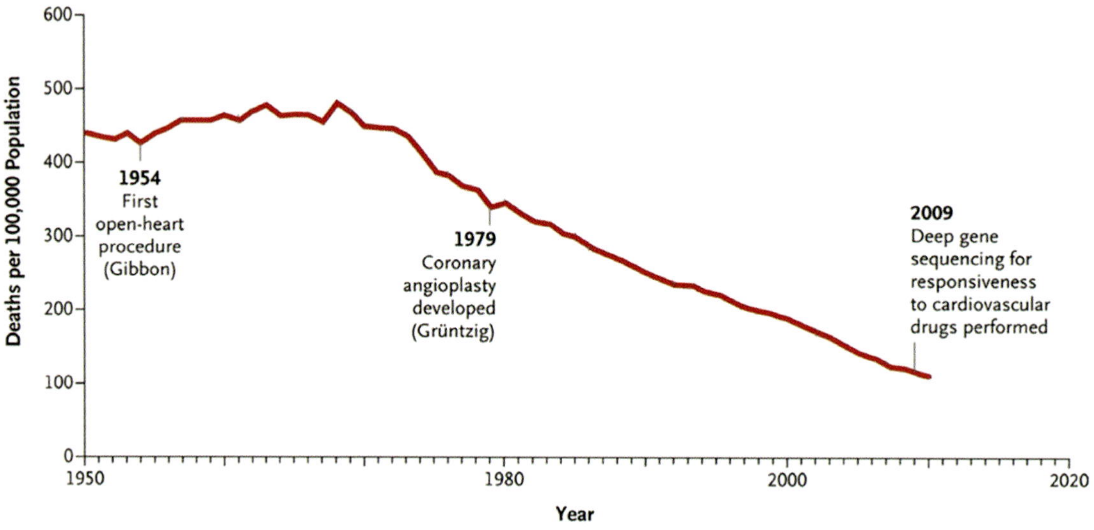

Figure 20.1: Cardiovascular death rates in relation to scientific advances. Adapted from EG Nabel and E Braunwald.[2]

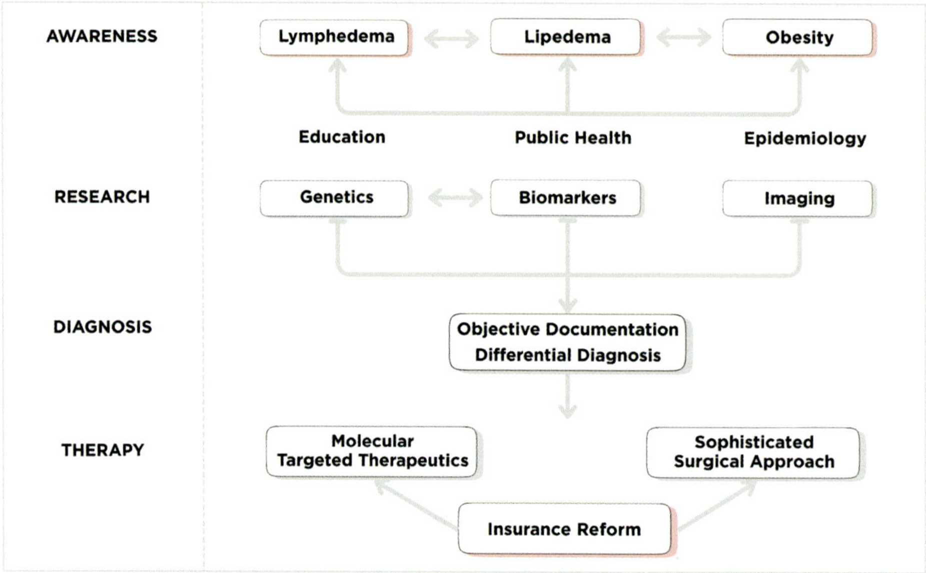

Figure 20.2: A hypothetical framework for the future of lipedema healthcare delivery.

to the promise that the biomedical sciences hold for the future in addressing lipedema. These advances, along with the objectivity that will ensue, are expected to bring about the much-needed insurance reform necessary to make appropriate healthcare universally accessible.

In an era where personalized medicine is increasingly sought, it is somewhat regrettable that treatment for lipedema is often withheld, whether consciously or unconsciously. When administered, lipedema therapeutics are most often delivered in a 'one size fits all' manner. However, the future is bright: the biomedical progress that promises sophisticated future diagnosis and disease stratification also augurs a new era of tailored surgical intervention and sophisticated molecular approaches to a complex disease process with remarkably heterogeneous clinical presentation.

In short, this book all but promises the coming 'golden age' for lipedema. It is exciting to imagine a future generation of healthcare providers well-versed in the clinical presentation of lipedema and optimally prepared to establish an accurate diagnosis, leading to personalized and sophisticated interventions designed to minimize the disease's impact and optimize quality of life for these patients.

References

1. Allen EV. Lymphedema of the extremities: classification, etiology, and differential diagnosis: A study of 300 cases. *Arch Intern Med.* 1934 Oct 1;54(4):606–24. DOI: https://doi.org/10.1001/archinte.1934.00160160125008
2. Nabel EG, Braunwald E. A tale of coronary artery disease and myocardial infarction. *N Engl J Med.* 2012 Jan 5;366(1):54–63. DOI: https://doi.org/10.1056/NEJMra1112570
3. Bilancini S, Lucchi M, Tucci S, Eleuteri P. Functional lymphatic alterations in patients suffering from lipedema. *Angiology.* 1995 Apr;46(4):333–9. DOI: https://doi.org/10.1177/000331979504600408
4. Forner-Cordero I, Szolnoky G, Forner-Cordero A, Kemény L. Lipedema: an overview of its clinical manifestations, diagnosis and treatment of the disproportional fatty deposition syndrome – systematic review. *Clin Obes.* 2012;2(3–4):86–95. DOI: https://doi.org/10.1111/j.1758-8111.2012.00045.x
5. Klimentidis YC, Chen Z, Gonzalez-Garay ML, Grigoriadis D, Sackey E, Pittman A, et al. Genome-wide association study of a lipedema phenotype among women in the UK Biobank identifies multiple genetic risk factors. *Eur J Hum Genet.* 2023 Mar;31(3):338–44. DOI: https://doi.org/10.1038/s41431-022-01231-6
6. Ishaq M, Bandara N, Morgan S, Nowell C, Mehdi AM, Lyu R, et al. Key signaling networks are dysregulated in patients with the adipose tissue disease, lipedema. *Int J Obes.* 2022 Mar;46(3):502–14. DOI: https://doi.org/10.1038/s41366-021-01002-1
7. Morgan S, Reid I, Bendon C, Ishaq M, Shayan R, Pope B, et al. A family-based study of inherited genetic risk in lipedema. *Lymphat Res Biol.* 2024 Apr 1;22(2):106–11. DOI: https://doi.org/10.1089/lrb.2023.0065
8. Kaftalli J, Bonetti G, Marceddu G, Dhuli K, E Maltese P, Donato K, et al. AKR1C1 and hormone metabolism in lipedema pathogenesis: a computational biology approach. *Eur Rev Med Pharmacol Sci.* 2023;27(6 Suppl.):137-47. Available from: https://usiena-air.unisi.it/handle/11365/1261114

INDEX

Note: Page numbers in **bold** refer to Figures and/or Tables. Index entries are in letter-by-letter order.

Note: Page numbers in **bold** refer to Figures and/or Tables. Index entries are in letter-by-letter order.

Note: Page numbers in **bold** refer to Figures and/or Tables. Index entries are in letter-by-letter order.

Note: Page numbers in **bold** refer to Figures and/or Tables. Index entries are in letter-by-letter order.

Note: Page numbers in **bold** refer to Figures and/or Tables. Index entries are in letter-by-letter order.

Note: Page numbers in **bold** refer to Figures and/or Tables. Index entries are in letter-by-letter order.

Note: Page numbers in **bold** refer to Figures and/or Tables. Index entries are in letter-by-letter order.

Note: Page numbers in **bold** refer to Figures and/or Tables. Index entries are in letter-by-letter order.

Note: Page numbers in **bold** refer to Figures and/or Tables. Index entries are in letter-by-letter order.

Note: Page numbers in **bold** refer to Figures and/or Tables. Index entries are in letter-by-letter order.

Also from Hammersmith Books...

Two new books that accompany and support
Lipedema: Principles and Practice of Diagnosis and Treatment:

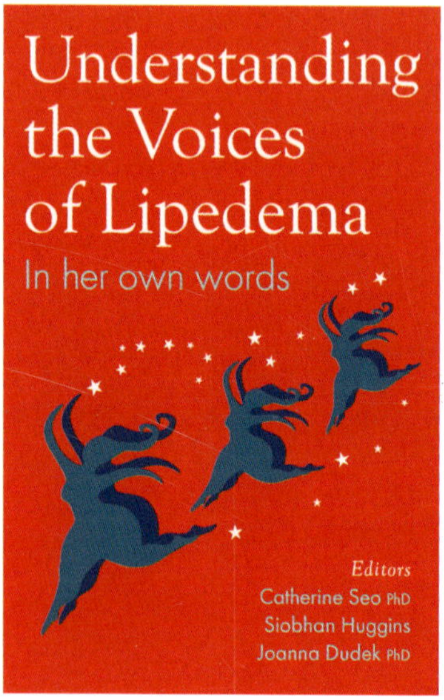

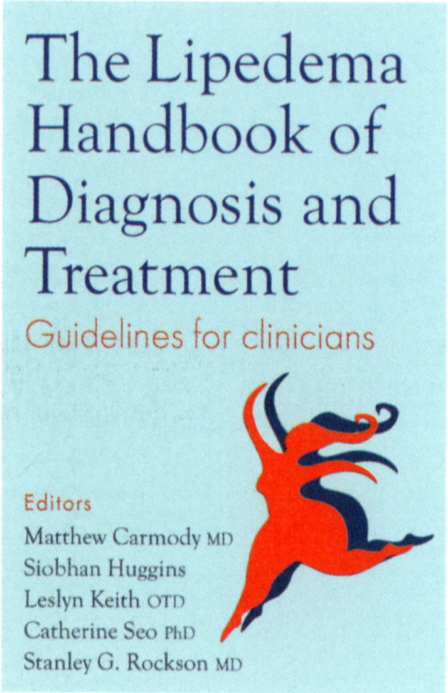